The Ethics of Surgery

The Ethics of Surgery

CONFLICTS AND CONTROVERSIES

Edited By Robert M. Sade, M.D.
DEPARTMENT OF SURGERY, INSTITUTE OF HUMAN VALUES IN HEALTH
CARE, MEDICAL UNIVERSITY OF SOUTH CAROLINA, CHARLESTON

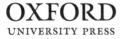
OXFORD
UNIVERSITY PRESS

Oxford University Press is a department of the University of Oxford.
It furthers the University's objective of excellence in research,
scholarship, and education by publishing worldwide.

Oxford   New York
Auckland   Cape Town   Dar es Salaam   Hong Kong   Karachi
Kuala Lumpur   Madrid   Melbourne   Mexico City   Nairobi
New Delhi   Shanghai   Taipei   Toronto

With offices in
Argentina   Austria   Brazil   Chile   Czech Republic   France   Greece
Guatemala   Hungary   Italy   Japan   Poland   Portugal   Singapore
South Korea   Switzerland   Thailand   Turkey   Ukraine   Vietnam

Oxford is a registered trademark of Oxford University Press
in the UK and certain other countries.

Published in the United States of America by
Oxford University Press
198 Madison Avenue, New York, NY 10016

© Oxford University Press 2015

Library of Congress Cataloging-in-Publication Data
The ethics of surgery: conflicts and controversies/edited by Robert M. Sade.
p.; cm.
Includes bibliographical references.
ISBN 978–0–19–020452–5 (paperback: alk. paper)—ISBN 978–0–19–020453–2 (hardcover: alk.
paper)
I. Sade, Robert M., 1938–, editor.
[DNLM: 1. General Surgery—ethics—Collected Works.   2. Physician-Patient Relations—
ethics—Collected Works.   3. Physicians—ethics—Collected Works.   4. Surgical Procedures,
Operative—ethics—Collected Works. WO 21]
RD27.7
174.2'97—dc23
2014024382

9 8 7 6 5 4 3 2 1
Printed in the United States of America
on acid-free paper

I dedicate this book to two mentors early in my professional life, who not only encouraged and supported my development as a surgeon, but also were the finest practitioners of the art and science of surgery I have known: Aldo R. Castañeda and the late M. Judah Folkman.

CONTENTS

Contributors   xi
Preface   xvii
Acknowledgments   xix

Introduction   1
ROBERT M. SADE

Section 1: The Problem of Surgical Ethics
ROBERT M. SADE

1. **Ethics Gap in Surgery   19**
ROBERT M. SADE, TIMOTHY H. WILLIAMS, DAVID J. PERLMAN,
CYNTHIA L. HANEY, AND MARTHA R. STROUD

2. **Ethics in Cardiothoracic Surgery: A Survey of Surgeons' Views   26**
THOMAS A. D'AMICO, MARTIN F. McKNEALLY, AND ROBERT M. SADE

Section 2: Professional Integrity
ROBERT M. SADE

3. **Deceiving Insurance Companies: New Expression of an Ancient Tradition   37**
ROBERT M. SADE

4. **Hepatitis C Virus–Infected Resident: End of Residency, End of Career?   47**
CAROLYN M. DRESLER, MICHAEL S. KENT, RICHARD I. WHYTE,
AND ROBERT M. SADE

5. **Must Surgeons Tell Mitral Valve Repair Candidates About a New Percutaneous Repair Device That Is Only Available Elsewhere?   58**
ERIC R. SKIPPER, KEVIN D. ACCOLA, AND ROBERT M. SADE

6. **The Surgeon's Work in Transition: Should Surgeons Spend More Time Outside the Hospital?   69**
JAMIE DICKEY, ROSS M. UNGERLEIDER, JOSEPH S. COSELLI,
LORI D. CONKLIN, AND ROBERT M. SADE

7. **Should Sleep-Deprived Surgeons Be Prohibited from Operating Without Patients' Consent?   80**
CHARLES A. CZEISLER, CARLOS A. PELLEGRINI, AND ROBERT M. SADE

8. Are Thoracic Surgeons Ethically Obligated to Serve as Expert Witnesses for the Plaintiff?   94
   DONALD C. WATSON, JR., FRANCIS ROBICSEK, AND ROBERT M. SADE

Section 3: Relationships with Patients—Autonomy and Consent
   ROBERT M. SADE

9. Should a Jehovah's Witness Patient Who Faces Imminent Exsanguination Be Transfused?   107
   KEITH S. NAUNHEIM, CHARLES R. BRIDGES, AND ROBERT M. SADE

10. No Heroic Measures: How Soon Is Too Soon to Stop?   118
    THOMAS A. D'AMICO, MARK J. KRASNA, DIANE M. KRASNA, AND ROBERT M. SADE

11. Should Surgical Errors Always Be Disclosed to the Patient?   130
    CONSTANTINE MAVROUDIS, CONSTANTINE D. MAVROUDIS, KEITH S. NAUNHEIM, AND ROBERT M. SADE

12. Another Surgeon's Error: Must You Tell the Patient?   141
    SUSAN D. MOFFATT-BRUCE, CHADRICK E. DENLINGER, AND ROBERT M. SADE

13. Impending Loss of Insurance Coverage Is an Indication to Proceed with Complex, Expensive Surgery   151
    ANTHONY L. ESTRERA, SHARON IKONOMIDIS, JOHN S. IKONOMIDIS, AND ROBERT M. SADE

14. Ethical Obligation of Surgeons to Noncompliant Patients: Can a Surgeon Refuse to Operate on an Intravenous Drug–Abusing Patient with Recurrent Aortic Valve Prosthesis Infection?   163
    J. MICHAEL DIMAIO, TOMAS A. SALERNO, RON BERNSTEIN, KATIA ARAUJO, MARCO RICCI, AND ROBERT M. SADE

Section 4: Innovation and Uses of Technology
   ROBERT M. SADE

15. Surgical Innovation: Too Risky to Remain Unregulated?   181
    HAAVI MORREIM, MICHAEL J. MACK, AND ROBERT M. SADE

16. Who Should Adopt Robotic Surgery and When?   194
    JESSICA K. SMYTH, KAREN E. DEVENEY, AND ROBERT M. SADE

17. Should Access to Transcatheter Aortic Valve Replacement Be Limited to High-Volume Surgical Centers?   204
    JOSEPH E. BAVARIA, PHILIP GREEN, GREGG F. ROSNER, MARTIN B. LEON, ALLAN SCHWARTZ, AND ROBERT M. SADE

18. Should the Use of Transcatheter Aortic Valve Implantation
Be Rationed?   214
JOHN E. MAYER, JR., GRAYSON H. WHEATLEY III, AND ROBERT M. SADE

Section 5: Organ Donation and Transplantation
ROBERT M. SADE

19. Heart Donation Without the Dead-Donor Rule   231
FRANKLIN G. MILLER AND ROBERT M. SADE

20. Saving Lives Is More Important Than Abstract Moral Concerns: Financial
Incentives Should Be Used to Increase Organ Donation   238
BENJAMIN HIPPEN, LAINIE FRIEDMAN ROSS, AND ROBERT M. SADE

21. Prisoners on Death Row Should Be Accepted as Organ Donors   250
SHU S. LIN, LAUREN RICH, JAY D. PAL, AND ROBERT M. SADE

Section 6: Conflicts of Interest in Surgery
ROBERT M. SADE

22. Politely Refuse the Pen and Note Pad: Gifts From Industry to
Physicians Harm Patients   265
KENNETH V. ISERSON, ROBERT JAMES CERFOLIO,
AND ROBERT M. SADE

23. Should the Financial Link Between Industry and Physician
Consultants Be Severed?   276
STEPHEN J. IMMELT, VINCENT A. GAUDIANI, AND ROBERT M. SADE

24. Full Disclosure—Should Presentations and Publications Include Dollar
Amounts and Duration of Surgeon-Industry Relationships?   286
J. PETER MURPHY AND ROBERT M. SADE

Section 7: Ethical Issues in Health-Care Policy
ROBERT M. SADE

25. Medical Ethics Collides with Public Policy: LVAD for a
Patient With Leukemia   301
PATRICK M. McCARTHY, RICHARD D. LAMM, AND ROBERT M. SADE

26. Should Coronary Artery Bypass Grafting Be Regionalized?   311
BRAHMAJEE K. NALLAMOTHU, KIM A. EAGLE, VICTOR A. FERRARIS,
AND ROBERT M. SADE

27. A Clash of Rights: Should Smoking Tobacco Products in Public Places
Be Legally Banned?   324
CAROLYN M. DRESLER, MARK J. CHERRY, AND ROBERT M. SADE

28. **Should a Medical Center Deny Employment to a Physician Because He Smokes Tobacco Products?**   **335**
JAMES W. JONES, WILLIAM M. NOVICK, AND ROBERT M. SADE

Index   345

CONTRIBUTORS

Kevin D. Accola, MD: Florida Heart Institute, Cardiovascular Surgeons, PA, Orlando, Florida

Katia Araujo, PsyD: Jackson Memorial Hospital, Miami-Dade County Attorney's Office, Kaplan University, School of Criminal Justice, Miami, Florida

Joseph E. Bavaria, MD: Division of Cardiovascular Surgery, Hospital of the University of Pennsylvania, Philadelphia, Pennsylvania

Ron Bernstein, JD: Miami-Dade County Attorney's Office, Kaplan University, School of Criminal Justice, Miami, Florida

Charles R. Bridges, MD: Division of Cardiovascular Surgery, Hospital of the University of Pennsylvania and the Pennsylvania Hospital, Philadelphia, Pennsylvania

Robert James Cerfolio, MD: Department of Cardiothoracic Surgery, University of Alabama at Birmingham, Birmingham, Alabama

Mark J. Cherry, PhD: Department of Philosophy, St. Edward's University, Austin, Texas

Lori D. Conklin, MD: Department of Anesthesiology and Chief, Division of Vascular Anesthesia, University of Virginia, Charlottesville, Virginia

Joseph S. Coselli, MD: Texas Heart Institute, Baylor College of Medicine, Houston, Texas

Charles A. Czeisler, PhD, MD: Division of Sleep Medicine, Department of Medicine, Brigham and Women's Hospital, and Division of Sleep Medicine, Harvard Medical School, Boston, Massachusetts

Thomas A. D'Amico, MD: Division of Thoracic Surgery, Duke University Medical Center, Duke University Health System, Durham, North Carolina

Chadrick E. Denlinger, MD: Division of Cardiothoracic Surgery, Medical University of South Carolina, Charleston, South Carolina

Karen E. Deveney, MD: Department of Surgery, Oregon Health and Science University, Portland, Oregon

Jamie Dickey (Ungerleider), MA, MSW-LCSW, PhD: Family and Community Medicine, Center for Integrative Medicine, Student Wellness Center, Wake Forest Baptist Health, Winston-Salem, North Carolina

J. Michael DiMaio, MD: Department of Cardiothoracic Surgery, University of Texas Southwestern Medical Center, Dallas, Texas

Carolyn M. Dresler, MD, MPA: Center for Tobacco Products, Food and Drug Administration, Rockville, Maryland

Kim A. Eagle, MD: University of Michigan Cardiovascular Center, Ann Arbor, Michigan

Anthony L. Estrera, MD: Department of Cardiothoracic and Vascular Surgery, University of Texas Medical School, Houston, Texas

Victor A. Ferraris, MD, PhD: Division of Cardiovascular and Thoracic Surgery, Linda and Jack Gill Heart Institute, University of Kentucky Chandler Medical Center, Lexington, Kentucky

Vincent A. Gaudiani, MD: Pacific Coast Cardiac and Vascular Surgeons, California Pacific Medical Center Heart Institute, and Cardiac Surgery, Community Hospital of the Monterey Peninsula, Redwood City, California

Philip Green, MD: Division of Cardiology, Department of Medicine, Columbia University Medical Center, New York, New York

Cynthia L. Haney, JD: Division of Legislative Counsel, American Medical Association, Washington, DC

Benjamin Hippen, MD: Metrolina Nephrology Associates and Carolinas Medical Center, Charlotte, North Carolina

John S. Ikonomidis, MD, PhD: Division of Cardiothoracic Surgery, Department of Surgery, Medical University of South Carolina, Charleston, South Carolina

Sharon Ikonomidis, MS, PhD: Department of History, Humanities and Political Science, Trident Technical College, Charleston, South Carolina

Stephen J. Immelt, JD: Hogan Lovells, LLP, Baltimore, Maryland

Kenneth V. Iserson, MD, MBA: Arizona Bioethics Program, University of Arizona, Tucson, Arizona

James W. Jones, MD, PhD: The Center for Medical Ethics and Health Policy, Baylor College of Medicine, Houston, Texas

Michael S. Kent, MD: Division of Thoracic Surgery and Interventional Pulmonology, Beth Israel Deaconess Medical Center, Boston, Massachusetts

Diane M. Krasna, CRNA: Meridian Cancer Care, Jersey Shore University Medical Center, Neptune, New Jersey

Mark J. Krasna, MD: Meridian Cancer Care, Jersey Shore University Medical Center, Neptune, New Jersey

Richard D. Lamm, LLB, CPA: Institute for Public Policy Studies, University of Denver, Denver, Colorado, Former Governor of Colorado

Martin B. Leon, MD: Center for Interventional Vascular Therapy, Columbia University Medical Center/New York-Presbyterian Hospital, New York, New York

Shu S. Lin, MD, PhD: Departments of Surgery, Immunology, and Pathology, and the Duke Lung Transplant Program, Duke University Medical Center, Durham, North Carolina

Michael J. Mack, MD: Cardiovascular Research and Cardiovascular Medicine, Heart Hospital Baylor Plano, Baylor Healthcare System, Baylor Plano, Plano, Texas

John E. Mayer, Jr., MD: Department of Cardiac Surgery, Children's Hospital Boston, and Harvard Medical School, Boston, Massachusetts

Constantine Mavroudis, MD: Congenital Heart Institute, Florida Hospital for Children, Orlando, Florida

Constantine D. Mavroudis, MD, MSC: Penn Surgery, Cardiac Surgery Direct Program, University of Pennsylvania, Philadelphia, Pennsylvania

Patrick M. McCarthy, MD: Division of Cardiothoracic Surgery, Northwestern University, Feinberg School of Medicine, Chicago, Illinois

Martin F. McKneally, MD, PhD: Toronto General Hospital, Department of Surgery and Joint Centre for Bioethics, University of Toronto, Toronto, Ontario, Canada

Franklin G. Miller, PhD: Department of Bioethics, National Institutes of Health, Bethesda, Maryland

Susan D. Moffatt-Bruce, MD, PhD: Department of Surgery, The Ohio State University Medical Center, Columbus, Ohio

Haavi Morreim, JD, PhD: College of Medicine, University of Tennessee, Health Science Center, Memphis, Tennessee

J. Peter Murphy, MD: Department of Cardiovascular Surgery, Missouri Baptist Hospital, St. Louis, Missouri

Brahmajee K. Nallamothu, MD, MPH: Division of Cardiovascular Medicine, Department of Internal Medicine, University of Michigan Medical School, Ann Arbor, Michigan

Keith S. Naunheim, MD: Division of Cardiothoracic Surgery, St. Louis University Health Sciences Center, St. Louis, Missouri

William M. Novick, MD: University of Tennessee Health Science Center, Memphis, Tennessee

Jay D. Pal, MD, PhD: Department of Cardiothoracic Surgery, University of Texas Health Science Center, San Antonio, Texas

Carlos A. Pellegrini, MD: Department of Surgery, University of Washington, Seattle, Washington

David J. Perlman, PhD: School of Nursing, Center for Bioethics, University of Pennsylvania, Philadelphia, Pennsylvania

Marco Ricci, MD: Division of Cardiothoracic Surgery, University of New Mexico Health Science Center, Albuquerque, New Mexico

Lauren Rich, RN, BSN: Departments of Surgery, Immunology, and Pathology, and the Duke Lung Transplant Program, Duke University Medical Center, Durham, North Carolina

Francis Robicsek, MD, PhD: Department of Thoracic and Cardiovascular Surgery, Carolinas Heart Institute and Carolinas Medical Center, Charlotte, North Carolina

Gregg F. Rosner, MD: Division of Cardiology, Department of Medicine, Columbia University Medical Center, New York, New York

Lainie Friedman Ross, MD, PhD: Departments of Pediatrics, Medicine, and Surgery, MacLean Center for Clinical Medical Ethics, University of Chicago, Chicago, Illinois

Robert M. Sade, MD: Department of Surgery, Institute of Human Values in Health Care, Medical University of South Carolina, Charleston

Tomas A. Salerno, MD: Department of Surgery and Division Cardiothoracic Surgery, University of Miami Miller School of Medicine and Jackson Memorial Hospital, Miami, Florida

Allan Schwartz, MD: Division of Cardiology, Department of Medicine, Columbia University Medical Center, New York, New York

Eric R. Skipper, MD: Department of Thoracic and Cardiovascular Surgery, Sanger Heart and Vascular Institute, Carolinas Medical Center, Charlotte, North Carolina

Jessica K. Smyth, MD: Department of Otolaryngology, University of North Carolina, Chapel Hill, North Carolina

Martha R. Stroud, MS: Division of Cardiothoracic Surgery, Medical University of South Carolina, Charleston, South Carolina

Ross M. Ungerleider, MD: Pediatric Cardiac Surgery, Brenner Children's Hospital, Wake Forest University Baptist Medical Center, Winston Salem, North Carolina

Donald C. Watson, Jr., MD: Pediatric Cardiovascular Surgery, Asheville, North Carolina

Grayson H. Wheatley III, MD: Department of Cardiovascular Surgery, Arizona Heart Institute, Phoenix, Arizona

Richard I. Whyte, MD, MBA: Division of Thoracic Surgery and Interventional Pulmonology, Beth Israel Deaconess Medical Center, Boston, Massachusetts

Timothy H. Williams, MD: Cardiothoracic Surgery, St. Francis Hospital, Greenville, South Carolina

PREFACE

This book was not created de novo but evolved as a consequence of the growing interest in biomedical ethics as it applies to surgery. Although it is set in the context of cardiothoracic surgery, the ideas, conflicts, and controversies that it addresses are applicable to all surgical specialties. The evolution of certain ideas and events ultimately led to the creation of the book itself.

In the mid-1990s I came across a paper that piqued my interest. It compared the frequency of discussion of bioethical issues in medical compared with surgical journals. The study found that ethical topics were discussed more than four times more frequently in medical than in surgical journals. In an attempt to identify the causes of this "ethics gap," I conducted a pilot survey within my own institution, the Medical University of South Carolina in Charleston. Although the study provided no clear explanation for the discrepancy, its findings were of sufficient interest that it was accepted for presentation at a surgical conference in 1999. This paper, "The Ethics Gap in Surgery," was published the next year in a surgical journal and is reproduced as the first chapter of this book. The presentation and publication of this pilot study led to two important outcomes.

Immediately after the oral presentation, I discussed the implications of the ethics gap for both surgical practice and surgical education with the newly appointed editor of the *Annals of Thoracic Surgery* (the *Annals*), Dr. L. Henry Edmunds. He considered and then accepted the idea that oral and written discussion on ethical topics in the context of surgery could be valuable. Subsequently, Hank appointed me as ethics editor of the *Annals*, the official journal of the Society of Thoracic Surgeons (STS) and the Southern Thoracic Surgical Association (STSA). This post had not existed previously. From that position, I was able to facilitate the publication of a series of articles on ethical issues in surgery, many of which are found in this book.

The second significant outcome came several months after the publication of the ethics-gap paper. Dr. Martin McKneally and I, both members of the Society of Thoracic Surgeons Standards and Ethics Committee at the time, explored the possibility of creating an organization for providing ethics education for cardiothoracic surgeons. As a result, the Ethics Forum (the Forum) was created. (The name was recently changed to the Cardiothoracic Ethics Forum, but Ethics Forum was used throughout previously published material in this book, so I use it in this book rather than the new name whenever referring to the Forum.) Martin and I invited a few surgeons who were interested in ethics to join us, and this group subsequently met regularly to plan programs on ethical issues for presentation at national meetings of surgical societies. It gradually evolved to comprise the entire membership of the ethics committees of the STS and the American Association for Thoracic Surgery (AATS), as well as a few former members of those committees who had sustained an interest and scholarly involvement in surgical ethics.

Eventually, discussions of ethical issues became a permanent fixture in the programs of the annual meetings of the STS, the AATS, and the STSA. To expand the audience for these programs beyond those in attendance at the meetings, their proceedings were published in the *Annals* and the *Journal of Thoracic and Cardiovascular Surgery* (the *Journal*), thus reaching a readership of thousands. Some of the ethics-related writings in these journals did not originate in conference presentations but came from solicited manuscripts on ethical issues.

Between 2000 and the end of 2013, more than forty ethics programs were presented at the annual meetings of cardiothoracic surgical societies, and members of the Forum had published more than 300 articles on topics in ethics, nearly all in surgical journals, mostly in the *Annals* and the *Journal*.

I have selected articles that I have written or coauthored from the *Annals* and the *Journal*—they comprise most of this book's content—in hopes of further augmenting the educational value of the Forum's efforts by presenting them to an expanded audience of surgeons and surgical trainees. This book is not intended to cover the field of surgical ethics comprehensively; rather, it focuses on issues that have been determined by the members of the Forum (nearly all of whom are practicing surgeons) to be controversial and of current relevance to surgeons and surgeons in training.

The book has two goals. The first is to provide educational materials in surgical ethics for the enjoyment and enlightenment of practicing surgeons and other physicians, surgical residents, and medical students. The second is to make surgeons aware that ethics is not a static, stable discipline; rather, it is a dynamic field that is animated by varying perspectives on important controversies, perspectives that arise from diverse training backgrounds, from differences in personal value systems, and sometimes from fundamentally differing worldviews. If these goals are achieved, I believe that surgical practice will be better for it, to the ultimate benefit of the patients we treat.

ACKNOWLEDGMENTS

The publication of a book is the culmination of the efforts not of one person but many. Most of the material in this book came about as a result of the collaboration of dozens of individuals. In the beginning, Martin McKneally, MD, my colleague and friend, and I germinated the idea of developing an educational program for the field of thoracic surgery. We worked together to create the Ethics Forum, members of which over the past fourteen years are listed below (records were poorly kept or missing in the early days, and I apologize to anyone in that group whom I inadvertently omitted).

From the beginning, L. Henry Edmunds, MD, editor of the *Annals of Thoracic Surgery*, was enormously helpful and supportive of the publication of much ethics-related material in his journal. Special thanks goes to Heide Pusztay, managing editor of the *Annals of Thoracic Surgery*, who has been extraordinarily effective in support of our publication efforts. The editors of the *Journal of Thoracic and Cardiovascular Surgery*, Andrew Wechsler, MD, and subsequently Lawrence Cohn, MD, have also been encouraging by publishing ethics papers in their journal. Enthusiastic support for the activities of the Forum has come from the leadership of both the Society of Thoracic Surgeons (STS) and the American Association for Thoracic Surgery, most particularly from Robert Wynbrandt, STS executive director, and Grahame Rush, the STS director of information services.

On the home front, my work over many years has benefited greatly from the support of my administrative assistants, most recently and notably Ms. Megan Fier. The Department of Surgery and Division of Cardiothoracic Surgery of my home institution, the Medical University of South Carolina (MUSC), have provided both financial and moral support over many years, in particular Fred Crawford and John Ikonomidis, both of whom I am fortunate to count as friends as well as colleagues. My move from the active practice of pediatric cardiac surgery into the field of bioethics was greatly facilitated many years ago by discussions, encouragement, and financial support from Layton McCurdy, who was dean of the MUSC college of medicine at the time.

Many thanks are due to my editor, Peter Ohlin, senior editor of Oxford University Press, for his guidance through the process of bringing the materials in this book from a nascent idea to final publication, with the assistance of Lucy Randall, Associate Editor. Stephen Hoffius was of great help in editing the final manuscript.

A huge thank-you goes to the many coauthors of the papers that compose the bulk of this work. We have learned a great deal from one another, and we have had a lot of fun putting together the talks and debates at annual surgical society meetings and carrying them through to publication. Members of the Ethics Forum are noted below. Coauthors of the essays in this book are listed in the pages following.

Members of the Ethics Forum, 2000–2014

Cary Akins, MD	Martin McKneally, MD, PhD
Mark Allen, MD	Eric Mendeloff, MD
Lawrence Bonchek, MD	Walter Merrill, MD
Charles Bridges, MD, ScD	Bryan Meyers, MD, MPH
David Campbell, MD	Lynda Mickleborough, MD
Thomas D'Amico, MD	John Mitchell, MD
Jennifer Ellis, MD	Scott Mitchell, MD
Richard Engelman, MD	Susan Moffatt-Bruce, MD, PhD
Kathleen Fenton, MD	Gordon Murray, MD
Mark Ferguson, MD	Keith Naunheim, MD
Richard Freeman, MD, MBA	Kenneth Oberheu, MD
David Fullerton, MD	Mark Orringer, MD
Stephen Guyton, MD, MHA	Lorraine Rubis, MD
John Hammon, MD	Richard Sanderson, MD
Lynn Harrison, Jr., MD	Mark Slaughter, MD
Wayne Isom, MD	Scott Stuart, MD
James Jaggers, MD	Gregory Trachiotis, MD
James Jones, MD, PhD	Ross Ungerleider, MD, MBA
Leslie Kohman, MD	Donald Watson, MD
Nicholas Kouchoukos, MD	Andrew Wechsler, MD
Jeffrey Kramer, MD, MBA	Winfield Wells, MD
Sidney Levitsky, MD	Richard Whyte, MD
Michael Mack, MD	Walter Wolfe, MD
Constantine Mavroudis, MD	Joseph Zwischenberger, MD

Introduction

Robert M. Sade

Health-care ethics is a broad field that includes many overlapping subcategories: bioethics (concerned broadly with health-care issues, including public policymaking), clinical ethics (concerned with decision-making at the bedside), medical ethics (concerned with the appropriate behavior of physicians), organizational ethics (concerned with choices made by health-care organizations among available options), and surgical ethics (a subcategory of medical ethics, focusing on issues of special significance to surgery). Ethics in general aims to provide justifications for judging a particular action right or wrong or for choosing and acting upon the best among competing options.

Theoretical approaches to answering questions of how to make the best choice among several options for action have been controversial ever since the earliest deliberations on the morality of human action. Dozens of distinct approaches have been proposed and used in ethical analysis, but most fall into one of three general categories: deontological (rule-based), consequentialist (outcome-based), and teleological (virtue-based). Each of these is associated with conceptual problems. To apply rules in choosing a particular action, one has to decide which rules to follow, and there is little agreement on which rules or rule systems are most easily defensible or best justified. Choosing an action based on consideration of its consequences while hoping for the outcome that best optimizes human welfare is made difficult or impossible by the problems of identifying the full range of effects and consequences of the action options. While the virtues that are best suited for human welfare have been well described over millennia, there has been little agreement as to which of them are most important for human happiness or excellence.

Like all physicians, surgeons have many different roles at various stages of their careers. Their dominant role, of course, is caring for patients, but they may also be teachers of medical students, residents, and other trainees, as well as of each other; innovators and researchers seeking to improve patient care or adding to the foundations of scientific knowledge; and administrators, contributing to the administration of medical centers. In each of those roles, surgeons are guided by the ethics relevant to the role. I do not mean that there are different ethics for different functions within the health-care system, only that I believe the Code of Medical Ethics of the American Medical Association is misleading when it says

> Assuming a title or position that removes the physician from direct patient-physician relationships does not override professional ethical obligations.... Adherence to professional medical standards includes ... placing the interests of patients above other considerations, such as ... employer business interests.[1]

To back up a bit, the ethical principles that guide clinicians, educators, administrators, and researchers are the same as they are for all human beings. Our human nature requires a common set of responses to the challenges we face every day. Although the principles apply to all of us, they have a hierarchy of importance that is critically different in each of the roles, because in different roles, the surgeon faces different sets of challenges.

Human beings make thousands of choices every day, starting, for instance, with a health-related decision whether to have bacon and eggs or oatmeal with berries for breakfast, ranging up to high-impact decisions, such as whether to recommend medical treatment versus major surgical intervention for patients with severe coronary artery disease. Virtues are habits of mind that become engrained and automatic when an individual analyzes specific situations intelligently and chooses the correct response repetitively over long periods of time. For example, we have the virtue of honesty because we choose to tell the truth rather than to lie in order to gain a transient advantage, and we do this time after time. We have the virtue of integrity because the actions we choose from among many options are consistent with our personal beliefs and values, time after time.

We use those virtues, which serve as principles of action, to guide us in making important decisions. Some of the virtues that are particularly important for physicians are these: respect for the right of all patients to decide what is done to them; integrity, by which I mean consistency between our beliefs and our actions; honesty in all of our interactions with patients and colleagues; cognitive and technical competence in making accurate diagnoses and carrying out correct treatments; and compassion for the suffering of our patients. These are important virtues for all human beings, as well as for physicians in our various roles. Their rank order changes, however, depending on the nature of the job we are doing and the goals we strive toward as clinicians, educators, administrators, and researchers. I explain what I mean by changes in rank order.

The first goal of physicians in a clinical setting is to serve the good of the patient. Patients must trust that their physicians are acting in their best interest in order for the healing relationship to have successful outcomes—patients who do not trust their physicians are unlikely to follow directions or accept their physicians' advice. Two aspects of the patient's good must guide the virtue of fidelity to the patient's interests. First, serving the *biological* good of the patient requires scientific objectivity and competence in technical skill and medical knowledge. Second, serving the *subjective* good of the patient from the patient's viewpoint requires the virtues of respect for the patient's personal values and preferences, honesty in disclosing relevant information for the patient to make good decisions, and compassion for the patient's situation. This can be summed up as a single virtue: trustworthiness, which encompasses all of the above. Yet physicians may strive to earn the patient's trust but may not always be worthy of it. For example, patients harmed by mistakes made during their treatment have a right to know what happened, and it is the surgeon's responsibility to tell them, but only half of 1,300 physicians who responded to one survey believed that a serious error should be disclosed to the patient.[2] Also, many physicians condone lying to insurance companies to benefit patients,[3] yet deceptions of this kind undermine the possibility of developing the virtue of honesty and thereby challenge the patient's trust.

As educators, the first goal of physicians is to transmit to their students and trainees accurate and unbiased knowledge and skills that are required in their future practices, with integrity, avoiding abuse of the asymmetry of power between teacher and student. The road to those goals is not always smooth. The Association of American Medical Colleges surveys all recent medical graduates with its Medical School Graduation Questionnaire. In the 2012 survey, a section dealt with mistreatment of students, citing fifteen serious abuses. No less than 47.1% (about 6,000 of the more than 12,000 respondents) experienced at least one of those abuses.[4] There are no data on mistreatment of students and trainees by specialty, but in the view of many, surgeons top the list of transgressors.

Many surgeons serve as administrators in one form or another during their careers. Hospital administrators are in the business of maintaining hospitals, and the central goal of a businessperson is to preserve the hospital's long-term success. In doing so, they have to be concerned with the financial balance sheet and must develop and administer policies that support the hospital's mission. Administrative failures, however, have led to scandals that have damaged the reputations of university medical centers, such as Emory University, Harvard University, the University of Pennsylvania, and the University of Wisconsin.[5]

Another role that many physicians fill is that of research scientist. The primary goal for the investigator is to discover new knowledge that will improve the care of patients. Scientists must operate with the virtues common to all human beings, including respect for their subjects' self-determination, cognitive and technical competence, and compassion for the humanity of their subjects. The ethical principles that are most important to achieve the goals of science, however, are integrity and honesty, because without them the very foundations of science will be seriously undermined. Yet research misconduct is surprisingly widespread in biomedical research. In a recent study of thousands of biomedical scientists, 33% admitted that they had violated at least one of ten egregious scientific transgressions, such as fabricating or falsifying research data, in the previous three years.[6]

Most physicians do the right thing most of the time in each of the various roles they fill during their professional lives. Yet there is clearly room for improvement in reinforcing the virtues that are required for success in each of the roles they fill.

What Sets Surgical Ethics Apart?

Surgical ethics differs from other categories of ethics because of special aspects of surgery. Several examples of the differences come to mind: vulnerability and trust, absence of complete information at the moment decisions must be made, a requirement for manual dexterity, the widespread use of medical devices in surgery, and distinctive aspects of surgical research.

VULNERABILITY AND TRUST

The foundation of the patient-physician relationship is trust, because without it patients are unlikely to take the physician's advice seriously, may make choices that are inimical to their best interests, will not return for follow-up visits, and, when trouble occurs, are likely to blame the physician and perhaps even pursue a lawsuit. Physicians promote trust in many ways: through clear explanations, projection of empathy, and honesty in all aspects of dealing with patients.

Respecting confidences and privacy are of special importance in medicine because of the unique intimacy of the patient-physician relationship. Patients share a great deal of private financial and business information with their lawyers, emotional and other private information with clergy, and a wide range of deeply personal information with their spouses. Yet none of those confidantes is privy to all of the details that patients share with their physicians, and none has access to every part of the patient's body as does the physician in the course of a physical examination.

Within medicine, the degree of intimacy between patient and physician varies, but nowhere is access to physical privacy greater than in the field of surgery. The informed-consent process requires that the surgeon gain insights into the patient's emotional state and personal values, as is true in nearly all medical disciplines. But, in addition to this personal information, the patient also knows that at the time of surgery she will be anesthetized and devoid of all resources to protect herself—she will be entirely dependent on the surgeon's knowledge, skills, and professional integrity. These facts place surgical patients at the top of the scale of trust, and the corresponding responsibility makes extraordinary demands on the surgeon, exacting the highest level of professionalism.

Finally, among all the medical specialists, surgeons are the most accountable for their patients' outcomes. There are many reasons for this, but the most important is the underlying expectation of success—cure or palliation—before a surgeon operates. Charles Bosk put it in this way:

> If a surgeon operates on an eighty-three-year-old patient with gallbladder problems and the patient dies, then the surgeon cannot very well make the claim that the patient died of old age. He must first explain how and why the patient received a scar on his abdomen. Now, an internist medically managing the same gallbladder problem with the same result can legitimately claim that the patient died of old age. Deaths and complications present different questions to different specialists. When the patient of an internist dies, the natural question his colleagues ask is, "What happened?" When the patient of a surgeon dies, his colleagues ask, "What did you do?"[7]

SURGICAL DECISION-MAKING

Uncertainty is an omnipresent feature of medical practice. Before we can help a patient, we must accurately determine the nature of the problem. We accomplish this using many modalities, such as the patient's medical history, the history of the current illness, a well-executed physical examination, and a wide variety of diagnostic examinations and tests. Although we often can determine the precise nature of the patient's illness, there is usually some degree of uncertainty. For surgeons, the problem of incomplete information is greatly magnified by the short time frames between the arrival of the patient and the need for intervening to treat the problem. This is especially the case in urgent or emergency situations, when the surgeon often must act without all the evidence he needs. Acquiring diagnostic information takes time, and balancing the need for information against the urgency of intervention may force difficult choices driven by limited time.

Unexpected events during the course of an operation place considerable pressure on the surgeon to make the right decision, often when he does not know precisely what the problem is. In such situations, the patient's welfare is at stake. Because surgeons must maintain a high level of alertness throughout operations in order to execute technical maneuvers accurately and to deal with unexpected situations, they must maintain a level of self-awareness beyond those needed by nonsurgeons. Surgeons, like all human beings, have stresses in their personal lives that can interfere with their professional functioning. They must control their reactions to such stresses in order to avoid distractions and concentrate on what they are doing. One example of such a stress is sleep deprivation, raising ethical questions of whether an operation should be done in the face of inadequate sleep in the hours before the scheduled procedure.

Surgeons are sometimes called upon to make decisions that pit their professional obligations against the patient's instructions. For example, during the course of a usually safe operation, a surgeon operating on a patient who is a Jehovah's Witness may unexpectedly face a rare exsanguinating hemorrhage. Because years of training have instilled a deep dedication to turning death aside whenever possible, the surgeon may feel an obligation to save the patient's life with banked blood that is immediately accessible, against the patient's express refusal of transfusions. Moral distress often accompanies such situations.

MANUAL DEXTERITY

Medical education and training aim to produce physicians who are competent to perform the tasks relevant to their professional roles. All clinical physicians must be competent to evaluate patients' problems and act appropriately for the patients' benefit. Board examinations at all levels of education and training are designed to ensure adequacy of requisite knowledge, that is, to ensure cognitive competence. Surgeons, however, require a range of skills beyond those required of nonsurgeons, namely, skills related to manual dexterity. During their training, surgeons spend thousands of hours in operating rooms for the purpose of acquiring those skills; acquiring and refining manual skills remain important tasks throughout the years of practice. Learning new and better maneuvers while performing operations is a process that virtually never ends for the conscientious surgeon.

Evaluating cognitive competence is a matter of asking relevant questions and measuring the correctness of the physician's responses (viz., the board examinations that are familiar to all physicians). Measuring manual dexterity is much more difficult; a variety of such measures have been developed, but none has been widely utilized. Determination of readiness of surgical trainees to move to the next stage of graded operative responsibility is generally subjectively determined by faculty members' observations when they operate with trainees. This places ethical responsibilities on both the evaluator and the trainee. For example, because relatively rigid work schedules depend on the availability of trainees, faculty may be tempted to advance residents to the next level despite misgivings about their technical readiness to move on. Trainees must do their utmost to learn the necessary skills to evolve into competent surgeons.

A difficulty that most training programs occasionally face is dealing with the recognition that the readiness of a resident to enter independent practice is questionable. Alternative responses may include requiring an additional year or more of training, recommending (in egregious cases) that the resident enter a field of medicine other than surgery, or taking an optimistic view by writing a letter of approval for independent practice. Deciding the proper course of action in such cases, which fortunately are not common, can be ethically challenging.

Additional ethical dilemmas may occur as a surgical career nears its end. Manual dexterity declines with age, and the rate of deterioration varies widely. Some surgeons no longer have sufficient manual dexterity to operate safely on patients by the time they are fifty-five or sixty years old, while others may not reach that point until they are in their mid-seventies. No good evaluation tools are available to determine when the time to quit has arrived, and surgeons, like all human beings, can easily fail to recognize their own declining capacities because of the all-too-human defense mechanism of denial: I'm just as good as I ever was. We must rely on the advice and subjective judgments of colleagues regarding deteriorating operative outcomes, increasing complication rates, and softer signs that the end of a career is approaching or has arrived. Deciding to end one's career on the basis of declining competence is perhaps the most difficult decision a surgeon faces and too often evades.

DRUGS AND DEVICES

Dr. William Silen, former surgeon-in-chief at Boston's Beth Israel Hospital, used to quip, "A surgeon is an internist who has completed his education." Surgeons must have broad knowledge of general medicine in order to make correct diagnoses and accurately manage patients before and after operations. We use the same drugs in managing various illnesses and surgical complications as internists and pediatricians, but we also use a large variety of artificial devices in repairing body parts. Surgeons interact with drug-company representatives as do nonsurgeons, but we also interact with personnel of device companies—detail representatives and technical experts—which adds a layer of complexity to surgeons' relations with industry.

Some of these multifaceted interactions are similar to those seen in medicine, such as conflicts of interest involving exchanges of sums of money for using or promoting a company's products, including drugs and devices. But some interactions are unique to surgery. For example, the use of innovative devices such as cardiac-assist pumps and robotic-surgery technologies have been utilized for marketing rather than primarily for the benefit of patients. Innovation generates ethical questions of when and how new technologies should be incorporated into surgical practice.

Many surgical technologies and devices are expensive. For example, implantation of a left ventricular assist device intended to permanently replace the function of the heart in a patient with severe cardiac failure generally costs about $250,000 for the device, procedure, hospitalization, and management for the first postoperative year. More than $150,000 is required each year thereafter for managing the patient and his or her artificial heart. Because of the uncertain but probably shortened life expectancy after implantation of these devices, such large expenses raise substantial questions of resource allocation.

SURGICAL RESEARCH ETHICS

Ethical issues are present at every step of the research process, from conception to publication.

Conception and Design

At the stage of conception and design, proper methodology must be followed. In clinical studies, for example, in order to test a new drug or device in a randomized controlled trial (RCT), clinical equipoise must exist. The concept of equipoise was adopted as the resolution of a fundamental conflict: the goals of clinical medicine versus the goals of research, that is, the conflict between holding the patient's interests as paramount versus the search for truth as paramount. In order to enter patients into a clinical study, clinical equipoise must exist; there is an ethical requirement for uncertainty as to whether the study treatment is better than or at least as good as standard treatment or no treatment.[8]

Recruitment

In the recruitment phase of a study, inclusion and exclusion criteria must be followed closely in order to ensure the integrity of the study results. The informed-consent process is critically important in recruiting subjects. Although the informed-consent document is carefully written and thoroughly reviewed by an institutional review board to ensure that the benefits of the investigation outweigh the risks to subjects, informed consent does not exist on a form but comprises conversations with the potential subjects to ensure that they understand what is being proposed in the study so they have sufficient information to decide whether to participate.

Execution

During the execution of a study, the protocol must be followed precisely; otherwise the study's data cannot support valid conclusions. As data accumulate, they are reviewed by a data safety and monitoring board, which further ensures the safety of subjects in the study and integrity of the process. Changes in the balance of benefits and risks that become apparent during a study must be conveyed to the subjects so that they can decide whether to continue to participate.

Analysis

Ethical difficulties often arise during the analysis of the data. Because of pressures to produce grants and publications, there are many temptations to manipulate data to produce results that are clearer or more positive than *prima facie* interpretation.[6] Some of the most sensational scandals in the past two decades have come from fabrication and falsification of data that led to the destruction of careers of eminent scientists.[9] The same kinds of pressures may lead to inflation of the conclusions that are reached or the inferences that are drawn from the results.

Presentation

As research studies are being prepared for presentation at meetings, bias can result from similar pressures to produce positive results that will lead to grants and publications. In addition, however, funding sources such as industry or foundations can provide undue influence motivated by the desire for certain results. To deal with these issues, the Accreditation Council for Graduate Medical Education has created a series of guidelines for presentations at continuing medical education events, such as review of the presentation in advance by a third party who is responsible for detecting bias; if any is found, the sponsoring organization must manage the conflict of interest in an appropriate manner.[10]

Publication

During the publication process, additional ethical difficulties appear. Who should be listed as an author? Guidelines have been created by the International Council of Medical Editors that are followed by many journals.[11] Some publications require a signed statement that discloses any conflicts of interest and, in some cases, a signed statement that the investigator had freedom of investigation, that is, had complete access to the data and freedom from outside influences to decide what information to include in the publication and when it should be published.

These problems apply to the entire range of clinical-research ethics, but surgical research has distinctive characteristics that single it out for special concern. For example, the gold standard of research methodology is the RCT. Patients are randomized into one of two or more arms of a research project in order to discover whether a new treatment is as good as or better than existing treatments. RCTs are carried out far less frequently in surgery than in other fields of medicine, for which surgeons have been criticized, but there are good reasons for this discrepancy. A well-designed RCT requires that neither the patient nor the physician knows what treatment the patient is receiving; in other words, the trial should be double-blinded. This is clearly not possible in surgery because the surgeon always must know what he is doing. Moreover, RCTs require a large enough cohort of subjects to avoid statistical errors associated with inadequate numbers. Many surgical conditions do not occur frequently enough to supply a sufficient number of subjects to avoid such errors. This difficulty can be overcome by doing multi-institutional studies, but this introduces a different kind of error: nonstandard treatment because of differences in surgical methods at different institutions and among different surgeons.

Furthermore, a medication of a certain dose is constant no matter who prescribes it, but a surgical procedure is executed differently by different surgeons. Moreover, the same surgeon is unlikely to do an operation the same way twice, because it is in the nature of surgery that its practitioners continuously make small adjustments of technique. In this way, surgeons improve a particular operation incrementally, resulting in greater benefit to present and future patients. As a result, surgical operations are moving targets, unlikely to satisfy the requirement of treatment standardization that is necessary for RCTs.

Although many ethical dilemmas facing surgeons are similar to those confronting other physicians, the differences of surgical practice from other medical disciplines lead to ethical issues that are largely confined to surgical practice. For this reason, surgical ethics is worthy of consideration apart from other categories of health-care ethics, and understanding the reasoning underlying the special ethical issues in surgery can be of considerable value to practicing surgeons, surgical trainees, and medical students.

HOW THIS BOOK CAME ABOUT

Ethics discussions have historically taken place far less frequently in the surgical literature than in the medical literature,[12] so in 2000 a group of cardiothoracic surgeons who were interested in surgical ethics decided to introduce more discussion of ethical issues into national meetings of cardiothoracic surgical societies and to publish these presentations in surgical journals. The topics for discussion are chosen for their currency and intensity of controversy by the Ethics Forum (the Forum), a joint committee of the American Association for Thoracic Surgery and the Society of Thoracic Surgeons.

The Forum's chosen topics generally do not address the grand, high-profile, sometimes sensational issues commonly explored in the print and electronic communication media, such as human cloning, genetic enhancement, and the role of health professionals in prisoner abuse; rather, they focus on controversial issues selected from the day-to-day experiences of the surgeons who comprise the Forum. Thus the topics are of immediate interest to those who are actively involved in caring for surgical patients.

All of the essayists in these sessions are professionals, but most are not professional ethicists or philosophers—they are, for the most part, practicing surgeons, with an admixture of philosophers, social scientists, and attorneys, among others. Along with the common ethical dilemmas that have been the foci of the presentations, the predominance of surgeons as essayists has grounded the oral presentations and the associated publications in the real world of surgery.

The proceedings of sessions presented orally at annual meetings have been published in one of two major peer-review surgical journals, the *Annals of Thoracic Surgery* and the *Journal of Thoracic and Cardiovascular Surgery.* Though the discussions are situated in cardiothoracic surgery, the topics are not specific to that field—they are relevant and of interest to practicing surgeons, surgical trainees, and students in every surgical field.

Most of the papers selected for this book take the form of debates or point–counterpoint discussions, but a few of them are free-standing pieces such as editorials. I have organized and moderated all of the oral debates and have authored or coauthored all of the corresponding articles that are included in this collection.

We chose the debate format for addressing ethical issues not only for identification and discussion of important ethical issues in surgery but also for enabling the reader to understand varying viewpoints. Much of the bioethics literature gives the impression that important questions in ethics have been settled, but this view is far from accurate. The broad field of biomedical ethics is riddled with controversy. The diversity of viewpoints and analytical methods of bioethics have produced deep rifts in the field of bioethics, amply illustrated by the wide divergence of views published by President Bill Clinton's left-leaning National Bioethics Advisory Commission, President George W. Bush's right-leaning President's Council on Bioethics, and President Barack Obama's left-leaning Presidential Commission for the Study of Bioethical Issues.[13] No doubt future presidents will appoint ethics panels that reflect their own political positions and Weltanschauungen. The debate format has at least two purposes: By eluding prescriptive solutions to ethical dilemmas, this structure may help readers understand that there is often more than one good answer to vexing ethical dilemmas, and it may enable them to explore and better understand their own views.

The previously published papers in this book, which have been designated chapters, have their own introductions, arguments, and conclusions, but I have added a small amount of introductory material to each section to provide background, identify important ethical areas, and highlight key positions and arguments. I have deleted redundant or superfluous material from most of the papers, and have denoted deletions with bracketed ellipses [. . .].

I have also deleted some of the literature citations, retaining those that are most germane to the discussion. The full articles, of course, are available from their original sources in the surgical literature.

The twenty-eight chapters in the book are divided into seven thematic sections: The Problem of Surgical Ethics, Professional Integrity, Relationships with Patients—Autonomy and Consent, Innovation and Uses of Technology, Organ Donation and Transplantation, Conflicts of Interest in Surgery, and Ethical Issues in Health-Care Policy. Each section contains several chapters, which are expository papers that make important points regarding ethical issues in surgery. The chapters that are in the debate format generally, with a few exceptions, have a specific structure: an introduction of the issue to be debated, the positive viewpoint, the negative viewpoint, and closing commentary pointing to strong and weak aspects of the discussions, as well as points that may have been understated, misstated, or missed by the essayists.

Many different, often competing methods of ethical analysis have been developed over centuries. The ancient form of ethical analysis, teleological or virtue ethics, is exemplified by the works of Plato and Aristotle and is still widely used.[14] Deontology, best embodied in the works of Immanuel Kant, judges ethical actions based on their adherence to certain rules describing duties or obligations.[15] Consequentialism bases ethical judgments on a calculus of benefits and harms, judging those actions best that will maximize human welfare; this approach is perhaps best exemplified by the utilitarianism of Jeremy Bentham and John Stuart Mill.[16] A widely used contemporary method of ethical analysis is the principlism of Tom Beauchamp and James Childress, introduced in 1979, based on four principles: respect for autonomy, beneficence, nonmaleficence, and justice.[17] Many other contemporary forms of ethical analysis are less widely used. The least acceptable form of ethical discourse, in general, is argument from authority. Quoting persons whose underlying philosophy is well known, such as "Kant asserts that X is true" or "Bentham argued Y," is usually a reasonable strategy. It is less acceptable to use isolated quotes, such as, "John Doe said Z," from persons whose views are not well known, without an additional basis or explanation. Most of the discussions in the papers presented in this book use one or more of the traditional methods of analysis, but occasionally arguments from authority will be found; these should be viewed with skepticism.

This book—indeed, any book on ethics—cannot be considered definitive or authoritative because there are no truly authoritative sources of secular ethical wisdom. Nevertheless, it contains much thoughtful consideration of ethical issues that are important and of daily concern to surgeons. It should prove useful and instructive to practitioners, trainees, and students in all surgical fields.

References

1. Council on Ethical and Judicial Affairs. Opinion 8.021, Ethical obligations of medical directors. Code of Medical Ethics, 2012–2013 ed. Chicago: American Medical Association; 2012:218–9.
2. Loren DJ. Risk Managers, Physicians, and Disclosure of Harmful Medical Errors. *Joint Commission Journal on Quality and Patient Safety.* March 2010;36(3): 102–8.
3. Sade RM. Deceiving insurance companies: new expression of an ancient tradition. *Ann Thorac Surg.* 2001;72(5):1449–53.
4. Association of American Medical Colleges. Medical School Graduation Questionnaire, 2012. https://www.aamc.org/download/300448/data. Accessed May 19, 2014.
5. Volpe M. Dr. Charles Nemeroff and Emory University's culture of corruption. *The Provocateur.* July 10, 2009. http://theeprovocateur.blogspot.com/2009/07/dr-charles-nemeroff-and-emorys-culture.html. Accessed May 19, 2014.
6. Martinson BC, Anderson MS, de Vries R. Scientists behaving badly. *Nature.* 2005;435(7043):737–8.
7. Bosk CL. *Forgive and Remember: Managing Medical Failure.* Chicago: University of Chicago Press; 1979.
8. Djulbegovic B. Uncertainty and equipoise: an interplay between epistemology, decision making and ethics. *Am J Med Sci.* 2011;342(4):282–9.
9. Kumar G, Ryan J. Embattled Professor Marc Hauser will resign from Harvard. *Harvard Crimson.* July 19, 2011.
10. Accreditation Council for Continuing Medical Education. Standards for Commercial Support: Standards to Ensure Independence in CME Activities. http://www.accme.org/requirements/accreditation-requirements-cme-providers/standards-for-commercial-support. Accessed April 2, 2014.
11. International Council of Medical Editors. Defining the role of authors and contributors. http://www.icmje.org/recommendations/browse/roles-and-responsibilities/defining-the-role-of-authors-and-contributors.html. Accessed May 17, 2014.
12. Sade RM, Williams T, Haney C, Perlman D, Stroud M. The ethics gap in surgery. *Ann Thorac Surg.* 2000;69(2):326–9.
13. Eckenweiler LA, Cohn FG, eds. *The Ethics of Bioethics: Mapping the Moral Landscape.* Baltimore: Johns Hopkins University Press; 2007.
14. Kuczewski MG, Polansky R. *Bioethics: Ancient Themes in Contemporary Issues.* Cambridge, MA: MIT Press; 2000.
15. Kant I. Critique of Pure Reason, In: Guyer P and Wood AW, ed. *The Cambridge Edition of the Works of Immanuel Kant.* New York: Cambridge University Press; 1998.
16. Bentham J, Mill JS. *Utilitarianism and Other Essays (Classics).* Ed. Ryan A. New York: Penguin Putnam; 2004.
17. Beauchamp TL, Childress JF. *Principles of Biomedical Ethics,* 7th ed. New York: Oxford University Press; 2012.

SECTION 1

The Problem of Surgical Ethics
Robert M. Sade

> The difference between surgeons and internists is that
> surgeons practice ethics, while internists mainly talk about it.
>
> —Ward O. Griffen, Jr., MD, PhD

The very idea of surgical ethics is problematic. Surgeons are often seen as
technical experts who do not expend a great deal of effort understanding
issues that are deeper than identifying a surgical problem and doing
whatever is needed to fix it. So surgery has an image problem: the surgeon
as unthinking automaton or shallow technician. The problem goes deeper
than image, however, because nonsurgical physicians do not understand
how surgeons approach clinical problems and what is required of a surgeon
to evaluate a patient's illness, convey information to the patient, reach
a mutual decision on the best therapeutic option, execute the required
procedure, and manage the postoperative course.

This lack of understanding originates and is intensified by important
differences in the way surgical and medical physicians go about
their business, at least in an academic environment, which is where
physicians-in-training develop their professional modi operandi and their
attitudes toward other specialists. Medical residents generally make their
working/teaching team rounds on patients in the early morning followed by
teaching rounds with the attending physician and conferences that last to
or through lunch. Most of the afternoon is spent getting clinical work done
before late afternoon team rounds on patients.

Routines on the surgical services are entirely different. The operating
schedule starts early, often around 7:00 AM, so early morning rounds at
5:30 to 6:00 are mainly working rounds, finished in an hour to an hour and

a half, then off to the operating room. The junior residents are left on the wards to get the work done, and those efforts continue until late afternoon rounds, which occur after most of the operating schedule has been completed. Teaching on surgical services is generally more diffuse than on medical services, taking place ad hoc at the bedside, in the operating room, and at early morning or late afternoon teaching conferences.

The paucity of the daily formal group teaching rounds and conferences that characterize medical services gives the impression of relatively superficial routines in caring for surgical patients, but this is far from the truth. Surgical training does not suffer from less thoughtful teaching and learning—it is simply organized differently.

Chapters

There might actually be a problem of surgical ethics beyond perception: a relative dearth of open discussion of ethics in surgical journal articles has been documented. **Chapter 1** is the report of a pilot study we designed to uncover the reasons for this discrepancy.[1] The study surveyed a medical school faculty with two clinical vignettes that posed a dilemma: Given four possible answers, respondents were asked to choose the one they considered to be ethically best and the one they thought legally most acceptable. Analysis of the responses stratified by medical, pediatric, and surgical specialties showed no difference between the ethical choices of the three groups; minor differences were found among legal choices. The proportion of faculty who chose legally and ethically unacceptable options, however, was surprisingly high.

Although this small study did not answer the question of why the ethics gap existed, it led to the creation of an educational program, developed by the Ethics Forum, that has produced ethics discussions at annual meetings of surgical societies and numerous publications on ethical issues in surgical journals. After several years of producing these programs and publications, we wondered whether they had any effect on surgical practice. We sought an answer to this question with another survey, this one directed to the membership of the Society of Thoracic Surgeons and the American Association for Thoracic Surgery. The survey described in **chapter 2** explores surgeons' views about the value of ethics education in clinical practice and the usefulness of including ethics questions on surgery certification and recertification board examinations.[2] The results are encouraging. Most respondents agreed that better understanding of ethical issues would improve their own practices and those of surgeons in general. They also believed that demonstration of adequate understanding of ethical issues should be part of the American Board of Thoracic Surgery certification and maintenance of certification processes. Fully 79% of the respondents believed the debate format to be an effective educational structure, and only 4% of those who attended ethics presentations at annual meetings believed that the sessions did not improve their understanding of complex ethical issues. Ten percent believed that the sessions did not affect their surgical practices.

Taken together, these two studies demonstrate that ethics education for surgeons in the form of debates and other presentations at annual meetings and in journal publications is both relevant to clinical practice and effective in improving the care of patients. The implications of these studies and the educational efforts resulting from them motivated the production of this book.

References

1. Sade RM, Williams TH, Perlman DJ, Haney CL, Stroud M. Ethics gap in surgery. *Ann Thorac Surg.* 2000;69:326–9.
2. D'Amico TA, McKneally MF, Sade RM. Ethics in cardiothoracic surgery: a survey of surgeons' views. *Ann Thorac Surg.* 2010;90(1):11–13.

1

Ethics Gap in Surgery

Robert M. Sade, Timothy H. Williams, David J. Perlman, Cynthia L. Haney, and Martha R. Stroud*

Introduction

Over the last few decades, new technologies have made possible levels of life support that were previously unavailable. Renal dialysis, organ transplantation, ventilators for respiratory support, and cardiac support devices have contributed to longer and better quality of survival than was previously possible for many patients suffering from vital organ failure. For many others, however, these technologies have led to survival with a poor quality of life, particularly in patients with brain injury or inadequacy of other major organs. Quandaries involving the way in which decisions are made led to a growing emphasis on the notion of autonomy: namely, the moral and legal right of patients to make decisions regarding their own bodies and their own healthcare. The idea of informed consent and informed refusal of care is relatively new, having grown from case law early in this century, then from the dialogue between ethicists, policymakers, physicians, and others over the past few decades.

Clinicians have also paid increasing attention in recent years to many other ethical issues, such as privacy and confidentially, truth telling and disclosure, and surrogate decision making. This attention has been reflected in medical periodicals and books, but the extent to which such discussions take place has varied among medical specialities. Surgeons in particular have been singled out as participating in discussion of ethical issues less frequently than other specialists.

A recent survey compared the surgical literature with the medical literature over a 1-year period, the 1992 publication year.[1] The authors carried out a detailed Medline search using key words related to ethics and bioethics in

*Sade RM, Williams TH, Perlman DJ, Haney CL, Stroud M. Ethics gap in surgery. *Ann Thorac Surg.* 2000;69:326–9. Copyright the Society of Thoracic Surgeons, republished here with permission.

12 surgical and 15 medical journals. The authors found that discussions of bioethical issues occurred much less frequently in the surgical literature than in the medical literature. Of 2,645 articles identified in 12 surgical journals, 17 (0.6%) contained substantive discussion of an ethical issue. Of 11,239 articles identified in 15 medical journals, 307 (2.7%) had ethics commentary. Thus, the medical literature contained over four times the frequency of ethics discussions than the surgical literature. This has been referred to as the "ethics gap" in surgery.

The reasons for the ethics gap are unclear, but several possibilities have been suggested[1]: (1) Surgeons may ascribe less importance to ethical considerations than internists do, so talk about them less. (2) The traditional beneficence model of medical ethics (doing what is best for the patient), a fundamental surgical principle, sometimes conflicts with the contemporary autonomy model (patient self-determination, which may include refusing medically indicated treatment). For this reason, surgeons may feel alienated from contemporary bioethical discourse[1,2] (3) There is evidence that surgeons are more authoritarian than other physicians, perhaps because of their professional training and the nature of surgical practice.[3,4] If this is true, surgeons may be more likely than other physicians to make paternalistic decisions and fail to recognize ethical problems when they appear. (4) Ethical principles may be so deeply ingrained in surgeons through training and practice that discussion of the principles may seem redundant.[5] One surgical educator has explained the ethics gap in this way: "The difference between surgeons and internists is that surgeons practice ethics, while internists mainly talk about it" (Griffen WO, personal communication).

We have observed that a type of case that seemed particularly subject to potential conflict and to differing perceptions among specialties was patient incapacity requiring surrogate decision making. We therefore undertook a small pilot study using two cases of this type to try to elucidate reasons for the ethics gap, as well as to investigate physicians' understanding of their legal obligations in such circumstances.

Material and Methods

We surveyed our academic medical center faculty by soliciting their views of ethical and legal options available to the physician in each of two cases of surrogate decision making. The standard for ethical acceptability was derived from published guidelines for surrogate decision making from six medical organizations, only one of which was surgical.[6-11]

Finding a standard for legal acceptability was not as straightforward, because the outcome for any particular legal challenge is not predictable. Rather than labeling the options as legal or illegal, we used the terms "acceptable-unacceptable" or "prudent-imprudent," based on whether a reasonable attorney would be likely to advise that a particular option had a greater or lesser likelihood of being upheld in a court of law. We solicited legal opinion regarding which of the options would be legally prudent or imprudent on grounds of liability risk.

Case 1 was that of a young woman suffering from severe brain injury with potential for only minimal recovery at best, whose parents wanted to withdraw feeding, based on comments made by their daughter in the past. Case 2 was that of a newborn infant with hypoplastic left heart syndrome and Down syndrome, whose parents asked that prostaglandin be discontinued.

Four options for responses by the physician were provided for each case. Three were ethically acceptable options in both cases: accede to the parents' wishes, withdraw from the case and transfer the care of the patient to another physician, and seek a court order to continue life support. The fourth option was the only one that was ethically unacceptable; continue treatment despite objection by the surrogate decision maker. The published opinions or policies regarding surrogate decision making of nearly all six organizations explicitly supported this classification of options; none expressed an opinion at variance with it.

The legal status of the four options, according to our legal counsel, was exactly parallel to their ethical acceptability: the first three options were deemed to be legally prudent, while the fourth was legally imprudent.

The survey requested that each option be rated as either ethically acceptable or unacceptable, and that the options be ranked in order of ethical preferability. It also requested that each option be rated as either legally acceptable or unacceptable, and that the options be ranked in order of legal preferability.

In case 2, we also asked whether the respondent would have changed their ratings or rankings of the options if the child did not have Down syndrome.

We searched our data for evidence to support the several possible explanations for the ethics gap cited above. If surgeons ascribe less importance to ethical considerations than internists do, or feel alienated from contemporary biomedical discourse, they perhaps would have not responded to the survey as frequently as others, so we measured the response rate to the survey. If surgeons fail to recognize ethical problems because they are more paternalistic than other physicians, then their responses should reflect more authoritarian attitudes than those of other physicians. We, therefore, combined two options as authoritarian (willingness to treat over parents' objections, and seeking a court order to override the parents) and two options as nonauthoritarian (willingness to accept parents' decision to withdraw treatment or transferring the patient to another physician who was willing to withdraw treatment). We then compared the most highly ranked options of surgeons with those of other physicians to determine their relative levels of authoritarian and nonauthoritarian choices. Finally, if ethical principles are so deeply ingrained in surgeons that their discussion seems redundant, there should be more agreement in choice of options among surgeons than among other specialty groups. We measured this by recording the proportion of physicians in each specialty who agreed on the acceptability of each ethical option. [. . .]

Results

The survey was mailed to 407 faculty physicians, and 133 (33%) responded. Responses were grouped into surgery (including all surgical specialties), internal medicine (including all medical specialties), pediatrics, and others (eg, pathologists, radiologists). For interspecialty comparisons, only the surgeons, internists, and pediatricians had sufficient numbers for statistical comparison. The response rates for those groups were: surgeons, 31 of 74 (42%); pediatricians, 18 of 44 (41%); and internists, 51 of 173 (29%); surgeons' response rate was significantly higher than that of internists (p < 0.05).

ETHICAL RESPONSES

Many faculty members mistakenly believed it to be ethically acceptable to override the wishes of the parents (case 1, 88 of 132, 67%; case 2, 57 of 132, 42%). That ethically unacceptable option was ranked as the first choice among all options by 33 of 133 (26%) of faculty members. Every commentator on ethical standards for treatment of disabled individuals has held that disability, including mental disability, should not be the sole grounds for making treatment withdrawal decisions. Nevertheless, 44 of 115 (38%) faculty members would have made a different treatment decision if Down syndrome had not been present in case 2.

When we compared the specialties for their ethical choices, surgeons did not either rate or rank any ethical option differently from either internists or pediatricians.

Authoritarian responses were ranked the first choice more often by pediatricians (9 of 18, 50%) than by surgeons (3 of 28, 11%) or internists (11 of 51, 22%) (p < 0.05). The survey revealed uniformity of ethical views among the three groups: no differences were detected in the proportion of identical ratings of options by surgeons (76%), internists (74%), and pediatricians (71%).

LEGAL RESPONSES

Among the general faculty, the only legally imprudent response, to continue treatment over the objections of the parents, was mistakenly believed to be legally prudent in case 1 by 73% of our faculty, and, in case 2, by 39%. It is legally unacceptable to treat children with Down syndrome differently from other children, yet 44 of 115 (38%) of our faculty would have treated case 2 differently if Down syndrome had not been present; there were no differences among specialties.

Several differences appeared when comparing the legal responses of specialty groups. Pediatricians (61%) were less likely than surgeons (84%) and internists (85%) to recognize that it was legally acceptable to discontinue feeding at the parents' request in case 1 (p < 0.05). Pediatricians (78%) were also less likely than surgeons (92%) and internists (98%) to recognize in case 2 that challenging the parents in court was legally acceptable (p < 0.05). Surgeons (19 of 31, 62%), however, were more likely than internists (18 of 51, 35%) or pediatricians (4 of 18, 22%) to believe, mistakenly, that operating on the baby in case 2 without parental consent was legally acceptable (p < 0.05).

AGE AND GENDER

Univariate and multivariate analyses showed no difference in any ethical or legal measure by gender (male 5 = 98, female 5 = 25) and only two differences by seniority. By multivariate analysis, senior faculty members were more likely than junior faculty members to mistakenly rate discontinuing feeding in case 1 as ethically unacceptable (10 of 51 [20%] vs. 9 of 82 [11%], respectively, p < 0.05). Senior faculty members were also ethically more authoritarian than junior faculty members (23 of 51 [45%] vs 21 of 82 [26%] in case 1, and 17 of 51 [34%] vs 14 of 82 [17%] in case 2, respectively, both p < 0.05).

Comment

The surgical literature contains fewer discussions of ethical issues than the medical literature. Moreover, in searching for official positions taken by a wide range of medical organizations on surrogate decision making, we found only one by a surgical society, the American Academy of Otolaryngology, and five by other medical organizations. These facts speak to a paucity of ethical discourse among surgeons. We chose to limit this pilot study to a single type of ethical issue, surrogate decision making, because we have observed substantial differences and vehemently held positions on this topic in our institution.

Our main objective was to elucidate the reasons for the surgery ethics gap. Several authors have speculated on causes of the gap, but no speculation was confirmed by this survey. Within the limits of our study, the high rate of response to the survey by surgeons suggests that they consider ethical deliberation to be as important as do other specialists, and that they are not alienated from ethical discourse. Surgeons may be no more paternalistic than others, because they chose authoritarian options no more often; in fact, pediatricians gave priority ranking to authoritarian options more often than did either surgeons or internists. The speculation that discussion of ethics may seem redundant to surgeons because ethical principles are deeply ingrained in surgeons through training and practice seems undermined by our finding that surgeons do not agree with each other on rating of options any more often than do other specialists. Thus, we are left with no clear explanation of the ethics gap in surgery.

Comparisons of the specialists for their ratings of legal acceptability of the options revealed an interesting finding. Pediatricians were less likely than either internists or surgeons to recognize the legal acceptability of discontinuing feeding the newborn at the parents' request, and the acceptability of challenging the parents' decision to discontinue feeding their daughter. Perhaps most surprising, however, was the finding that surgeons were the most likely, by a large margin, to believe that operating on the baby without parental consent was legally prudent. This observation may flag an important educational problem for all faculty, particularly surgeons.

The survey provides interesting insights into the way our general faculty understands ethical and legal issues in surrogate decision making. Surprisingly often, faculty members mistakenly rated as acceptable the ethically unacceptable and legally imprudent option to override the wishes of the parents in both cases. Indeed, this unacceptable option was ranked as the first choice of more than a quarter of the responding faculty. Finally, it is clear that using mental disability as a factor in clinical decision making is both ethically and legally unacceptable; yet, a third of our faculty would have changed their choices among the options if the newborn did not have Down syndrome. These observations may flag additional educational needs for all faculty members.

It was interesting, though perhaps not surprising, that senior faculty were more authoritarian in their choices than junior faculty. This may be a reflection of the trend in recent decades toward increasing recognition of the importance of patients' exercise of autonomy in making clinical decisions. The training of older physicians took place before 1978, when physician authority over most clinical decisions was only beginning to wane. Younger physicians were trained in an era when patient autonomy had taken hold more securely in clinical decision making.

This pilot study has several shortcomings. The population we studied was small, and the 33% of our faculty who responded may not have been representative of the entire group. Moreover, the cases we presented narrowly focused on a single area of bioethics, decisions for incapacitated patients. Other areas of potential ethical conflict may have produced greater differences in choices by specialty groups. The precise form of the cases we presented and the questions we asked may have had some ambiguities, lending uncertainty to some responses. Finally, the study was a pilot, so the format was not designed to elicit the respondents' reasoning underlying their choices, which might have helped to explain our findings better.

We suggest, however, that more detailed studies that avoid these short-comings are needed, because it is incumbent on us to understand the reasons for the ethics gap. Surgeons have a strong sense of personal responsibility for patients' welfare, and it is important that this ethic be transmitted to medical students and residents. This goal can be addressed in many ways, but one route certainly is to discuss and write about ethics more than we do. Moreover, our analysis of the legal aspects of the survey suggests that physicians have important lapses in their understanding of legal obligations. Perhaps more importantly, the results suggest that a significant gap may also exist between surgeons and other physicians in understanding health law.

References

1. Paola F, Barton SS. An "ethics gap" in writing about bioethics: a quantitative comparison of the medical and surgical literature. *J Med Ethics.* 1995;21:84–8.
2. Jonsen AR, Siegler M, Winslade WJ. *Clinical Ethics,* 3rd ed. New York: McGraw-Hill;1992:37–84.
3. Schenk WG, Jr. Is there a surgical personality? *Curr Surg.* 1988;45:1.
4. Zimny GH, Thale TR. Specialty choice and attitudes toward medical specialties. *Soc Sci Med.* 1970;4:257–64.
5. Lytle G. Surgical education—an ethics gap? *Focus on Surg Educ.* 1996;13:22.
6. American Thoracic Society Bioethics Task Force. Withholding and withdrawing life-sustaining therapy. *Am Rev Resp Dis.* 1991;144:726–31.
7. Council on Ethical and Judicial Affairs. Code of Medical Ethics: current opinions with annotations. Chicago: American Medical Association; 1997.
8. American College of Physicians. American College of Physicians Ethics Manual, Third Edition. *Ann Intern Med.* 1992; 117:947–60.
9. Ethics Committee of the Society of Critical Care Medicine. Consensus statement of the Society of Critical Care Medicine's Ethics Committee regarding futile and other possibly inadvisable treatments. *Crit Care Med.* 1997;25:887–91.
10. Ethics Committee of the American Academy of Otolaryngology—Head and Neck Surgery. Chapter 2: Patient rights and surrogacy. *Otolaryngol Head Neck Surg.* 1996;115:186–90.
11. Committee on Bioethics, American Academy of Pediatrics. Ethics and the care of critically ill infants and children. *Pediatrics.* 1996;98:149–52.

2

Ethics in Cardiothoracic Surgery

A SURVEY OF SURGEONS' VIEWS

Thomas A. D'Amico, Martin F. McKneally,
and Robert M. Sade*

Before 2000, topics in medical ethics were discussed or mentioned far less often in the surgical than in the medical literature and appeared less often in surgical than in medical meeting programs.[1] The source of this difference was not clear, but it seemed reasonable to conclude that increasing the frequency of ethics discourse among cardiothoracic surgeons could add value to the overall educational efforts of our cardiothoracic organizations. [...]

The Ethics Forum's [...] educational efforts have taken the form of debates and other presentations at annual meetings and publication of the presentations as well as editorial commentaries in the official journals of the two organizations, *The Annals of Thoracic Surgery* (*ATS*) and the *Journal of Thoracic and Cardiovascular Surgery* (*JTCVS*). The effectiveness of these various efforts has been unknown, yet understanding their effects on cardiothoracic surgeons and their practices would be helpful in determining how valuable they have been and how they might be improved in the future. A survey of the views of cardiothoracic surgeons was therefore undertaken.

Material and Methods

A 17-question survey was developed to assess the effects of the Ethics Forum's educational agenda on its target audience, cardiothoracic surgeons, and to seek guidance in developing future projects for ethics education. The survey

*D'Amico TA, McKneally MF, Sade RM. Ethics in cardiothoracic surgery: a survey of surgeons' views. *Ann Thorac Surg.* 2010;90(1):11–3. Copyright Society of Thoracic Surgeons, republished here with permission.

contained questions related to ethics presentations at annual meetings and publications in *ATS* (32 articles in the last 5 years) and *JTCVS* (14 articles in the last 5 years). In addition, the survey sought views on inclusion of ethics education in training programs, board certification, and maintenance of certification. The membership of the STS and the AATS, including senior and international members, was contacted by sending the survey by electronic mail to the STS membership list (3,705 cardiothoracic surgeons), which includes nearly all members of the AATS. Three weeks after the initial distribution of the survey, we sent a second request for response to the survey instrument.

Results

Responses to the survey were returned by 578 of 3,705 surgeons (15.6%). The distribution of time in practice ranged from 16% in practice less than 10 years to 34% in practice 25 years or more. Among the respondents, 92% were in clinical practice (academic 55%, and private 37%). Most respondents endorsed the importance of ethics education and improved understanding of complex ethical issues in cardiothoracic surgery; 69% agreed that their own practices would be improved by such education, and 83% believed that cardiothoracic surgeons in general would benefit. In addition, 61% of respondents believed that demonstration of an adequate understanding of ethical issues should be part of the American Board of Thoracic Surgery (ABTS) initial certification process, and 60% believed that it should also be included in the ABTS maintenance of certification process.

In the last 5 years, 66% of respondents attended at least two STS annual meetings and 68% attended at least one AATS annual meeting. Of those who attended national meetings, 51% attended at least one cardiothoracic surgery-related ethics session. Among those who attended none of the sessions the reasons for not attending were scheduling conflicts (46%) and not knowing that the sessions were available (29%). Among those who attended one or more of the ethics sessions, 64% agreed or strongly agreed that the sessions improved their understanding of ethical issues in cardiothoracic surgery, 32% were neutral, and only 4% disagreed. In addition, 79% confirmed that the debate format is an effective educational format, and only 10% stated that the sessions did not affect their practices.

Of the 32 ethics-related articles that have been published in *ATS* since 2004, 88% of the respondents read at least one and 33% read eight or more. Of the 14 ethics articles that have been published in *JTCVS* since 2004, 74% read at least one and 17% read six or more.

The final survey item requested suggestions for topics to be presented or discussed at ethics sessions at meetings or journal articles—159 individual suggestions were provided.

Comment

Ethics education for physicians has attracted considerable attention in recent years: curricula in medical schools focus increasingly on ethical issues, and the number of medical schools offering formal education in medical ethics grows.[2] However, the content, method and timing vary substantially, suggesting a lack of consensus about the optimal educational process.[3] Including surgery-specific ethics modules within the medical student surgery rotation has been reported, but adding ethics education to an already crowded and demanding curriculum might be difficult to generalize to other programs.[4] In addition, a recent review of the literature found that ethics education for surgical residents is valuable, but that the timing, methods and content of ethics education and training for residents is still a matter of debate.[5]

The role of ethics education specifically in cardiothoracic surgery has not been studied, to our knowledge. Ethics topics are not included in the weekly curriculum established by the Thoracic Surgical Directors Association (TSDA), an 88-week comprehensive teaching schedule that constitutes the didactic framework for many training programs in thoracic surgery.[6] Moreover, demonstration of an adequate fund of knowledge regarding complex ethical issues is not required on the ABTS qualifying examination, certifying examination, or maintenance of certification process.

The practice of cardiothoracic surgery, however, requires a sound fund of knowledge and judgment about ethical challenges. A substantial number of such challenges arise in cardiothoracic surgical practice, a pattern that was not well represented in the surgical literature before 2000. The Ethics Forum identified numerous contentious issues for debate or discussion at cardiothoracic meetings and in cardiothoracic journals every year over the last 10 years. There have been 34 such sessions at meetings from November 1999 through November 2009, and 48 ethics-related papers have been published in *ATS* and *JTCVS* from 2000 through 2009. (There is a link to lists of oral sessions and papers in the online version of this article.) The present survey was conducted to evaluate the effect of these educational efforts, but the survey was limited to recollections about the last 5 years because of concerns about diminishing reliability of memory with increasing chronologic distance from an event.

The distribution of practice duration among respondents corresponds roughly to the age distribution of cardiothoracic surgeons in the most recent cardiothoracic surgical manpower report,[7] so the responding sample of the survey appears to be fairly representative of cardiothoracic surgeons as a whole with respect to time in practice and age.

A majority of respondents endorsed the importance of education and improved understanding of complex ethical issues in cardiothoracic surgery.

This finding may be flawed by selection bias, however, because surgeons who are interested in ethics may be more likely to respond to an ethics survey than those who are less interested. The discrepancy between the number of surgeons who thought their own practices would be improved by ethics education (69%) and the number who believed that cardiothoracic surgeons in general would benefit (83%) suggests that some surgeons are either unaware of their own deficiencies or underestimate the knowledge base of others.

The ABTS certification and maintenance of certification processes have not included formal evaluation of knowledge or understanding of concepts in ethics, yet a substantial majority of respondents asserted that both processes should require demonstration of an adequate understanding of ethical issues in cardiothoracic surgery. Perhaps the ABTS should consider adding such an evaluation to certification processes.

The Ethics Forum sessions at the STS annual meeting have taken place at a consistent time for the past 4 years: the lunch break on Tuesday of the meeting. Because lunch is available for a fee of $25, registration for the session has been required, so numbers of registrants for those sessions are available: 94, 106, 86, and 147 attended in 2007, 2008, 2009, and 2010, respectively. The majority of respondents have attended at least one of the previous 5 STS and AATS annual meetings, and 51% of those who attended these meetings attended a cardiothoracic surgery-related ethics session. Of those, a clear majority agreed that the sessions improved their understanding of ethical issues; nearly 80% confirmed that the debate format is a valuable educational format, and only 10% believed that the sessions did not affect their practices. The ethics presentations at annual meetings seem to be perceived as educationally effective.

Of those who attended no ethics sessions, 46% cited scheduling conflicts as the reason they did not attend. The ethics debates at STS meetings are held during lunch, so it may be difficult to find an hour that is more convenient. However, because 29% did not know that the sessions were available and in view of the generally positive response to the value of the sessions, it seems reasonable to increase the publicity about ethics sessions in communications regarding meeting programs.

A large majority of respondents read one or more of the articles in ATS and one or more of the articles in JTCVS, and a significant minority read most of the articles in both journals. This suggests that published articles on ethical topics can provide an enduring educational experience, especially because the articles in ATS and JTCVS are available to all the members of the STS and AATS, respectively.

The most serious flaw of this survey is the relatively low response rate (15.6%). This rate is consistent with response rates to previous surveys of the STS membership, but generalization of the survey findings is nevertheless questionable. Still, the Ethics Forum has reason to be encouraged by the results, because they provide some indication that its efforts to bring controversial topics from the domain of medical ethics to the attention of cardiothoracic surgeons have had at least some beneficial effect and at best substantial influence on improving cardiothoracic surgical practice. [...]

References

1. Sade RM, Williams T, Haney C, Perlman D, Stroud M. The ethics gap in surgery. *Ann Thorac Surg.* 2000;69:326–9.
2. Lehman LS, Kassoff WS, Koch P, Federman DD. A survey of medical ethics education at U.S. and Canadian medical schools. *Acad Med.* 2004;79:682–9.
3. Eckles RE, Meslin EM, Gaffney M, Helft PR. Medical ethics education: Where are we? Where should be going? A review. *Acad Med.* 2005;80:1143–52.
4. Giligorov N, Newell P, Altilio J, et al. Dilemmas in surgery: medical ethics education in surgery rotation. *Mt Sinai J Med.* 2009;76:297–302.
5. Helft PR, Eckles RE, Torbeck L. Ethics education in surgical residency: a review of the literature. *J Surg Educ.* 2009;66:35–42.
6. TSDA weekly curricula. Chicago: Thoracic Surgery Directors Association. http://www.tsda.org/documents/PDF/weekly_curricula/Curricula%20Docs/88_Week_Curriculum_Topics.09-1. Accessed September 20, 2009.
7. Shemin RJ, Dziuban SW, Kaiser LR, et al. Thoracic surgery workforce: snapshot at the end of the twentieth century and implications for the new millennium. *Ann Thorac Surg.* 2002; 73:2014–32.

SECTION 2

Professional Integrity

Robert M. Sade

> It's not what we eat but what we digest that makes us strong;
> not what we gain but what we save that makes us rich; not what
> we read but what we remember that makes us learned; and not
> what we profess but what we practice that gives us integrity.
>
> —Francis Bacon (1561–1626)

Most people believe that integrity is synonymous with honesty—indeed, some dictionaries list the two words as synonyms. They are not synonymous, however. Consider the individual who is caught shoplifting and who readily admits that he took the product simply because he needed it and could not afford to pay for it, even though he knew and believed that shoplifting is wrong. That person certainly is honest, but does he have integrity? Clearly, he does not, so how are we to understand the meaning of this word?

The root of the word is from the Latin adjective *integer*, meaning whole or complete. In the context of ethics, the wholeness referred to is the single nature of one's beliefs and one's actions.

Consider the meaning of an antonym of integrity, hypocrisy, which generally denotes behavior that is inconsistent with one's beliefs. Our shoplifter is honest, but he is hypocritical because his beliefs and his actions are contradictory. Integrity is the opposite of this—it means acting in ways that are consistent with one's beliefs. This idea defines personal integrity, but how might it be related to professional integrity?

In medicine, the term "professional integrity" refers to physicians making choices and acting in a manner that is consistent with medicine's professed principles.

A profession is a vocation that requires a certain degree of special knowledge and skill, and professionals are those who pursue that vocation while "professing" commitment to the ideals and principles developed by the profession itself. The classical professions from ancient times are medicine, theology, and jurisprudence, each of which has its own standards of acceptable activities that are often expressed in a code of ethics. In contemporary medicine, many medical societies, including many surgical specialty societies, have adopted codes of ethics, and the one most widely cited by state licensure boards and courts of law in determining standards for ethical behavior of physicians is the American Medical Association's Code of Medical Ethics. The Code's Principles are encapsulated on a single page,[1] while the interpretation and practical application of those principles require a 500-page book.[2] In describing professional behavior, the Principles identify such characteristics as honesty, respect for human dignity and rights, maintaining competence, safeguarding confidences and privacy, commitment to lifelong education and training, and respect for the law.

The Ethics Forum has addressed several topics related to professional integrity, including various aspects of honesty in dealing with patients and colleagues, such as honest assessment of personal limitations, responsibility to society, and responsibilities to the legal system. The papers in this section address issues related to honesty as the paramount characteristic of professional integrity, obligations to patients when temporarily impaired, responsibilities for personal wellness, and obligations within the legal system.

Chapters

Chapter 3 is an essay rather than a debate. In it, I describe the history of honesty in medicine, starting with the Hippocratic instruction to physicians (deceive patients by withholding information that might be harmful to them) progressing to the relatively recent adoption of standards of honesty in all dealings with patients.[3] The newest form of dishonesty among physicians is a practice that has become widely accepted since the advent of managed care three decades ago: deceiving insurance companies in order to benefit patients. In this essay, I suggest that the motivation driving these deceptions is not purely the benefit of patients but also the benefit of physicians and the institutions in which they work. Indeed, lying to insurance companies is associated with several problems, including harms to the patient, the insurance industry, society, and, not least, the physicians themselves.

The vignette associated with **chapter 4** describes a resident who innocently acquires infection with hepatitis C virus.[4] He spends a year in treatment and recovery, and ultimately the infectious diseases consultants declare that his viral titer is so low that he poses no more risk to patients than uninfected surgeons. He fully resumes his clinical responsibilities. When he finishes his training program, he applies for positions as a surgeon, placing his program director in a difficult position. He must write letters of recommendation that could include mention of the resident's year-long leave of absence and the reason for it; however, the stigma of HCV infection could sharply limit willingness to hire him. Does honesty require the director to report this aspect of his resident's background?

Competition between medical centers has intensified in recent decades, leading to ethical dilemmas around the requirements for disclosure during the informed-consent process. The question of how much to disclose to a patient always arises in consent discussions, but an increasingly common problem is whether to tell a patient about a new technology that might be his or her best option but is available only at a competitor's institution. Is a surgeon ethically required to disclose the existence of the technology and, if requested, refer the patient to a competitor? That is the dilemma facing the surgeon in **chapter 5**, when a new device for percutaneous repair of a mitral valve is not available in his own practice.[5]

Chapter 6 addresses the imposition of the eighty-hour work week on graduate medical education over a decade ago; since then, controversy has surrounded the question of whether this limitation is appropriate for surgeons in training. Convincing arguments are made that the lives of all physicians, including surgeons, would be improved if a better balance were reached between work and leisure. It is argued to the contrary, however, that the special nature of surgery renders imposing time constraints on the availability of surgeons for their patients inappropriate; such constraints are counterproductive in the long run.[7]

Fatigue from lack of sleep impairs performance; this has been well documented in laboratory and clinical studies and was an important reason for the introduction of the eighty-hour work week for house officers. The facts of sleep-induced impairment recently have been marshaled to propose that attending surgeons be mandated to report lack of sleep and the possibility of impairment to patients who are about to undergo an operation. After a new informed-consent process, the patient must decide whether the surgeon should go ahead with the operation, cancel the operation, or ask another surgeon to do the procedure. **Chapter 7** presents a debate about the wisdom of this proposal.[8] The essayists are the sleep physiologist-neurologist who proposed the process and a senior officer of the American College of Surgeons who opposes it. In response to the neurologist's position, the surgeon does not challenge the data but argues that consent of the patient is the wrong solution to the problems of sleep deprivation. Many factors in addition to sleep influence a surgeon's performance, and it would be impractical and unwise to attempt reporting them all to patients. It should be left to the surgeon, as a matter of professional integrity and responsibility, to weigh the advisability of operating rather than burdening the patient with such a decision at a time when he or she is highly vulnerable, immediately prior to an operation.

Chapter 8 addresses a distinguishing feature of American medicine: the profound influence of malpractice litigation on medical practice.[9] Physicians who are sued for negligence face great expense and emotional turmoil in defending themselves and their reputations in a legal process that is likely to extend over several years. The threat of lawsuits has resulted, among other things, in defensive medicine, which is very costly and inappropriate, exposing patients to risks of diagnostic procedures they may not need. An outcome of this national litigious atmosphere is great antipathy by many physicians toward the trial bar—the attorneys who pursue malpractice suits against physicians. Physicians are generally willing to testify as expert witnesses in malpractice litigation, but because of antagonism toward plaintiff's attorneys, many of them feel strongly that they will testify only in the defense of physicians who are sued. Yet substantial ethical opinion suggests that physicians who are willing to testify for defendants should be equally willing to testify for plaintiffs. Two surgeons who have special interest and backgrounds in legal issues debate the question of whether there is an ethical obligation to testify for plaintiffs as well as defendants.

References

1. Council on Ethical and Judicial Affairs. Principles of medical ethics. Code of Medical Ethics of the American Medical Association, 2014–2015 ed. Chicago: American Medical Association; 2014:xv.
2. Council on Ethical and Judicial Affairs. Principles of medical ethics. Code of Medical Ethics of the American Medical Association, 2014–2015 ed. Chicago: American Medical Association; 2014.
3. Sade RM. Deceiving insurance companies: New expression of an ancient tradition. *Ann Thorac Surg.* 2001;72:1449–53.
4. Dresler CM, Kent MS, Whyte R, Sade RM. HCV infected resident: end of residency, end of career? *Ann Thorac Surg.* 2013;95(3):779–86.
5. Skipper ER, Accola KD, Sade RM. Must surgeons tell mitral valve repair candidates about a new percutaneous repair device that is only available elsewhere? *Ann Thorac Surg.* 2011;92(4):1163–9.
6. Kouchoukos NT, Cohn LH, Sade RM. Are surgeons ethically obligated to refer patients to other surgeons who achieve better results? *Ann Thorac Surg.* 2004;77:757–60.
7. Dickey J, Ungerleider RM, Coselli JS, Conklin LD, Sade RM. The surgeon's work ethic in transition: should surgeons spend more time outside the hospital? *Ann Thorac Surg.* 2004;77:1145–51.

8. Czeisler CA, Pellegrini CA, Sade RM. Should sleep-deprived surgeons be prohibited from operating without patients' consent? *Ann Thorac Surg.* 2013;95(2):757–66.
9. Watson DC, Jr, Robicsek F, Sade RM. Are thoracic surgeons ethically obligated to serve as expert witnesses for the plaintiff? *Ann Thorac Surg.* 2004;78:1137–41.

3

Deceiving Insurance Companies

NEW EXPRESSION OF AN ANCIENT TRADITION

Robert M. Sade*

> *Perform these duties calmly and adroitly, concealing most*
> *things from the patient while you are attending to him …*
> *revealing nothing of the patient's future or present condition.*
> —*Hippocrates of Cos (460–377 BC)*

Two divergent threads of thought regarding truth telling have persisted since ancient times. Examples taken from Plato and Aristotle may illustrate this dichotomy, although ideas from elsewhere in their writings suggest that their views were not as opposed as these excerpts suggest. Plato held that lying in general is to be avoided, but with certain exceptions. "The lie in words is in certain cases useful and not hateful, in dealing with enemies—that would be an instance, or again when those who we call our friends in a fit of madness or illusion are going to do some harm, then it is useful and is a sort of medicine or preventive."[1] In fact, the ideal society Plato describes in the Republic is a fabric woven from lies told to ordinary citizens by philosopher-kings, who alone are capable of understanding truth.

Aristotle, however, is most concerned with the effects of lying on personal character:

[The truthful person] is truthful both in what he says and how he lives simply because that is his state of character. Someone with this character seems to be a decent person. For a lover of the truth, who is truthful even when nothing is at stake will be still keener to tell the truth when something is at stake, since he will avoid falsehood as shameful when something is at stake, having already avoided it in itself when nothing was at stake. And this sort of person is praiseworthy.[2]

---

*Sade RM. Deceiving insurance companies: new expression of an ancient tradition. *Ann Thorac Surg*. 2001;72:1449–53. Copyright Society of Thoracic Surgeons, republished here with permission.

According to Aristotle, lying undermines character and, in the long term, makes achievement of the good life more difficult.

Over the centuries since ancient times, these two approaches—Platonic justification of some deception for short-term gain and Aristotelian insistence on honesty to make possible long-term goals—have each had advocates among philosophers and theologians. Nearly all have generally supported telling the truth, but a dichotomy has persisted between those who maintain that deception and lying are always or nearly always wrong and those who find frequent exceptions to this requirement. This dichotomy persists today in the debate over how best to respond to denial of payment by insurance companies in contemporary health care.

Deception in Medicine, Recent Shift to Honesty

For purposes of this discussion, I distinguish between deceiving and lying, after Sissela Bok: To deceive is to communicate messages intended to make others believe something the deceiver does not believe to be true, including omission of relevant information. To lie is to speak or write an intentionally deceptive message. Thus, lying is a subtype of deception.[3]

The use of deception by physicians has deep roots. The tradition of deceiving patients "for their own good" was well established in ancient times, as noted above, and remained integral to medical practice until the latter part of the 20th century. Gradually over the last several decades, traditional practices of deceiving patients with the intent to reduce their suffering has given way to attitudes of truth telling to facilitate patients' self-determination. New emphasis on respect for patient self-determination in this country has led to a level of truthfulness not seen before in dealing with patients.

This trend is reflected in the American Medical Association (AMA) code of medical ethics. When the code was first written in 1847, based largely on Thomas Percival's earlier writing (1803), deception was generally accepted: "The life of a sick person can be shortened not only by the act, but also by the words or manner of a physician. It is, therefore, a sacred duty to guard himself carefully in this respect, and to avoid all things which have tendency to discourage the patient and depress his spirits."[4] This exhortation to avoid the harmful effect of words on patients in the AMA's first ethical code, reminiscent of the Hippocratic view expressed in the epigraph above, is absent from the current strongly worded principles of medical ethics, adopted by the AMA in 1980: "A physician shall deal honestly with patients and colleagues...."[5] This principle is developed further in opinion 8.12: "Patients have a right to know their past and present medical status and to be free of any mistaken beliefs concerning their conditions."[6] This opinion also contains a specific warning that acting for personal protection should not override honesty: "Concern regarding legal liability ... should not affect the physician's honesty with the patient." This view is a considerable departure from the Hippocratic and early AMA view of deception.

These guidelines reflect, to some extent, the realities of recent medical practice. For example, a survey in 1961 asked physicians whether cancer patients should or should not be told that they have cancer; 88% thought they should not be told.[7] By 1979, a striking shift had occurred: a survey using questions nearly identical to those of the earlier study found that 98% of physicians believed patients should be told they have cancer.[8]

The New Deception: Lying to Insurance Companies

Despite this recent apparent change in attitude toward telling patients the truth, a new manifestation of deceit in medicine has appeared recently: misrepresentation of patient information to insurance companies. Consider the following case:

> A 60-year-old man has severe emphysema for which no treatment other than an operation for lung volume reduction is beneficial. This relatively new operation is considered experimental, is being studied under a National Institutes of Health protocol, and is not covered by the patient's private insurance policy. The attending surgeon completes the required operation, and asks the surgical resident who assisted during the operation to dictate the operative note. The surgeon asks the resident not to use the term "lung volume reduction," but to stress the few blebs seen on the surface of the lung, naming the operation "resection of emphysematous blebs." The resident initially hesitates, and the attending surgeon angrily states, "Well, then, I'll dictate it myself!" On discussing this incident with colleagues, the resident is surprised to learn that some attending surgeons usually dictate their own operative notes in order to assure that no statements are made or operative procedures recorded that might result in denial of insurance coverage. On occasion, the resident is told, some surgeons alter an admission diagnosis to gain insurance coverage for their patients. The resident wonders how long it will take to learn all these tricks of the trade.

The practice of lying to insurance companies appears to be widespread among physicians. A recent survey asked internists whether they would support a fellow physician who deceived a third-party payor to secure coverage for a specified group of services. The physician would not gain from the transaction. The proportion of physicians who approved of such deception varied according to the perceived severity of threat to the patient if a service were denied: for example, coronary bypass operation (58%), arterial revascularization (56%), mammography (48%), emergency psychiatric referral (32%), and cosmetic rhinoplasty (3%).[9] In another study, 70% of physicians admitted that they would choose to misrepresent a patient's symptoms in order to convince an insurance company to fund a routine mammogram, if the company would otherwise refuse to pay for the procedure.[10]

In a third study, when asked why they miscode, many physicians reported that they consider doing so is necessary to "provide high-quality health care today."[11] Participants in these studies were most likely to approve of deception when the condition was life threatening, and approval was related to the clinical severity of the condition. This finding suggests that study participants were not likely to choose miscoding as a first option, but that they would do so if they believed that serious harm would result to the patient if coverage were denied. Rates of willingness to miscode decline for palliative care and sink even lower for diagnostic procedures. In each of these situations, there are more options for care, less urgency to provide the care immediately, and more time available to pursue an appeal. Few physicians were willing to miscode to secure cosmetic procedures for their patients, suggesting that their willingness to deceive does not extend to serving a patient's vanity. Most physicians who advocated miscoding in at least one of the vignettes also reported feeling torn between their professional obligation to act as an advocate for their patients, and their contractual obligations to preserve the integrity of the insurance system.

The data from these studies are consistent with the view that physicians miscode because they are committed to acting as advocates for their patients. On this view, miscoding only manipulates a tool, insurance coverage, to promote the well-being of patients.

The Insurance Company as the Enemy

The AMA code of medical ethics advocates dealing honestly with patients and colleagues, as noted above. The code, however, goes further than this, extending the principle of honesty to dealing with insurance companies: "Physicians shall make no intentional misrepresentation to increase the level of payment they receive or to secure noncovered health benefits for their patients."[12] Truth telling is clearly held in high regard by many ethicists. Why, then, as pointed out in the studies cited previously, are physicians generally so willing to deceive insurance companies? For Plato, some lies are justified for their immediate practical benefits. He gave the example of the utility of lying to an enemy. In Platonic terms, many believe that insurance companies of modern times have become the enemy, so, according to this line of reasoning, deceiving them is fully warranted. They are the enemy because they prevent the patient from receiving needed care, which the physician is morally obligated to ensure the patient will receive.

Is the insurance company truly the enemy? The flaws, inefficiencies, and perversities of our current health care financing system make this belief appear to be true.[13] Health insurance for most residents of the United States is obtained through their employers, largely because of public policy developed over the last several decades. Health insurance is tax deductible, and therefore substantially less expensive when purchased by an employer than when purchased by an individual. The employer, however, is acting as the patient's agent. When a health insurance policy is purchased, patients or their agents (the employers) choose a policy based in part on higher or lower cost. Lower premiums are generally associated with fewer or less costly benefits. Employers tend to choose policies that are less expensive because of the financial savings to them. Employees are free to buy a more comprehensive health insurance policy on their own, but seldom do so because of the large additional financial burden. They almost always choose instead to accept the insurance selected and purchased for them by their employer. Thus, when an insurance company denies payment for a procedure because it is not covered, patients are getting what they (or their agent) have paid for.

Some argue that insurance companies use deceptive practices in selling policies or keep details of coverage purposely vague, so purchasers do not really know the precise terms of their insurance coverage. On this view, patients should not be held rigidly to seemingly arbitrary decisions of their insurance companies, and lying to the companies is justifiable as an antidote to their deceptions. There is no doubt that many companies do not reveal the details of covered illnesses and procedures, sometimes defending this practice as protecting proprietary competitive information (much as Coca-Cola keeps secret its formula for Coke). Some may even engage in corporately sanctioned deceptive sales practices. But when an insurance company deceives purchasers, there are legal remedies for fraud. When a company protects information as proprietary, we may not like that practice, but the company is legally entitled to do so. We can, and do, decry such practices as reprehensible. Employers and employees are free to take their business elsewhere to more reliable companies, or to make efforts to change the insurance laws. Lying to the insurance company, however, does little to rectify the problem the company has created for its policy holders.

Deception Serving Self-Interest

Some kinds of deception are clearly self-serving and unrelated to benefiting patients, such as upcoding removal of a sternal wire to "sternal debridement," or embellishing an incidental single suture closure of a patent foramen ovale by naming it "repair of atrial septal defect." I confine my discussion here, however, to the morally more ambiguous case of miscoding ostensibly for the benefit of the patient.

It is not altogether clear when a surgeon lies to an insurance company for the benefit of a patient that it is his or her only motivation. The surgeon also stands to benefit himself or herself and his or her organizations in several ways. By obtaining insurance coverage for the patient, the surgeon and others (eg, practice partners, hospitals of affiliation) secure payment that otherwise would have been uncertain. Time and energy do not have to be expended in appealing to an insurance company. When a surgeon deceives a third party, the motivation may be partly to serve the interests of the patient, but also may be partly to serve the surgeon's financial self-interest.

An interesting illustration of deception serving self-interest can be seen in the case of the resident physician being asked to dictate an operative note in a deceptive manner, cited above. That case was hypothetical, and I have used it in teaching exercises with surgery residents and attending surgeons. When asked if the sort of deception the case describes is acceptable, all but a small minority respond affirmatively. I then point out that the operation has already taken place, so nearly all of the benefits from the lie will accrue to the surgeon and the hospital, in the form of assuring payment of their bills. No medical benefit accrues to the patient, who has already had his operation (though the patient may be spared the bother of negotiating payment of the bill). On a second showing of hands, the consensus among the physicians hearing the case does not change: they still believe the deception to be acceptable. This poll suggests that no bright line separates the perception of morality in actions that benefit patients from those that benefit physicians, at least for the dictation of operative notes.

Benefits and Harms of Deception

The paramount ethical consideration in the practice of clinical medicine traditionally is balancing benefits and harms.[14] In evaluating a proposed action, benefits should outweigh harms. How does this balance play out in considering lying to insurance companies? Both short and long-term effects of deception must be considered.

In the short term, when surgeons lie to insurance companies, benefits accrue to both the patient and the surgeon. The patient receives an operation or service he or she might not have received if insurance coverage were denied, for example, if the hospital would not allow the patient to be admitted without assurance of payment, which the patient cannot afford. If the patient would have received the operation even without coverage, he or she is spared the necessity of negotiating with providers to pay the bills. The surgeon benefits by being paid a fee, which might not have occurred without insurance coverage. The surgeon also avoids the inconvenience and loss of time an appeal to the insurance company would consume. Moreover, the surgeon avoids the discomfort and anger he or she might feel at having to deal with an adversarial insurance company. There seem to be little immediate harm. In the short term, benefits to both patient and surgeon appear to outweigh substantially the harms of lying to the insurance company. Deception is expedient.

But what of the long term? Does the balance of benefits and harms change? Long-term benefits of misrepresenting patient information include the patient being appropriately cared for, and the surgeon being financially better off. There are noteworthy long-term harms as well, however. There is a practical risk to the surgeon that the deception will be detected and therefore he or she is vulnerable to the charge of fraud (which may, in fact, be true), with all its social and legal consequences. Moreover, by practicing deception routinely, the physician undermines his or her own character and future wellbeing. David Hume, the 18th century philosopher, made the point in this way:

> Honesty, fidelity, truth are praised for their immediate tendency to promote the interest of society; but after those virtues are once established on this foundation, they are also considered as advantageous to the person himself, and as the source of that trust and confidence, which can alone give a human any consideration in life. One becomes contemptible, no less than odious, when he forgets the duty, which, in this particular, he owes to himself, as well as to society.[15]

If a physician lies for a patient, how is the patient to know that the same physician is not willing also to lie to him or her? Mutual trust and confidence inevitably may be eroded when deception enters the relationship, even if it is directed externally. Loss of trust is a critically important harm because trust comprises the very foundation of the physician–patient relationship.[16]

Deception may lead directly to harming the patient in the long term, because of the potential for future confusion and misdiagnosis.[17] This concern may be particularly pertinent for the most socially and economically vulnerable, because they have the least access to health care insurance, and are the most likely to switch insurance providers and to lose health care coverage. Each of these outcomes compromises continuity of care. One can readily imagine how miscoding could be undetected by the future physicians of these patients, and how such miscoding could easily lead to misdiagnosis. In such a situation, a well-intentioned earlier decision to assist a patient might lead to harmful future consequences that the surgeon cannot predict. [. . .]

Another long-term harm is systematic: whereas miscoding might serve an individual patient in a given situation, it does nothing to change a flawed health care system, miscoding serves only to perpetuate the problem. Moreover, miscoding is arbitrary and capricious, insofar as it best serves patients who have a personal relationship with their surgeons—those patients for whom one cares about enough to undertake risks. This might exclude substantial portion of a surgeon's patient population, including the very patients who could benefit most from health care reform.

Beyond its harmful effects on individual surgeons and patients, when deception of insurance companies becomes as widespread as it is now known to be, the entire profession suffers from undermining of the trust that is essential to the physician–patient relationship. This will especially be the case when the media bring to light, as is ultimately likely, the extent to which surgeons personally benefit from deceiving third parties under the cloak of protecting the patient's interests.

Society as a whole is harmed as well. The dishonesty of surgeons who assist patients to gain what does not rightfully belong to them undermines the actuarial foundation of the insurance industry, making it more difficult for patients, their employers, and insurance companies to control the cost of health care. Also, in helping one patient by lying to an insurance company, the surgeon harms large numbers of others, specifically, other policyholders who pay premiums.

By dealing dishonestly with insurance companies, surgeons fail to put the real problem squarely on the table for open consideration by the insurance company, the employer, and society. The problems related to denial of needed care remain hidden and unresolved. It would be better for surgeons to try to obtain coverage by advocating openly and honestly for the patient, requesting coverage by the insurance company through the appeal mechanisms many companies have in place. This course may be the best way to preserve the trusting relationship of individual patients with their physicians and of all patients with the medical profession.

Undoubtedly, surgeons are in the difficult position of wanting to serve the patient's best interest, but being unable to do so because of an agreement the patient (or the patient's agent) has made with an insurance company. The remedy for this situation, however, is not for the surgeon to deceive the insurance company, but rather, to work toward changing the system so that such deception is not needed. There are a number of ways to achieve reform, ranging from creating a single-payor, nationalized health insurance system to creating a competitive insurance market through tax reforms that would encourage patients to choose, purchase, and own their own insurance policies. I do not intend to enter that debate at this point, having done so in the past.[13] My intention is only to point out that dishonesty may not be the best solution to the difficulties surgeons face daily in caring for patients. Indeed, dishonesty may contribute to the perpetuation of a profoundly unsatisfactory health care financing system.

Conclusion

Surgeons have many motivations to deceive insurance companies. Some of them serve the patient's interests, whereas some serve the surgeon's interests. Clearly defining the relative power of the several motivations is difficult. Personal conversations with colleagues have persuaded me that many believe their only motivation in misrepresenting patient information to an insurance company is to help the patient. Often, they believe this in the face of clear evidence to the contrary (e.g., when lying is the only way they will receive payment for their services).

Many physicians not only find it to be acceptable to deceive insurance companies, but do so with a feeling of pride, believing it to be a praiseworthy act. The loss of a sense of wrongdoing when lying is perhaps the most baleful consequence of deceiving insurance companies. It may sometimes be necessary to deceive in order to achieve a good or prevent an evil so great that it overrides the harmful effects of deception on trustworthiness and trusting relationships. In my view, however, such lies should be necessary rarely, if ever, and should never be a cause for rejoicing or complacency. This point was stated well by Dorotheus of Gaza in the fifth century: "If one does not lie with fear and sorrow, then one does wrong even when one lies for good and necessary cause."[18]

References

1. Plato. *The Republic*, II:382, translated by B. Jowett. The dialogues of Plato: Vol. 1. New York: Random House; 1937:646.
2. Aristotle. *Nichomachean Ethics*, iv:4.93, translated by T. Irwin. Indianapolis, IN: Hackett Publishing; 1985:110–1.
3. Bok S. Lying. Moral choice in public and private life. New York: Vintage Books; 1999:13–16.
4. Baker R, Emanuel L. The efficacy of personal ethics: the AMA code of ethics in historical and current perceptive. *Hastings Cent Rep.* 2000;30(Suppl.):S13–7.
5. Council on Ethical, and Judicial Affairs, American Medical Association. Code of Medical Ethics: current opinions with annotations, 2000–2001 ed. Chicago: American Medical Association; 2000:xiv.
6. Council on Ethical, and Judicial Affairs, American Medical Association. Opinion 8.12, Code of Medical Ethics: current opinions with annotations, 2000–2001 ed. Chicago: American Medical Association; 2000:174–5.
7. Oken D. What to tell cancer patients: a study of medical attitudes. *JAMA.* 1961;175:120–8.

8. Novack DH, Plumer R, Smith RL, Ochitill H, Morrow GR, Bennett JM. Changes in physicians' attitudes toward telling the cancer patient. *JAMA*. 1979;241:897–900.
9. Freeman VG, Rathore SS, Weinfurt KP, Schulman KA, Sulmasy DP. Lying for patients: physician deception of third party payors. *Arch Intern Med*. 1999;159:2263–70.
10. Novack DH, Detering BJ, Arnold RM, Forrow L, Ladinsky M, Pezzullo JC. Physicians' attitudes toward using deception to resolve difficult ethical problems. *JAMA*. 1989;26:2980–5.
11. Wynia MK, Cummins DS, VanGeest JB, Wilson IB. Physician manipulation of reimbursement rules for patients: between a rock and a hard place. *JAMA*. 2000;283:1858–65.
12. Council on Ethical, and Judicial Affairs, American Medical Association. Opinion 9.132(2), Code of Medical Ethics: current opinions with annotations, 2000–2001 ed. Chicago: American Medical Association; 2000:229–30.
13. Sade RM. Health care reform: implications for clinical medicine. *Ann Thorac Surg*. 1994;57:792–6.
14. Fletcher JC, Miller FG, Spencer EM. Clinical ethics: history, content, and resources. In: Fletcher JC, Lombardo PA, Marshall MF, Miller FG, eds. *Introduction to clinical ethics*, 2nd ed. Frederick, MD: University Publishing Group; 1997:13.
15. Hume D. *Enquiries concerning the human understanding and concerning the principles of morals*, 2nd ed. Oxford, UK: Clarendon Press; 1957:238.
16. Pellegrino E. The commodification of medical and health care: the moral consequences of a paradigm shift from a professional to a market ethic. *J Med Philos*. 1999;24:243–66.
17. Morreim EH. Gaming the system, dodging the rules, ruling the dodgers. *Arch Intern Med*. 1991;151:443–7.
18. Dorotheus of Gaza. Instructions, 9.96–103. Cited in B. Ramsey, Two traditions on lying and deception in the ancient church. *The Thomist*. 1985;49:504–33.

4

Hepatitis C Virus–Infected Resident

END OF RESIDENCY, END OF CAREER?

Carolyn M. Dresler, Michael S. Kent,
Richard I. Whyte, and Robert M. Sade*

Introduction
Robert M. Sade, MD

Every surgeon faces the possibility of becoming infected by a bloodborne pathogen during the course of an operation. Cardiothoracic surgeons are among those with the highest risk because of the confined, deep spaces in which we operate. The possibility of cross-infection between surgeon and patient has been recognized since the existence of bloodborne viruses has been known, but came into high relief in the early days of the human immunosuppressive virus epidemic of the 1980s.

Hepatitis C virus (HCV) is the most common such infection, affecting 2.7 to 3.9 million Americans (approximately 1% to 1.5% of the US population).[1] The number of cardiothoracic operations carried out annually is well over 300,000, suggesting that cardiothoracic surgeons face roughly 3,000 potential exposures every year. The number of surgeons who become infected is unknown, is probably low, but definitely occurs.[2] The Centers for Disease Control (CDC) has no guidelines for surgeons who become infected with HCV, but recommends standard precautions for all health care personnel—this would seem especially important in the operating room where the risk of transmission is particularly high. Once infected, a surgeon can transmit the virus to a patient during surgery, but this risk is apparently very low.

---

*Dresler CM, Kent MS, Whyte R, Sade RM. HCV infected resident: end of residency, end of career? *Ann Thorac Surg.* 2013;95(3):779–86. Copyright Society of Thoracic Surgeons, republished here with permission.

The consequences of infection with a bloodborne pathogen are most notably worrisome when the infected surgeon is a resident in training, because the stigma of such an infection may affect the chances of the resident finding a position when his training is completed. We present a case of an infected resident and a difficulty faced by his residency director: he must write a letter of recommendation (LOR) to accompany the resident's job applications.

THE CASE OF THE UNLUCKY RESIDENT AND THE PERPLEXED DIRECTOR

A resident becomes infected with HCV, probably from an incidental sharp injury during a routine cardiac surgery operation. He is later found to have high HCV RNA titers and cannot participate in the training program for a year while being treated with interferon. His titers fall over the course of the year to a level that the infectious diseases consultants declare to be compatible with the resident resuming his place on the cardiothoracic surgery team, including in the operating room.

The well-liked and respected resident completes his residency successfully, and the cardiothoracic faculty believes he is clinically well-prepared and technically competent to start working independently in either private practice or an academic setting. He still has a low HCV titer, and is deemed by the infectious diseases consultants to be able to operate safely, posing minimal risk to his patients.

His residency director is writing a LOR for job applications. The director believes that anyone who learns that the applicant is HCV positive is unlikely to hire him, perhaps to the point that he cannot get a job at all as a cardiothoracic surgeon. He also believes that the information about the resident's HCV status is relevant to his job application, so perhaps should be disclosed in the letter he is writing. Should the director disclose the resident's HCV status?

Pro
Carolyn Dresler, MD, MPA

I was 14 years old when I decided that I wanted to find the cure for lung cancer— as a result of a strong family history and heavy smoking. After medical school, I trained for 10 years to develop the expertise to address the research, clinical, and surgical treatment of lung cancer. I had high expectations of my thoracic surgical career. Somewhere during my chief residency in general surgery and the surgical oncology fellowship, before my cardiothoracic training, my liver function tests became asymptomatically elevated. I had been vaccinated for hepatitis B (HBV) and had been tested for human immunodeficiency virus (HIV)—I was glad that I had made it through training without these acquired diseases, but had no idea why the liver function tests were elevated in 1987.

Seven years into my real career in academia, which I thought was progressing well, I had blood tests performed for an insurance application. My world fell apart when I received the blood test results in the mail that said "HCV" and positive. This was the end of 1997—the HCV antibody test first became clinically available in 1991, about 2 years after I had finished my clinical training.

I did not know what to do or who to talk to or how to be treated. Of course I was worried about my health and prognosis, but I was petrified of what it meant to my career. I had trained for over 10 years, and I was just beginning my eighth year of practice. This was very unfair. I thoroughly researched the basic and clinical science, and searched for the best clinician to treat me. I decided I needed legal advice and sought a referral—without disclosing the reason why. I did not tell my employer. The legal advice stated unequivocally that I was required to disclose my HCV status to my employer and patients and that I must not operate. They said they would not represent me further if I did not agree. They also said that they could no longer represent me anyway, as their law firm also represented the Cancer Center in which I was employed, and the Cancer Center had a prior claim to their services. It was a disastrous time for me.

However, what guided my decisions reflected more my personal ethics than the legal opinion. I had decided from early in my surgical education, that I would always strive to treat patients how I personally wanted to be treated. In this case, it meant full disclosure of my HCV status, with an understandable explanation (exceedingly low risk of transmission, but possible, as anything in medicine is possible), and the decision would be mine (or my patient's) on whether to proceed based on my (their) values or assessment. With this personal opinion of what I believed was most ethical, I decided that my realistic options were to leave surgery in the United States or move to another country that did not have the surfeit of thoracic surgeons as was available in the United States who did not have a potentially transmissible infectious disease.

Thus, I enter this ethical discussion today with a strong personal opinion. Now, let us review some of the bioethical opinions from experts in the literature that would support the disclosure of the viral status of the cardiothoracic resident in the director's LOR. There are many bioethical models of ethics that can be drawn upon to support this recommendation.

"First do no harm" or, more precisely, "I will do no harm or injustice to them," derives from the Hippocratic Oath. This oath translates into the concept of nonmaleficence, meaning that physicians will not provide the patient any treatment or intervention that is intended to harm or injure them. Related to nonmaleficence is the concept of beneficence: One ought to prevent evil or harm. One ought to remove evil or harm. One ought to do or promote good. [...]

However, two other concepts within biomedical ethics must be considered: the balance between autonomy and paternalism. The importance of autonomy is best illustrated by the progressively focused attention on informed consent over the past decades. [...] Informed consent has become much more complicated and longer over the years. As a result, there is much interest and research into the understandability, literacy, competency, complexity, and so forth, that occur with the intent to obtain a valid informed consent.

Contrary to the idea of autonomous informed consent, and more pervasive historically and culturally, is the concept of paternalism. Basically, with a paternalistic approach, the physician makes the decision concerning the appropriate intervention for the patient [...]. Traditionally, paternalistic decisions were made because it was felt that the physician knew what was the best course of action for each patient and the concepts or issues might be too difficult, confusing, alarming, or not understandable by the patient. [...] It is critical to remember that the entire spectrum of decision making is to provide the most beneficent outcome for the patient—there is no intent of maleficence.

To understand the question of autonomy versus paternalism concerning disclosure of viral status, a national survey in 2000 queried 2,353 adults in the United States.[3] To the statement "It should be mandatory for doctors and dentists who are infected with HBV or HCV to tell their patients before they provide medical care," 82% of adults responded that they either strongly agree or agree. Americans want to know if their health care providers have a potentially communicable disease (89% wanted the HIV information). [...]

Next to consider in this bioethical discussion, is the approach to the compromised physician, whether by mental health diagnosis, alcohol or other substance abuse, or other diagnosis, such as a communicable infectious disease. [...] For communicable diseases, there are guidelines and recommendations for physicians with such diagnoses as HBV, HCV, or HIV. The Society for Healthcare Epidemiology of America (SHEA) in 2011 provided a comprehensive summary of such guidelines that should be considered within the context of all impaired physicians.[4] [...] To briefly summarize background information [...]:

- The prevalence of HCV is still rising.
- There is no vaccine for HCV.
- Provider to patient transmission is very uncommon (rate estimated at 0.13%).
- Rate of transmission of HCV is intermediate between HBV (higher) and HIV (lower).
- The rate "may be complicated by low rate of voluntary reporting."

◻ Of the known providers transmitting the disease to patients, 3 of 7 were cardiothoracic surgeons.

◻ There is no known level of HCV viral titer that predicts higher or lower rates of transmission. (There are such levels in HBV and HIV.)

◻ United Kingdom and European Consortium state that HCV-infected providers cannot perform exposure-prone procedures.

[…] Of pertinence to this discussion of the HCV-infected resident, if the viral load is 104 or less genome equivalents per milliliter, it is permissible for the surgeon to perform category I, II, and III (III being the most invasive, encompassing cardiac and thoracic procedures) with double glove technique and frequent glove changes. Five other recommendations to follow are similarly made, and include (1) not detected as having transmitted infection to patients; (2) advice from expert review panel about continued practice; (3) twice annual assessment of viral burden to confirm 104 or less genome equivalents per milliliter; (4) follow-up by expert personal physician; and (5) compliant with written contract concerning responsibilities. If the surgeon does have HCV viral titers above 104, he or she is not to perform category III (standard cardiothoracic procedures), despite usual infection control measures.

More recently, the CDC published their recommendations for HBV-infected health care providers.[5] This document […] reverses the 1991 recommendation that patients are informed of their health care provider's viral status, but reaffirms that viral positivity should not disqualify the health care provider from the practice of their profession. […]

What do these recommendations mean for our cardiothoracic resident completing his training and searching for a job? The resident underwent treatment and although the viral titers are not provided, his infectious disease program said that they were "low" and he was "deemed to be able to operate safely, posing minimal risk to his patients." […] Arguably, the director and the training program have not fully complied with the current recommendations—or the brief case presentation has not delineated them. […] Appropriate oversight and review of the adequacy of the mental health, addiction—or viral status—is critical. Per the concern in the SHEA guidelines, many physicians choose to not volunteer their positive viral status, owing to the very real concern over their viability to continue their practice, similar to the concerns from impairment from mental health or substance abuse. The director has a duty to fully represent the qualifications and limitations of the resident under his purview for conditions that may impact patient care, whether it is drug abuse or a communicable disease. This duty to disclose the resident's HCV status is based on a higher principle than a legal responsibility. Rather, it is an issue of honesty and transparency with an eye toward the director's fiduciary responsibility to both the resident and future patients—to train not only a technically facile surgeon but an ethical one as well. [...] The director needs to disclose in his letter of recommendation that the resident is HCV positive and delineate how the program has instituted measures to ensure patient safety.

This answers the question posed by the case study. However, to go further, the resident has a duty to provide beneficent treatment in the context of an autonomous, namely, fully informed consent, which includes disclosure of his HCV viral status to his patients. This disclosure is not supported by the SHEA or CDC recommendations. However, as discussed above, the surgeon undertaking the highest category of exposure-prone procedures has a duty to fully inform his patients of the risks, inclusive of the information of the extremely low risk of transmission of the virus, despite its low risk. This "deliberative model" of surgeon-patient decision making is therefore a collaborative effort, fully exploring the patient's fears and concerns not only of the significant surgical procedure but also of the surgeon's transmission risk, and is based on trust. The surgeon does not have the right to make the paternalistic decision that she or he knows the values and judgments of the patient better than the patient does. To decide otherwise denigrates the competency of the patient and is destructive to the fiduciary relationship that is so critical to physician-patient relationships. Profound empathy for the resident should not cloud the bioethical path of disclosure.

Con

Michael S. Kent, MD, and Richard Whyte, MD

Approximately 180 million people worldwide are infected with HCV. The sequelae of chronic infection are significant: end-stage liver disease, hepatocellular carcinoma, and death. As a result, HCV infection is the most common indication for liver transplantation in the United States and Europe.

The most common pathway for transmission of HCV is intravenous drug use, followed by sexual contact. However, iatrogenic transmission of HCV is well recognized, specifically through blood transfusion or in dialysis centers. Transmission from infected patients to health care workers, and from health care workers to patients, as described in this case, are distinctly uncommon. However, so-called exposure-prone procedures, defined as invasive procedures in which the blood of patient and health care worker may come into contact, are a well-recognized pathway for transmission of HCV.

Cardiac surgery is the prime example of an exposure-prone procedure, and several case reports have documented transmission of HCV from patients to surgeons, and from the infected surgeon to subsequent patients.[6] Given the high prevalence of blood-splash and needle stick injuries during open-heart surgery, it is no surprise that cardiothoracic surgeons are more likely to transmit HCV to patients than other health care workers. Indeed, in a retrospective investigation of a HCV-infected cardiac surgeon, the risk of transmission to a patient during open-heart surgery was 6%.[6] In contrast, the risk of a health care worker having infection after percutaneous exposure to HIV-infected blood is only 0.3%.[7]

The risk of transmission of HCV from a cardiothoracic surgeon to a patient need not, however, be this high. For example, the rate of needle-stick injuries is known to be higher among less-experienced surgeons. In addition, the risk of transmission will depend on the specific operation in question. [...]

Two other issues are relevant to the current case. The first regards the significant recent advances in treatment for HCV. For years, the standard treatment involved the use of interferon alpha in combination with ribavarin. Standard treatment led to cure rates in treatment naive patients of 40% to 50%.[8] Treatment time was lengthy (48 weeks) and associated with significant toxicity and low rates of compliance. However, in 2011, two new drugs (telaprevir and boceprevir) were approved for HCV patients. These agents impair viral replication and are associated with a sustained virologic response (i.e., cure) in as many as 75% of patients treated.[9] [...] Several other agents are expected to be available for commercial use within the next few years, with early studies indicating cure rates approaching 100%.

The final issue concerns the official policy of health care workers infected with HCV. In Europe, guidelines vary widely. [...] In the United States, the CDC website states "There are no CDC recommendations to restrict a health care worker who is infected with HCV. The risk of transmission from an infected health care worker to a patient appears to be very low. All health care personnel, including those who are HCV positive, should follow strict aseptic technique and standard precautions, including appropriate hand hygiene, use of protective barriers, and safe injection practices."[10] In the United States, therefore, there is no mandate that a HCV-infected surgeon limit his or her practice, or inform patients of their health status.

THE PRESENT CASE

In the present case, we are asked to determine whether the residency director should disclose the HCV status of a highly regarded cardiothoracic resident in a LOR. It is clear that disclosure of this information will likely result in the resident becoming unemployable as a cardiothoracic surgeon.

We strongly believe that this information should not be disclosed in a LOR. It is important to note that we are not being asked to render an opinion on the national policy for health care workers infected with HCV. [...] The question in this case revolves around the specific obligations of the residency director in writing a letter, and whether confidential health information should be disclosed.

There are no official guidelines regarding LORs for surgeons concluding their training and seeking employment. However, guidelines do exist for
medical school dean's letters,[11] and for applicants to emergency medicine resi-
dencies.[12] These guidelines indicate that a writer of such a letter has an ethical duty to be honest and accurate, and to limit and acknowledge bias. The
writer does not have an obligation to write a flattering letter, although that
may be the expectation of the resident. However, the writer clearly has an
obligation to his or her profession, and to the institution to which the resident
is applying. In this particular case, the residency director will surely wonder
whether writing a LOR that allows the resident to begin a cardiothoracic
practice will put future patients at risk for HCV infection.

The resident in this case is both a physician seeking employment and
a patient. As a patient, his HCV status is private health information and is
protected by the Health Insurance Portability and Accountability Act. It is
reasonable to assume that the resident would not want this information disclosed, and as a patient he has every right to expect this.

However the residency director is not the resident's health care provider,
and he is asked to write a letter regarding the resident's capacity to practice cardiothoracic surgery. Given the obligations of letter writers discussed
above, we would argue that in certain circumstances confidential health
information should be disclosed in a LOR. For example, if the resident contracted HCV by illicit drug use, or was noncompliant with antiviral therapy,
the residency director would be ethically bound to discuss this. These health
issues reflect on the professionalism of the resident, and have a direct impact
on patient safety.

But in this case, there are no issues that would put patients at risk.
The resident is widely regarded as professional and technically competent,
and contracted HCV while providing patient care. In fact, the resident was
deemed safe to operate on patients at the institution of the program director. Given this, it seems inconsistent, if not hypocritical, that the resident
would be allowed to care for other physicians' patients while in training,
but not his own.

Furthermore, there is no national policy regarding health care workers infected with HCV. Surgeons with HCV infection are not restricted
from practicing, nor do they need to disclose their health status to patients.
In general, private health information should not be disclosed in a LOR,
unless there is a compelling reason to do so. In this case there is no such
compelling reason.

There is a reason why health information is protected by law. Patients
may be denied rights or face discrimination as a result of such disclosures.
In this case, the HCV resident is likely to be rendered permanently unemployable as a cardiothoracic surgeon. And the reason for this is the person

reviewing the resident's letter, whether it be a physician or an administrator, is likely to know very little about HCV infection, its treatment, or policies regarding infected health care workers. [...]

It is important to note that the resident also has a responsibility to disclose his HCV status, when appropriate. Hopefully this well-trained resident will find employment, and this information will be disclosed to the occupational health office at his new institution. [...] Those in the occupational health office will know the policies regarding HCV-infected health care workers, and in specific that infected physicians are not proscribed from engaging in exposure-prone procedures. Appropriate precautions, whether this be periodic surveillance serology or some other measure, will certainly be taken.

Given the advances in treatment for HCV, there is a high likelihood that the resident either has been cured, or will be, with new agents now available. There is no reason to think that patients cared for by the resident will be placed at unnecessary risk. Inappropriate disclosure of his HCV status in a LOR will preclude the resident from finding employment, even though he was considered safe to operate while in training. The residency director should understand the consequences of such disclosure, and respect the resident's right to privacy.

Concluding Remarks
Robert M. Sade, MD

The central issue of this debate is whether the director of the residency program should report the resident's HCV status to potential employers. A substantial part of both discussions concerns ethical and scientific issues that are not directly relevant to this point; rather, they are related to the reasons why the patient should or should not know of the surgeons HCV status, the obligations of the resident to his present and future patients, and recent improvements in the treatment of HCV infections. [...]

The essayists miss some important points, however. Dresler does not mention the stigma attached to HCV infection and the likelihood that future employers will consider the opportunity cost of learning the implications of a surgeon's HCV infection to be too high so will simply reject the application. More importantly, however, she does not consider an important limitation of her argument: viral infections are known to be transmitted from patients to surgeons and from surgeons to patients, the rates of which have been estimated to be very low but are not known accurately. Moreover, the incidence of HCV infection is estimated to be 1% to 1.5% in the U.S. population,[1] so it seems likely that 1 or 2 of the approximately 125 cardiothoracic residents finishing their training each year (not to mention many attending surgeons) are HCV positive and do not know it. The likelihood that a surgeon is unknowingly HCV positive and therefore poses a risk to his patients is unknown; it is quite possible that the resident in this case poses no greater risk to his patients than is posed by other residents who have cryptic infections—both risks are extremely small. If Dresler's arguments are correct, we could protect patients more fully by identifying the surgeons who are HCV (and HBV and HIV) positive, accomplished by requiring blood tests on all residents who are about to finish their training (or, by extension, on all practicing surgeons); that would be overly intrusive, however, with low cost-benefit balance. The CDC has considered such questions and has decided not to address them because of the paucity of reliable data upon which to base recommendations.

Kent and Whyte argue that the opportunity cost of seeking information about the implications of a surgeon's HCV infection is likely to be avoided by future employers, resulting in immediate rejection of the resident's job application, and therefore is a reason not to mention the resident's viral status. They do not, however, consider the possibility of disclosing the resident's HCV status in the LOR, in the interest of honesty and transparency, and explaining that the resident, on the advice of infectious diseases consultants, safely operates without limitation (save perhaps oversight by an expert review committee) on patients in his training institution's cardiothoracic surgical service. Given that information, some might reject the resident's application out of hand, but it seems likely that some would not, considerably reducing the likelihood that the resident would be unable to find a job. The authors also do not consider a practical implication of withholding information: the possibility that the reputation of both the director and his program will be damaged if the resident's HCV status is not disclosed and is later discovered by the program that hires him. Reputations for honesty and reliability have suffered because of similar situations.

Unfortunately, the data that could settle some of these questions are not available, and we are left with the need to strike a balance between risks of viral transmission to patients that are very low and the risk of joblessness for the resident that is not certain but seems far from zero. Surgeons have many obligations, but caring for their patients is their paramount (though not absolute) responsibility. They also have a responsibility, albeit a lesser one, to ensure that years of training of the persons under their purview are not wasted and that a well-trained surgeon is not lost to the domain of surgical manpower. It seems that neither side in this debate has won decisively—the director must weigh the many factors supporting both horns of the dilemma and make his decision.

References

1. CDC. Recommendations for the identification of chronic hepatitis C virus infection among persons born during 1945–1965. *MMWR Morbid Mortal Weekly Rep.* 2012;61(RR04):1–18.
2. Thorburn D, Roy K, Cameron SO, Johnston J, et al. Risk of hepatitis C virus transmission from patients to surgeons: model based on an unlinked anonymous study of hepatitis C virus prevalence in hospital patients in Glasgow. *Gut.* 2003;52:1333–8.
3. Tuboku-Metzher J, Chiarello L, Sinkowitz-Cochran RL, Casano-Dickerson A, Cardo D. Public attitudes and opinions toward physicians and dentists infected with bloodborne viruses: results of a national survey. *Am J Infect Cont.* 2005;33:299–303.
4. Henderson DK, Dembry L, Fishman NO, Sepkowitz KA, Weber DJ. SHEA guideline for management of healthcare workers who are infected with hepatitis B virus, hepatitis C virus and/or human immunodeficiency virus. *Infect Cont Hosp Epi.* 2010;31:203–32.
5. Holmberg SC, Suryaprasad A, Ward JW. Updated CDC recommendations for the management of hepatitis B virus-infected health-care providers and students. *MMWR Morbid Mortal Weekly Rep.* 2012;61(RR03):1–12.
6. Olsen K, Dahl PE, Paulssen EJ, et al. Increased risk of transmission of hepatitis C in open heart surgery compared with vascular and pulmonary surgery. *Ann Thorac Surg.* 2010;90:1425–31.
7. Ippolito G, Puro V, Heptonstall J, et al. Occupational human immunodeficiency virus infections in health-care workers: worldwide cases through September 1997. An overview. *Clin Infect Dis.* 1999;28:365–83.
8. Fried MW, Shiffman ML, Reddy KR, et al. Peginterferon alfa-2a plus ribavarin for chronic hepatitis C infection. *N Engl J Med.* 2002;347:975–82.
9. Jacobson IM, McHutchinson JG, Dusheiko G, et al. Telaprevir for previously untreated chronic hepatitis C infection. *N Engl J Med.* 2011;364:2405–16.
10. Centers for Disease Control and Prevention website. http://www.cdc.gov/hepatitis/hcv/hcvfaq.htm#f4. Accessed August 4, 2012.
11. Hunt DD, Maclaren CF, Scott CS, et al. Characteristics of dean's letters in 1981 and 1992. *Acad Med.* 1993;68:905–11.
12. Larkin GL, Marco CA. Ethics seminars: beyond authorship requirements: ethical considerations in writing letters of recommendation. *Acad Emerg Med.* 2001;8:70–3.

5

Must Surgeons Tell Mitral Valve Repair Candidates About a New Percutaneous Repair Device That Is Only Available Elsewhere?

Eric R. Skipper, Kevin D. Accola,
and Robert M. Sade*

Introduction
Robert M. Sade, MD

One of the persistent problems in achieving informed consent for surgical patients is the question of what should be covered in the disclosure component of the consent process. Certainly, one need not tell patients about every conceivable complication or about every possible alternative therapy that might be available for their specific illnesses. So what must be included? In particular, what alternative therapies should be described or must be described to patients? The problem has become a bit more complicated in recent years as the competitive aspects of cardiothoracic surgical practice have become more prominent and as some new technologies have been used as much for marketing surgical programs as for addressing patients' needs.

This issue was explored at the annual Ethics Forum session of the Southern Thoracic Surgical Association meeting in 2010. A case was built around an actual new device that was still investigational at the time of the meeting, but set in the future (November 2011) at a time when Food and Drug Administration (FDA) approval is presumed to have occurred. [Editor's note: The FDA approved the device in October 2013.]

*Skipper ER, Accola KD, Sade RM. Must surgeons tell mitral valve repair candidates about a new percutaneous repair device that is only available elsewhere? *Ann Thorac Surg.* 2011;92(4):1163–9. Copyright Society of Thoracic Surgeons, republished here with permission.

CASE

Richard Bishop, 60 years of age, has been known to have mitral insufficiency for 5 years, has recently developed shortness of breath, and his cardiologist at Lourdes Heart Center has found left ventricular dysfunction: ejection fraction 50%, end-systolic diameter 52 mm. He has referred Mr Bishop to his longtime colleague, Dr John Crowne, a cardiothoracic surgeon who has had excellent results with open mitral valve repair for more than 15 years.

A competing institution, St. Bernadette Medical Center, on the other side of town recently participated in a multi-center trial of a new device, the Evalve MitraClip, which is deployed percutaneously for mitral valve repair. It was approved for clinical use by the FDA 3 months ago, in August 2011. St. Bernadette has been using the device with considerable success for 3 years. Published studies indicate that the device is 98% successful in reducing moderately severe (3+) or severe (4+) regurgitation to mild or none at 30 days after than procedure, but there is no information about long-term durability. Many heart centers want to use MitraClip and are training personnel in the technique, but only the original investigating institutions are up and running with experience in use of the device, so Lourdes Heart Center does not yet have clinical access to it.

During his initial discussion with Mr Bishop, Dr Crowne realizes that no one in the cardiology department has mentioned the MitraClip to the patient, so he does not know what the patient's preferences might be. He has read the limited number of published papers about the device and knows that its early success rate is excellent, no long-term results are available, and the FDA believes it is safe enough for clinical use. He wonders whether he is ethically obligated to tell the patient about the MitraClip and to offer referral to St. Bernadette as a treatment alternative.

Pro
Eric Skipper, MD

The surgeon should inform his patient and offer referral. The impact of health care technology has generally been positive, with new and simplified procedures entering the medical field on an almost daily basis. All innovations come with "issues."[1] Early adoption of new technologies can be a double-edged sword, with beneficence pitted against nonmaleficence in the name of progress, thus creating conflict between physicians' most fundamental values.

This debate, however, is not about new technologies nor about their appropriateness. It is about full disclosure and, more generally, informed consent.

What exactly is informed consent? Certainly, it is more than a mere signed piece of paper. It is a process founded in ethical principles, and of paramount importance in the practice of medicine. In 1847, the American Medical Association (AMA) adopted the first national code of professional ethics in medicine. This was renamed "The Principles of Medical Ethics" in 1903. In 1985, the Judicial Council of the AMA became the Council on Ethical and Judicial Affairs (CEJA). The first Ethics Conference of the AMA was held in Philadelphia, the city of the AMA's founding, in 1997, thus establishing the AMA's Institute of Ethics.

The AMA's Code of Medical Ethics describes informed consent as a patient-physician communication that results in the patient's authorization or agreement to undergo a specific medical intervention. To obtain informed consent, the physician should disclose and discuss the diagnosis, nature, and purpose of a proposed treatment or procedure, risks and benefits thereof, alternatives, and risks/benefits of not receiving or undergoing a treatment or procedure.[2] This communication process is both an ethical obligation and a legal requirement spelled out in statutes and case law in all 50 states.

The AMA Council on Ethical and Judicial Affairs 2006 report states that with respect to informed consent, the physician's obligation is to accurately present the medical facts, make recommendations for management in accordance with good medical practice, and help make choices from among the therapeutic alternatives consistent with good medical practice.[3] [...]

The Code of Professional Conduct from the American College of Surgeons Statement on Principles states that informed consent is more than a legal requirement.[4] It is a standard of ethical surgical practice that enhances the surgeon-patient relationship, and a mechanism for presenting information fairly, clearly, accurately, and compassionately. The discussion conducted by the surgeon should include the nature of the illness and the natural consequences of no treatment. It should include the nature of the proposed operation, including estimated risks of mortality and morbidity. Common complications and benefits of the proposed operation should be disclosed. Alternative forms of treatment including nonoperative techniques should be divulged. A freedom of choice clause states that an ethical surgeon should not participate in a system that denies serving the best interest of the patient by refusing referral out of the system. Moreover, the doctor-patient relationship requires that the patient's interests supersede all other interests, including the personal and financial interests of the surgeon.

The Hippocratic Oath states, "I will prescribe regimens for the good of my patients according to my ability and judgment and never do harm to anyone." Historically the "Hippocratic tradition" fostered paternalism in which physicians were ethically obligated to promote the patient's welfare by providing care in accordance with their own judgment regarding the most appropriate course of treatment. They could opt not to share medical information with the patient if they believed that disclosure might prove detrimental to the patient's well-being.[5] Paternalism has long since been replaced with the contemporary concepts of patient autonomy and shared decision making.[3]

The lack of adequate information can preclude patients from receiving necessary medical attention or making optimal life decisions on the basis of their individual needs and personal values. The patient-physician relationship is founded on trust. The lack of candid disclosure can compromise this relationship. Thus, an act of deception intended to be benevolent can risk undermining both confidence and trust in the medical profession.[6]

CONCLUSION

The Society of Thoracic Surgeons, in its position statement regarding the off-label use of coronary artery stents states, "... patients must be better informed of treatment options and the relative risks and benefits of medical therapy, percutaneous coronary interventions and coronary artery bypass grafting (CABG)." Their recommendations to the FDA included, "... adequate informed consent to be given to patients regarding treatment options ... before catheter intervention is performed...."[7] As surgeons, we cannot have it both ways. One cannot argue successfully against full disclosure in this case; quite the contrary, full disclosure is the only right decision.

Con
Kevin Accola, MD

"Men in general are quick to believe that which they wish to be true."
— *Gaius Julius Caesar*

"When you have a new hammer, choose your nails wisely."
— *Meredith L. Scott, MD*

The surgeon has no obligation to inform or refer the patient. The simple and obvious answer to the central question of this debate is, no—Dr Crowne is not ethically required to discuss this new treatment option with the patient or to offer referral. Dr Crowne should proceed with conventional mitral valve repair surgery, as he is not obligated to discuss with the patient this new technology for mitral valve insufficiency, because the data are suspect, with few short- or long-term results upon which to make judgments, unless the patient is an inappropriate candidate for conventional surgery. Granted, if the patient asks Dr Crowne about alternative approaches, the surgeon is obligated to present the data that are available in an objective manner, before proceeding with open repair.

In my opinion, ethical concerns about new technologies should be more focused on the innovative institutions and individuals who pursue new treatment modalities than on the practicing surgeon. [...] The ethical course of action should be evidence based, using data and results obtained from organized trials of a particular treatment modality or investigational device. Many of the procedures or technologies that have come and gone were marketed as procedures that would end conventional surgery as we know it, and now are merely curiosities that are of historical value only. [...]

These considerations should lead us to ask a series of questions[, which I will address in detail below]. First, what is the surgeon's responsibility regarding new technologies as they relate to clinical standards of care? If we surgeons do not responsibly monitor innovative procedures or technologies with strict oversight, someone else will, and we can almost guarantee it will not be a cardiothoracic surgeon. A second question is how surgeons adopt new procedures and technologies—when does an innovative procedure or technology become accepted as a standard practice? A third question is about industry—what is industry's perspective and behavior relative to new technologies, and how do companies interact with cardiothoracic surgeons? Finally, how do Internet-based information and televised infomercials influence surgeons' responses to patient requests for "new technologies" in this Internet age? Patients are much better informed on medical matters than they were only a few years ago because of ready access to large amounts of information from self-help books, magazines, newspaper columns, and, most notably, the Internet. Much of this information, however, is not peer reviewed and is processed through an institutional marketing filter. Have we allowed patient-driven pursuit of new technology spawned by institutional marketing to displace our ethical responsibility to guide the patient through an evidence-based discussion of what procedure serves their best short-term and long-term interests?

SURGEONS' RESPONSIBILITY

What is the surgeon's responsibility to new technologies as these procedures or devices relate to clinical standards? Evidence-based medicine recommendations and protocols give us some guidance while these devices and procedures are becoming accepted. Evidence-based medicine seeks to assess the strength of evidence of the risks and benefits of treatments, including lack of treatment and diagnostic tests.[8] Evidence-based medicine aims to apply the best available evidence gained from the scientific method to diagnostic and therapeutic decisions. Evaluation of evidence can be challenging, but it remains the foundation of clinical decision making. [...]

Patients have become much better educated about health matters over the past 10 to 15 years, and rightly so. One major flaw and troublesome issue, however, is that this public information on technologies and procedures is not peer reviewed, has bias that may be subtle or obvious, and often is compromised by glaring conflicts of interest. Many cardiothoracic surgeons have been asked by patients if they perform procedures like "Institution X," or asked why are they not candidates for particular treatment modalities or new technologies. Physicians come under significant pressure from hospital systems to provide new technologies to keep pace with the major institutions or with competing hospital systems. Where this will eventually lead is somewhat problematic. It is clear, however, that we surgeons must take the responsibility to do our best for our patients by making decisions based on clinical data and resisting institutional pressures. If we do not accept this responsibility, someone else will, and we will be held accountable. The paucity of evidence about the efficacy (and perhaps safety) of the Evalve MitraClip makes it optional for Dr Crowne to include it among the alternative therapies he describes to Mr Bishop.

HOW SURGEONS COME TO ACCEPT NEW PROCEDURES OR TECHNOLOGIES

Most surgeons are cautiously optimistic in considering the uses of new technologies. The science behind behavioral patterns exhibited by purchasers of consumer products can be applied to the behavior of surgeons in using new technologies. The Law of Diffusion of Innovation describes a behavioral spectrum from "innovators/early adaptors" to "laggers"[9] (Figure 5.1). This law applies to a wide range of consumer products, such as the cell phone, for example. The innovators stand in line waiting to be the first to have a cell phone, and the early adapters quickly follow because they simply must have one as well. Once a product reaches a "tipping point" of 15% to 18% market penetration, the early and late acceptors adopt it because they have seen data

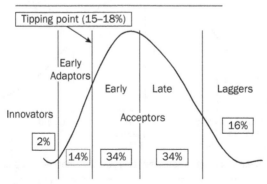

FIGURE 5.1 Law of diffusion of innovation.

and now believe that cell phones work and are dependable. The laggers are the few who no longer use rotary phones only because they cannot find any to buy. Once the tipping point of consumer acceptance is reached, the product gains the interest and acceptance of the early and late acceptors, market penetration escalates, and it becomes a household product (Figure 5.2). [...]

Many cardiothoracic procedures and technologies illustrate the accuracy of the Law of Diffusion of Innovation. For instance, HeartPort was a good idea, but because of an inappropriate launch and other factors, it was unsuccessful in changing the way heart surgery is done—the tipping point was never reached.[10] Another example is off-pump coronary artery bypass surgery, which some suggested should be applied to all coronary revascularizations.[11] It nearly reached a tipping point, but the early and late Acceptors wanted more proof of the efficacy and advantages of the procedure, and the proof never appeared, so the rate of off-pump bypass surgery increased from 15% early after its introduction[12] to only 20% 10 years later.[13]

An important point about the procedures mentioned above is that some are very beneficial for selected patients, but have not been widely accepted. That leads us to the next topic, the industry perspective.

INDUSTRY PERSPECTIVE

Cardiothoracic surgeons' collegial and collaborative relationship with industry has generated much industry funding and engineering expertise in

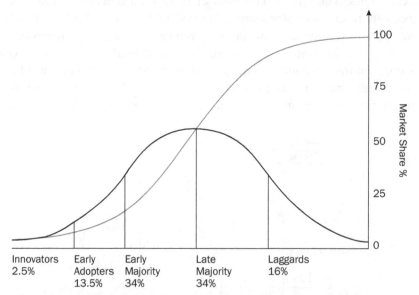

FIGURE 5.2 Once the tipping point of consumer acceptance is reached, the product gains the interest and acceptance of the early and late acceptors, market penetration escalates, and it becomes a household product.

support of research and development of new technologies. Without industry involvement, cardiothoracic surgical innovation could not occur at the levels achieved in the past. A corollary of this, however, is that marketing or promotion of these technologies is sometimes overwhelming and conflicting. Certainly, the need for promotion can be understood in the context of the huge economic impact on industry related to research and development, as well as launching new products.

In my experience, cardiothoracic surgeons are often approached with promotional pressures such as, "better do this before the other group in town or you will miss out," and "this procedure is sure to increase your referrals." Another inducement to use a new product is, "there is a CPT code for this, so you can bill for it."

A number of well-organized controlled clinical trials investigating new technologies are scientifically designed to document efficacy and safety with reliable data. Trials such as these may be persuasive to early and late acceptors, allowing these technologies to reach a tipping point that will result in widespread use, expanding our armamentarium of treatment modalities. Again, we as surgeons must take a responsible role in this process with objective oversight.

CONCLUSION

In conclusion, Dr Crowne is acting ethically and responsibly by proceeding with conventional mitral valve repair surgery without mentioning the Evalve MitraClip to the patient. The limited amount of information about this device does not satisfy the standards of evidence-based medicine, and the lack of peer-reviewed data along with his personal experience and surgical results support such a decision. Because Dr Crowne is under no obligation to discuss with Mr Bishop a new technique with such a sparse track record, he is also not ethically or morally obligated to refer the patient to another institution for amelioration of his mitral valve insufficiency.

Concluding Remarks
Robert M. Sade, MD

The three informational requirements to ensure that consent is informed are these: preconditions (the patient's competence and voluntariness), informational disclosure, and consent to undergo the chosen treatment. At issue in the case at hand is the second element, informational disclosure—how much information Dr Crowne is required to provide to the patient.

Dr Skipper has provided convincing evidence that providing information to the patient is necessary, but he has placed no upper or lower limit on the amount of information required. If Mr Bishop must be told about the

Evalve MitraClip, must he also be told about each of the dozen or so rings and annulus suture techniques, the many distinct methods of mitral valve repair, and the dozen or more types of valve prostheses that are currently available to treat mitral valve insufficiency? What boundaries, if any, delimit the information required for adequately informed consent? Skipper has not made as strong a case as perhaps he might.

Dr Accola has provided persuasive reasons for the surgeon to discount the importance of disclosing the existence and availability of the Evalve MitraClip, but we may ask whether the patient is truly incapable of processing the available information himself. Is the surgeon's skeptical interpretation of the data sufficient reason to withhold that information from the patient?

The informational requirements for informed consent are more complex than the discussants have appreciated. The concept of informed consent as we know it today has developed over more than 2 centuries. The evolution of informed consent, as is true of much else in the field of bioethics, has been driven more by lawyers and courts of law than by thoughtful analysis by philosophers. [...]

The law (and consequently ethics) has also seen evolution of the kinds of information that must be disclosed to the patient to ensure that consent is adequately informed. In 1957, the professional or "reasonable physician" standard of disclosure was established: a physician must disclose the amount of information that other reasonable physicians would disclose (also known as the Bolam principle, after the legal case).[14] The "reasonable patient" standard was established in 1972, in yet another legal case: all the risks and alternatives that a reasonable person would want to know must be disclosed.[15] A 1980 court decision established that the risks of not accepting a recommended course of treatment also must be disclosed to the patient.[16]

At this time, the predominant standard for informational disclosure is the reasonable patient standard, modified to include what the particular patient facing a decision would want to know. The latter, of course, requires that physicians gauge what they believe the patient wants to know, and also that they ask the patient whether he or she desires any additional information. The professional standard has not entirely disappeared; it is still used in some jurisdictions.

APPLYING INFORMATIONAL STANDARDS TO THE BISHOP CASE

Making the case for or against requiring Dr Crowne to disclose to Mr Bishop the availability elsewhere of a less invasive procedure to treat his mitral valve insufficiency requires exploring the question of whether a reasonable person would want to have that information, and whether Mr Bishop in particular would want it. From the vignette as presented, we do not have enough information to know what the patient would want, information that might have been gleaned from the details of communication, spoken and unspoken, during the disclosure conversation, but those details were not given to us.

We are left with the reasonable person standard—what information would a hypothetical reasonable person want? Would such a person want to know about a treatment for his problem that has the benefit of avoiding open-heart surgery, but also the uncertainties accompanying a sparse number of short-to medium-term studies and no long-term data? The surgeon could tell the patient that the device in question is safe and effective enough to have gained approval for clinical use by a federal regulatory agency, and provide such information as already exists about the results of the investigational studies, while carefully placing those results in the context of the well-established safety and effectiveness of the open procedure. It is perfectly acceptable, even laudable, for the surgeon to give the patient his opinion about the balance of benefits and harms associated with the two differing approaches, whether he believes that balance favors the open-heart operation or the newer transcatheter procedure. With all of the information laid out before him, the patient could then make an informed decision.

Certainly, the sheer volume of information might be confusing, but a carefully planned discussion, using language consistent with the patient's level of education and capability of comprehension, can help the patient to make a decision that is consistent with his own values and beliefs.

WHAT IS THE CORRECT CHOICE FOR THE PATIENT?

It would be wrong to assume that Mr Bishop will choose the less invasive procedure, no matter how appealing it seems at first glance. An open, honest relationship with a patient, reinforced by full disclosure of reasonable therapeutic alternatives in terms the patient can understand, establishes a level of trust that is not easily fractured. Most patients in a trusting relationship with their physicians will follow their doctors' advice.

The open-heart techniques and the transcatheter device both seem to be reasonable options. The patient's ultimate decision is likely to be substantially influenced by the degree of trust he has in his surgeon. If Mr Bishop had been referred to Dr Accola, after a frank and open discussion, the patient probably would choose open repair of his deformed valve. If he had been referred to Dr Skipper, he probably would choose the MitraClip and accept referral to another center that has access to that device. The patient will have made his decision based on his understanding of both options, and no matter which alternative he selects, it will have been the right choice for him.

References

1. McMahon K, McCarthy J, Goodson R, Stein J, O'Donnell D, Zyck K. Health care technology's impact on medical malpractice. Paper presented at the Crittenden Medical Insurance Conference, May 5–6, 2005. www.kfplegal.com/articles/InsuranceJournalArticle.pdf.
2. Council on Ethical and Judicial Affairs. E-8.08 informed consent. American Medical Association Code of Medical Ethics: current opinions with annotations, 2010–2011 ed. Chicago, American Medical Association; 2010:260–1.: http://www.ama-assn.org/ama/pub/physician-resources/medical-ethics/code-medical-ethics/opinion808.shtml. Accessed January 8, 1011.
3. American Medical Association report of the Council on Ethical and Judicial Affairs. CEJA report 2-A-06. Chicago: American Medical Association; 2006. http://www.ama-assn.org/ama/pub/about-ama/our-people/ama-councils/council-ethical-judicial-affairs/ceja-reports.shtml. Accessed October 26, 2010. Cited with permission.
4. American College of Surgeons statements on principles. Relation of the surgeon to the patient. Chicago: American College of Surgeons, 2008. http://www.facs.org/fellows_info/statements/stonprin.html#top. Accessed October 26, 2010.
5. Meisel A. The "exceptions" to the informed consent doctrine: striking a balance between competing values in medical decision making. *Wisc Law Rev.* 1979;413:460.
6. Bok S. Lies to the sick and dying. In: *Lying: Moral Choice in Public and Private Life.* New York: Vintage Books; 1979:28.
7. Grover FL. The bright future of cardiothoracic surgery in the era of changing health care delivery: an update. *Ann Thorac Surg.* 2008;85:8–24.
8. Elstein AS. On the origins and development of evidence-based medicine and medical decision making. *Am Res.* 2004;53(Suppl. 2):5184–9.
9. Sinek SO. *Start with Why: How Great Leaders Inspire Everyone to Take Action.* New York: Penguin Group; 2009.
10. King RT. Keyhole heart surgery arrived with fanfare, but was it premature? *Wall Street Journal.* May 5, 1999:A1.
11. Bergsland J, D'Ancona G, Karamanoukian H, et al. Technical tips and pitfalls in OPCAB surgery: the Buffalo experience. *Heart Surg Forum.* 2000;3:189–93.
12. Mack MJ. Coronary surgery: off-pump and port access. *Surg Clin North Am.* 2000;80:1575–91.
13. Sellke FW, Chu LM, Cohn WE. Current state of surgical myocardial revascularization. *Circ J.* 2010;74:1031–7.
14. *WLR Bolam v. Friern Hospital Management Committee*, 1957 (1 WLR 583).
15. *Canterbury v. Spence*, 1972 (464 F.2d 772 [d.c. 1972]).
16. *Truman v. Thomas*, 1980 (611 P.2d 902 [Cal 1980]).

6

The Surgeon's Work in Transition

SHOULD SURGEONS SPEND MORE TIME OUTSIDE
THE HOSPITAL?

Jamie Dickey, Ross M. Ungerleider, Joseph S. Coselli,
Lori D. Conklin, and Robert M. Sade*

Introduction
Robert M. Sade, MD

Libby Zion was an 18-year-old college student who died in a New York City
emergency room in 1984. Her father, a newspaper columnist and former federal prosecutor, sued the hospital and campaigned against long working hours
for residents. As a result, New York State passed the "Libby Zion Law" in 1989,
limiting work hours for house officers.[1] Ever since then, events have moved
steadily, albeit in fits and starts, toward a conclusion that now seems to have
been inevitable. The national 80-hour workweek mandated for house officers
by the Accreditation Council for Graduate Medical Education has begun, and
the disruption of traditional work schedules will be dealt with more or less
effectively in medical graduate training programs around the country.[2]

We do not know what effect these changes will have on the profession of
surgery, but most of us strongly suspect that it will not be good. At the very
least, surgeons of the future are likely to have a work ethic that is different
from the one we acquired during and after our training. In fact, a shift in
attitude toward work seems to be well underway already. [...] It appears that
the era of the "24/7" availability of surgeons and 16 to 18 hour workdays (only
4 to 8 hours on weekend days with an occasional weekend off) may be ending
and slowly fading into oblivion.

---

*Dickey J, Ungerleider RM, Coselli JS, Conklin LD, Sade RM. The surgeon's work ethic in
transition: should surgeons spend more time outside the hospital? *Ann Thorac Surg.* 2004;77:1145–
51. Copyright Society of Thoracic Surgeons, republished here with permission.

Assuming that this scenario of surgery's future is accurate, does it contain lessons for those of us still caught up in the old paradigm? Is there something to be said for or, perhaps, something to be gained from cardiothoracic surgeons joining the trend by adopting a more friendly family or personal lifestyle attitude toward the distribution of our waking hours?

The question of more time for surgeons outside the hospital was debated at the Southern Thoracic Surgical Association Annual Meeting in November 2002. The topic of the debate was "The surgeon's work in transition: surgeons should cut back on time in the hospital to spend more time with family and personal interests." [...]

Pro

Jamie Dickey, PhD, Ross M. Ungerleider, MD

Steve White was on vacation with his wife. They had left the cold, windblown climate of their upper Midwest town very early that morning. Steve always told his wife that thoracic surgeons do not mind getting up early. She always preferred to keep the blinds drawn so as not to awaken from the first light of dawn. However, when they traveled together he invariably booked them on the first fight out of town, thus requiring them both to wake up shortly after she, a night person, would ordinarily be going to bed. Steve had begun his practice 18 months ago after 9 grueling years of training. He and Meg met, courted, married, and had 2 children during his residency. Although Meg quit her job after their son was born, she remained occupied with raising the family, but Steve continued to spend time at the hospital. If they could just make it through Steve's residency, his nights on call, and the constant pressures to do things right for his attendings, then life would get better. They would find a job in a town where they could raise their children and have a more normal family lifestyle.

This was more than a year ago and as far as Meg could tell, there had not been much of a change. Steve now toiled for his partners, in order to uphold his share of the responsibility. He kept reminding his wife that life would improve once he was more established with his partners and they knew he was not a slacker. He always seemed to say "yes" to work, which according to her perspective meant he was saying "no" to her and the children. Just getting Steve to agree to this vacation was huge. He was, of course, delayed at the hospital the night before, so Meg had to go to the dry cleaners and the bank, which were the errands that he was supposed to handle on his way home. Ironically, she planned on that occurring, because Steve was always detained. [...]

This was Steve's first vacation since he had joined the practice. His role models in residency training at the university rarely seemed to take vacation time. [...] During his first year of practice he worked as though he were still a resident. He covered the practice whenever he was needed. He was, after all, the junior partner, and he had dues to pay. [...] For the first time that he could remember in months, they had fun together. They flew first class. They drank wine and talked about all the things they could do together without the kids. When they got off the plane it was sticky warm. After hours of being confined to a seat in an airplane, the tropical air relaxed them like it was a drug. The hotel had a driver waiting for them. [...] It was when they were checking into the hotel that he got the message.

"Dr. and Mrs White, welcome to our beautiful island paradise. We will do everything we can to make your stay wonderful. I noticed that there is a message for you. Let me retrieve it. It will only take a moment." [...]

The manager handed Steve an envelope addressed to Dr. Steven White. He opened it and read it: "Please call ASAP." The note was from his senior partner, Preston, and it included his cell phone number. Now all of the connection between Steve and Meg dissipated. He reached into his pocket for his cell phone.

Damn! No service on the island. Steve needed a phone. He found one in the lobby. Meg went to check into their room.

It was the mayor. He was unstable and needing urgent surgery for acute aortic insufficiency from endocarditis. Steve's partner was going to perform the operation, but he wanted Steve's help. Preston thought the mayor would benefit from a Ross procedure, an operation that Steve had acquired a lot of experience with when he was in his residency. Preston was still learning the Ross procedure, and with Steve's help, he was getting pretty good at it. However, he did not want to do this one alone, because this was the mayor for God's sake! This would be hugely important to their practice. Television and the Press would be following this story closely. Everything had to go well. He hated to ask, but this was so important. Besides, Steve had said he could come back if things got out of hand. Meg could enjoy the island for a few days and Steve could be back the day after surgery.

"Sure," Steve said numbly. It was not what he meant, not what he wanted, but it was what he said. "I will look into the flights back. I need to tell Meg. I will call you when I have some information." [...]

When he got to bungalow 15, he was not finished thinking. He was not sure what to say to Meg. He was not really sure what to say to himself. If it were not for Meg being here with him, he would have no problem with going back. [...] Meg would, once again, understand. She would understand. She would be disappointed, but she would understand. How many times could he disappoint Meg? She was incredible, but she was human. Listen to her in there singing. She is so happy to be here. I will not be asking her to leave. I will be back in a few days after I do the professional, dutiful thing. I will be proud of myself. [...] Meg will understand. I can suck it up. The air feels so good here. I want to take a walk on the beach and hold Meg's hand [...].

We will leave Steve here at the threshold of his bungalow, struggling with a no-win dilemma. In some form, we have all dealt with this dilemma. We have been "enculturated" to put our profession first before ourselves, our family, our being human. During training, thoracic surgeons are never taught balance. Can you be professional as a dutiful thoracic surgeon and be balanced?

How does Steve make the correct decision? In fact, is there a correct decision?

What is required of Steve is to create a life of balance and fluid movement among three important conceptual aspects in his personal system. For example, he must learn the importance of valuing and respecting himself, his relationship with Meg (family, or others), and his medical practice (partners, patients, and media, which are the context of his job). To ignore or consistently choose one system ingredient (self, other, or context) over another will create an unbalanced and rigid lifestyle, putting Steve, his wife, and his medical practice in jeopardy. It may be possible for one aspect in Steve's system to grow and thrive temporarily, if it is consistently being chosen over other aspects in the system; however, even the chosen aspect will eventually suffer if one or both of the other aspects is destroyed.

What is the price to us of not having balance? Steve makes the well-traveled decision and returns to work. Once again, Meg understands. The statistics are grim. If Steve continues to make the decision that work comes first before his needs, including his relationship with Meg and their children, he may end up chronically depressed or with a substance abuse problem, which has been recorded as high as 8% to 12% among physicians, or he may even end up with both problems. With a little additional stress, such as his health or finances, he could become suicidal. The risk of suicide is higher in physicians than in the non-medical population. Each year it would take the equivalent of one to two average-size graduating classes of medical school to replace the physicians who commit suicide. The risk seems especially high for those who are driven, ambitious, individualistic, and compulsive. The previous description represents the profile of a thoracic surgeon.[3,4] [...]

Perhaps Steve makes the decision that Meg will not understand and that if his marriage is to survive, he just cannot return to work. After a while, making decisions to placate Meg, Steve begins to resent her. She is holding him back. She used to understand and support him. If it were not for her demands, he would be happy. How did this happen—this gradual slide into unhappiness? He just cannot keep everybody happy anymore. When did this become his responsibility?

What about his happiness? Why is life so hard? What would Steve do for Steve if there were only Steve to satisfy? The unsettling reality is he has no idea. He has spent so long in a culture that has taught him to take care of others, often demanded him to take care of others, to the point that he has no idea of how to take care of himself. He has derived his happiness from serving the needs and demands of others. When his pager goes off, he has ambivalence. He hates to be bothered, but at least it creates something important and meaningful and he knows he has to respond. This is why he has not taken a vacation. During his years of training, he has lost his existence. No wonder he is out of balance.

We do not have solutions for Steve's current dilemma. There is probably not a single correct decision. Steve has a "schema" that he has learned very well from his training and from his mentors in thoracic surgery. His training has defined the rules and code of conduct for him as a surgeon, and he has embraced it so that it feels comfortable and familiar to him. For Steve, to break the patterned responses of this schema would make him feel uncomfortable and unfamiliar. He has learned to work hard, take his responsibilities of being a surgeon seriously, and put his need for self-care and his need to spend time with his family last. [. . .] [W]e could propose a schema that may be more helpful to Steve, a schema that emphasizes the importance of valuing one's self, others, and the context for making choices. Adoption of this schema would create a dynamic, fluid, and balanced process for living.

Virginia Satir[5] described this process of choice, which requires flexibility, balance and the ability to value one's self, others, and the context as "system congruence" or "system-esteem." It becomes possible to create stability in one's life when the triadic components of self, other, and context are kept in balance over time and there is fluid movement among these elements in relationship to choice and value.

[. . .] [The] important discussion is to identify the learned (patterned) responses to which an individual continually chooses: (1) self, and ignores the needs of others and the context; (2) others, and continually puts his or her own needs last; (3) context, in which work is consistently chosen over the needs of one's family and self; or (4) self and others, by completely ignoring the validity of the context. [. . .] Life becomes unbalanced when individuals repeatedly choose one or two aspects of the triad (self, other, or context) and ignore the others. System congruence and system-esteem are present when an individual (as well as the other members of the system) wholeheartedly choose to value and respect all three system components. [. . .]

It is unlikely that Steve would do too much damage to his relationship with Meg by decreasing their time together in the Caribbean, if she frequently (over the course of time) felt chosen and valued in her relationship with Steve. It is the repetition of never being chosen that creates the discord. Steve's schema of putting context first is more of a problem than the ethics of this one situation. [. . .]

Just as Steve's culture (surgical training and mentoring) produced and reinforced this schema, it may also have to change for Steve to be able to function comfortably within it. The possibility for change to this culture may have been handed to us by the Accreditation Council for Graduate Medical Education (ACGME) in the form of the 80-hour workweek for residents and the core competencies for education [...]. Rather than view these as obstacles for training competent thoracic surgeons, we can try to embrace them as an opportunity to begin emphasizing balance in the way our residents are trained. At the same time, we can begin examining how well we can make these changes for ourselves as we become the role models for the future.

Con

Joseph S. Coselli, MD, Lori D. Conklin, MD

In recent years, a number of substantive changes have occurred in the training and practice of medicine and surgery. The pace of change is always accelerating. As surgeons, we initially believed that we were immune to many of the evolving issues and concerns regarding resident work hours and lifestyle debates. However, now that has all changed and we find ourselves in transition, trying to balance our professional lives with personal and professional responsibilities. This essay will provide opinions on the direction that our profession is heading and why we should remain concerned and engaged.

In his 1963 presidential address to the Thirteenth Annual Student American Medical Association Convention, Dr. Michael E DeBakey proclaimed that "the demands of a physician's practice are so rigorous, requiring such exclusiveness on the part of the doctor that he must forego almost all other aspects of life"[6]. Four decades later, this philosophy continues to exist within organizations such as the American College of Surgeons whose members pledge "to pursue the practice of general surgery with honesty and to place the welfare and the rights of [the] patient above all else...."[7] However, healthcare within the United States has become a multibillion-dollar industry, and it is estimated that by the year 2007, American healthcare will cost more than 2 trillion dollars and will require 20% of the gross domestic product.[8] Jones pointed out that in order to function effectively in today's healthcare system we need guidelines to sustain a focus on the welfare of sick people and "to navigate in a trillion dollar industry, we need a compass: medical ethics."[9]

As surgeons, we are being forced to justify and balance three distinct areas of responsibility encompassing ethical, moral, and personal obligations in the face of escalating patient-care requirements. It is inarguable that surgeons should be able to spend more time with their families and pursue outside interests; however, the caveat lies within the word "should" and between "the devil and the details."

ETHICAL OBLIGATIONS

Ethical decision-making involves personal sacrifice and an unwavering conscience. As surgeons, our ethical obligations transcend self-interest, personal emergency, and social, political, and economic forces. We chose surgery as a profession for a myriad of different reasons; however, by doing so, we all agreed to function in a capacity that would be beneficial and helpful to our patients.

Developing an inner ethical being requires (1) a fundamental belief and a total and permanent commitment to an ideal; and (2) full dedication to the good of others and to help people who are in need.

MORAL OBLIGATIONS

Moral development involves personal sacrifice, effort, resolution, work, and discipline, leaving little room for incompetence, selfishness, or even legitimate personal concerns like fatigue, lack of time, or demands by the family. In his 2001 presidential address to the Western Surgical Association, Dr. J David Richardson reminded us that "unlike other disciplines able to rely upon alternative caregivers, surgery does not lend itself to care by proxy."[10] One cannot discharge moral responsibility by giving it to someone else; it is nontransferable, that is, "you can delegate authority, but not responsibility."[11]

PERSONAL OBLIGATIONS

Satisfying our daily personal obligations with surgical responsibilities represents one of the most difficult aspects of the surgical lifestyle, as we are often criticized for not spending enough time taking care of our families or ourselves. However, we believe the surgical profession offers a service of high significant personal value. To accomplish this goal, we must (1) reinstate the principle of "just doing what is right"; (2) work without ulterior motives; and (3) display commitment and availability with no questions asked.

Alexis Carrel once wrote, "To accomplish our destiny, it is not enough to merely guard prudently against road accidents. We must also cover before nightfall the distance assigned to each of us."[12] Winston Churchill said, "It is no use saying, 'we are doing our best.' You have got to succeed in doing what is necessary."[13] General Dwight D. Eisenhower very eloquently stated, "We succeed only as we identify in life, or in war, or in anything else, a single overriding objective, and make all other considerations bend to that one objective."[14]

COMMENT

Advocating these concepts represents a difficult challenge. It seems as though putting our patients first has become something of an archaic concept, even though, we have an ethical obligation to the patient and society to provide good care, which is referred to as the "social contract." Society moves in the direction in which needs exist, and as physicians we not only must meet the needs, but we must also preserve certain basic principles essential to the proper provision of medical care. The surgical profession must be allowed to return to its original mission and renegotiate the social contract in order to become more balanced, because as we all know, "good medical care is rarely cheap and cheap medical care is rarely good."[3]

From both theoretical and practical standpoints, surgical training and practice go beyond the realm of simple commitment and reside firmly in hard work. In observing current medical students and residents, many have noted that there is a political incorrectness to the hard work that is so necessary to fulfill the commitment. Even with the current resident work hour restrictions, the number of unfilled general surgery residency programs in the United States increased from 5 in 1997 to 41 in 2001.[15] Prior studies have noted that lifestyle, especially a "controllable lifestyle," is a major contributing factor in specialty choice by students. We are not arguing that a balance between purposeful hard work and personal responsibilities should be overlooked; however, many surgical problems demand immediate attention. We agree with Dr. Richardson when he stated that "lifestyle as a buzzword cannot be allowed to be a 'cop-out' for failure to have adequate surgeons and other physicians to meet societal needs"[10] or eventually, our society will be "served" by a medical community that is less talented and definitely less interested in providing medical services in the tradition of its predecessors. Great care must be taken to support and refresh those aspects of American medicine that have sustained it as the most noble of vocations, that have enriched our professional lives, and that have set us apart as the steadfast protector for the interests of our patients.

In conclusion, as surgeons we continue to work through the night, long past the time when our colleagues have gone home, because that is how we have been trained. Attitudes such as this should not be changed, but rather embraced, because to our patients, we represent "hope." In the words of Stephen Paget,Í "We serve three masters: our profession, our patients, and our own people. For if a doctor's life may not be a divine vocation, then no life is a vocation, and nothing is divine."[16]

Concluding Remarks
Robert M. Sade, MD

Should surgeons spend more time with family and personal interests and less time in hospitals? Drs. Coselli and Conklin and Drs. Dickey and Ungerleider have provided conflicting answers in their respective essays. Their views, taken together, however, do not exhaust all possibilities. Additional insights may be gained by considering fundamental aspects of human behavior as understood by ancient philosophers. To them, Aristotle in particular, the most important of the virtues was *phronesis*, which has been roughly translated as "prudence" or "practical wisdom," though neither term captures its essence. Phronesis is the wisdom that helps us recognize those particular goals and virtues, both professional and personal, that are of greatest value to us as individuals. By applying this wisdom, we can choose a path that will correctly align our personal goals and virtues so that our individual and unique human potentials can be most fully realized.[17] [. . .]

These two essays cover a great deal of territory. Yet we wonder whether either viewpoint identifies the right way for a surgeon to achieve a truly fulfilling life. As human beings we all share certain needs, such as nutrition, friendships, and health, yet each of us has a one-of-a-kind blend of specific needs, desires, talents, interests, and tastes. Therefore we each have a unique path to follow if we are to achieve full realization of our individual potentials as human beings, including both our professional and personal lives.

How should we interact with our patients, colleagues, hospitals, spouses, children, friends, and others? How much time should we spend on solitary activities or with others? How much time should we spend on our profession or personal interests? In other words, how should we best utilize our limited time, energy, and resources? Dr. Coselli's answer may be right for him, or not. Dr. Ungerleider's answer may be right for him, or not. We cannot make that judgment; only they individually have access to personal information and insights that make such judgments possible. [. . .]

As for the future of the surgical ethic, crystal balls are notoriously cloudy by nature, and mine is no more revealing than anyone else's. The trend toward shorter work schedules and a bigger share of our time for personal activities is evidenced by medical students' attitudes toward lifestyle[18] and mandatory work limitations for residents,[19] as well as advice such as that offered by Drs. Dickey and Ungerleider. The evidence for an imminent transition to a personal lifestyle-friendly surgical profession seems compelling. Yet, although the ghastly vision (ghastly for many of us at any rate) of a 40-hour workweek for surgeons may seem just around the corner, it may not come to pass, at least not in our lifetimes. It is not that the nature of surgery necessarily demands workaholic surgeons; surgeons in other countries and other cultures have well-controlled schedules and a work ethic that accommodates a life outside of surgery. It is more that dedication to the well-being of our patients, the intensely personal nature of surgery (e.g., how many internists or pediatricians have talked to a patient at dawn, held her heart in his hands in the morning, and talked to her again in the afternoon to tell her that her problem has been fixed), and our deeply embedded work ethic may combine to make the "24/7" surgeon a thing of the future, as well as the past. Drs. Coselli and Conklin's contribution suggests the possibility of continuing survival of the traditional surgical work ethic and also provides us with reasons to believe that it may even be a good idea.

What will the practice of surgery look like in the future? This is not clear, but there is one certainty: change is inevitable. We need to prepare for whatever shifts occur as best we can. We may even hope to guide the process of change, perhaps in our profession but certainly in ourselves. Drs. Dickey, Ungerleider, Coselli, and Conklin have helped us to imagine how we may be better surgeons and better human beings, and for that we are grateful.

References

1. Robins N. *The Girl Who Died Twice: Every Patient's Nightmare: The Libby Zion Case and the Hidden Hazards of Hospitals*. New York: Delacorte Press; 1995.
2. Lowenstein J. Where have all the giants gone? Reconciling medical education and the traditions of patient care with limitations on resident work hours. *Perspect Biol Med*. 2003; 46(2):273–82.
3. Gundersen L. Physician burnout. *Ann Int Med*. 2001;135: 145–8.
4. Miller MN, McGowen KR. The painful truth: physicians are not invincible. *South Med J*. 2000;93:966–74.
5. Satir V, et al. *The Satir Model*. Palo Alto: Science and Behavior Books, Inc.; 1991.
6. DeBakey ME. The role of the physician in our changing society. *The New Physician*. 1963;12:443–8.
7. American College of Surgeons Fellowship Pledge. www.facs.org. Chicago: American College of Surgeons. Accessed November 4, 2002.
8. Committee on Quality of Health Care in America, Institute of Medicine. *Crossing the Quality Chasm: A New Health System for the 21st Century*. Washington, DC: National Academy Press; 2001.
9. Jones RS. Medicine, government, and capitalism. *J Am Coll Surg*. 2002;194(2):111–20.
10. Richardson JD. Workforce and lifestyle issues in general surgery training and practice. *Arch Surg*. 2002;137:515–20.
11. Comisky SJ. Forever and ever. In: *A good lawyer: secrets good lawyers (and their best clients) already know*. McLean, VA: Chaos; 1997. http://www.agoodlawyer.com.
12. Carrel A. The rules of conduct. In: *Reflections on Life*. New York: Hawthorn Books, Inc.; 1952:102–9.
13. Churchill W. In: Tsouras PG, ed. *The Greenhill Dictionary of Military Quotations*. London: Greenhill Books; 2000.
14. Royle T. In: *Dictionary of Military Quotations*. New York: Simon & Schuster; 1990.
15. Gelfand DV, Podnos YD, Wilson SE, Cooke J, Williams RA. Choosing general surgery: insights into career choices of current medical students. *Arch Surg*. 2002;137:941–7.
16. Paget S. *Confessio Medici*. London: MacMillan & Co.; 1909.

17. Den Uyl DJ. *The Virtue of Prudence*. New York: Peter Lang; 1991:55–83.
18. Lowenstein J. Where have all the giants gone? Reconciling medical education and the traditions of patient care with limitations on resident work hours. *Perspect Biol Med*. 2003; 46(2):273–82.
19. Bland KI, Isaacs G. Contemporary trends in student selection of medical specialties: the potential impact on general surgery. *Arch Surg.* 2002;137(3):259–67.

7

Should Sleep-Deprived Surgeons Be Prohibited from Operating Without Patients' Consent?

Charles A. Czeisler, Carlos A. Pellegrini,
and Robert M. Sade*

Introduction
Robert M. Sade, MD

The effects of sleep deprivation on performance of physicians has been widely studied ever since the death of Libby Zion in 1984, the subsequent campaign by her parents and others to regulate physician work hours, and the passage of the so-called Libby Zion Law by New York State in 1989.[1] Impetus was added to investigations of the effects of sleep deprivation when the Accreditation Council for Graduate Medical Education (ACGME) adopted similar standards for accreditation of residency programs in the United States in 2003.[2] While sleep deprivation clearly affects mental and physical functioning, results of investigations of clinical outcomes have been mixed—some finding adverse effects on patient care, others finding no such effects.

The arguments for regulating work hours of residents have been extended to apply in a more limited way to attending surgeons. In a recent issue of the New England Journal of Medicine,[3] two medical ethicists and a sleep specialist published a paper that opened with this scenario: "A surgeon on overnight call responds to an 11 pm call from the hospital, where a patient has presented with an acute abdomen. After working up the patient for several hours, the surgeon decides to ... perform a bowel resection. By the time the procedure is completed ... it is time for morning rounds. The surgeon has not slept all night and is scheduled to perform an elective colostomy at 9 am."

---

*Czeisler CA, Pellegrini CA, Sade RM. Should sleep-deprived surgeons be prohibited from operating without patients' consent? *Ann Thorac Surg.* 2013;95(2):757–66. Copyright Society of Thoracic Surgeons, republished here with permission.

The sleep specialists followed the vignette with a series of questions:[3] Does the surgeon have an obligation to disclose to the patient the lack of sleep during the past 24 hours and obtain new informed consent? Should the surgeon give the patient the option of postponing the operation or requesting a different surgeon? Should the hospital have allowed the surgeon to schedule an elective procedure following a night he was scheduled to be on call? Should it allow a surgeon to perform elective surgery after having been awake for more than 24 hours? After discussion of the effects of sleep deprivation (fewer than 2 hours of sleep in the previous 24 hours), the researchers answered these questions in the affirmative, with these statements: "Patients awaiting a scheduled elective surgery should be explicitly informed about possible impairments induced by sleep deprivation and the increased risk of complications." "They should then be given the choice of proceeding with the surgery, rescheduling it, or proceeding with a different physician." "If patients decide to proceed, they should explicitly consent to do so—in writing, on the day of the procedure, in front of a witness, and ideally on a standardized form designed for this purpose."

In the same issue of the [journal], three leaders of the American College of Surgeons responded to that paper in a letter to the Editor,[4] agreeing that sleep deprivation could be a problem for surgeons, but disputing the necessity or wisdom of mandating a signed informed consent document. They argued that, instead, surgeons should be better educated about the effects of sleep deprivation as well as other factors that may affect performance, enabling them to weigh all issues to provide the best patient care. "A call for mandatory disclosure," they stated, "essentially eliminates the necessary judgmental latitude surgeons should possess to determine their fitness for providing optimal patient care."

In the essays that follow, two authors of those publications, Dr Charles Czeisler and Dr Carlos Pellegrini, present arguments on either side of the question of whether sleep-deprived surgeons should be required to obtain informed consent from patients before elective surgery.

Pro
Charles A. Czeisler, PhD, MD

More than 40 years ago, Drs Richard Friedman, Thomas Bigger, and Donald Kornfield from Columbia University College of Physicians and Surgeons in New York published a landmark paper as a Special Article in the New England Journal of Medicine.[5] In it, Friedman and colleagues reported that sleep deprivation—which was first reported to adversely affect human performance in a classic 1896 study of Patrick and Gilbert from the University of Iowa[6] and had already been documented to impair cognitive and emotional brain functioning in healthy human participants more than fifty years ago—also adversely affected clinical task performance of physicians during their first postgraduate year of training in internal medicine. [...]

Publication of the Friedman study [...] precipitated a major change in the scheduling of physicians in training—although ironically not the elimination of the routinely scheduled extended duration (24-hour) work shifts that the investigators found degraded the performance of physicians. Moreover, the publication did not precipitate the elimination of the 60- to 84-hour work shifts that resident physicians routinely worked, until at least 2003, on weekends at many institutions nationwide.[7] [...] Simply put, the main rationale used to justify more than 24-hour shifts at the time—which was later formally tested and disproven in a randomized controlled trial[8]—was that it was better for a patient to be cared for by a tired physician who has followed his or her care since admission to the hospital than by a more rested physician who may be less familiar with the course of the patient's most recent illness. Yet no such rationale can be invoked to justify beginning an elective surgical procedure on a new patient when a surgeon's performance is impaired by sleep loss. Moreover, surgeons are required by law to obtain informed consent before elective surgery, after having disclosed what a reasonable patient would consider to be the "material risks" associated with the procedure. To evaluate the premise that sleep-deprived surgeons should thus be required to disclose such sleep deprivation and then obtain a patient's informed consent before operating, it is important to consider the current evidence linking sleep deprivation to human performance in the context of the ethical and legal principles of informed consent for elective surgery. [...]

SLEEP LOSS AND PERFORMANCE IMPAIRMENT

A great deal of evidence links sleep loss with performance impairment. Many factors influence the ability of healthy persons to sustain effective waking neurocognitive performance: biological time of day (i.e., circadian phase), length of prior wakefulness, nightly sleep duration, and proximity of the last sleep episode.[9] While the effects of these circadian and homeostatic sleep regulatory processes can be modified by environmental conditions, physical activity, and pharmacologic agents (i.e., caffeine or nicotine during night wakefulness or hypnotics during day sleep), they cannot consistently overcome the impact of adverse circadian phase and sleep deprivation on performance. Repeated interruptions of sleep, such as is experienced by physicians when they are on call, can lead to sleep deficiency by degrading the restorative quality of sleep. [...]

Without sleep, alertness and neurocognitive performance exhibit a steady deterioration attributable to sleep loss, onto which a rhythmic circadian variation is superimposed.[10] During sustained wakefulness, 24 hours of sleep deprivation has been shown to greatly impair neurobehavioral performance and judgment,[11] to an extent that is comparable to a level of 0.10% blood alcohol concentration.[12] [...] As with alcohol intoxication, chronically sleep deprived persons tend to underestimate the extent to which their performance is impaired, despite increasing impairment evident in objective recordings of the rate of lapses of attention. Thus, it would be just as inappropriate to ask a sleep-deprived surgeon whether he or she is able to operate safely as it would be to ask an intoxicated patron whether she or he is able to drive home from a bar safely.

ATTENTIONAL FAILURES AND AUTOMATIC BEHAVIOR

Importantly, persons struggling to stay awake in the face of elevated sleep pressure—whether due to acute total sleep deprivation, chronic sleep restriction, or repeated interruption of sleep (due to external interruptions or the presence of a sleep disorder)—are not always able to do so. The instability of the waking state due to sleep loss is associated with the occurrence of so-called microsleep episodes (i.e., involuntary sleep episodes <15 s long) and sleep attacks (i.e., involuntary sleep episodes >15 s long),[13] both of which can be classified as attentional failures. [...] Of course, once a person has lost the struggle to stay awake and makes the transition from wakefulness to sleep, however briefly, driving performance is much worse than that of a drunk driver, as the person is unresponsive to the environment throughout the duration of the micro-sleep episode or the sleep attack.

[...] Sleep deprivation degrades reaction time, impairs judgment, memory and vigilance, reduces attention span, increases distractibility, and raises the risk of attentional failures, automatic behavior, falling asleep at the wheel, and motor vehicle crashes, with drowsy driving accounting for an estimated 20% of motor vehicle crashes and serious crash injuries.[14]

Cognitive performance is markedly degraded during the transition from sleep to wakefulness.[15] The extent to which this phenomenon, which is called sleep inertia, interferes with neurobehavioral performance is related to the depth of the prior sleep episode. Thus, agents that interfere with sleep, such as caffeine, can mute the effect of sleep inertia. The adverse impact of sleep inertia on performance can exceed the impact of total sleep deprivation. [...] Sleep inertia can greatly degrade the performance of on-call physicians or surgeons when they are called upon to perform clinical tasks immediately upon awakening.[15]

Young physicians in training who were randomized to work extended duration (>24-hour) shifts experienced twice as many attentional failures,[16] and on average made 36% more serious errors caring for patients in intensive care units, including 55% more serious medical errors that reached the patient and 468% more serious diagnostic mistakes, as compared with the same physicians when they were scheduled to have many more handovers in care while working no more than 16 consecutive hours in intensive care units. [...] When performing procedures during the daytime, these young physicians had a 73% increased risk of a percutaneous injury after their 20th hour of work than during shifts that averaged less than 12 hours in duration.[17] In another study, the impairment of physicians on schedules in which sleep was restricted to an average of 2 to 3 hours in the prior 24 hours was comparable to the effects of elevated blood alcohol concentrations.[18]

[...] Faculty attending surgeons performing elective procedures during the daytime who had a sleep opportunity of less than 6 hours between cases during the prior on-call night had a significantly increased rate (+170%) of procedural complications (i.e., adverse events occurring as a result of care during an operation and likely attributable to the performance of the attending surgeon).[19]

INFORMED CONSENT AND DISCLOSURE

The standard of risk disclosure is based on the principle of patient autonomy, which has been stated in this way: "Physicians must have respect for patient autonomy. Physicians must be honest with their patients and empower them to make informed decisions about their treatment. Patients' decisions about their care must be paramount, as long as those decisions are in keeping with ethical practice and do not lead to demands for inappropriate care."[20]

In most jurisdictions, over the past 30 years, the standard of risk disclosure regarding informed consent has shifted from what a reasonable physician would expect to know (the "reasonable physician" standard) to what a reasonable patient would expect to know (the "reasonable patient" standard).[21] The principle of patient autonomy is a fundamental principle underlying informed consent, and it requires that physicians respect the right of the patient to make voluntary and informed health care decisions. The patient-centered standard for informed consent "emphasizes patient autonomy by requiring that risk disclosure be conducted to satisfy what an ordinary reasonable person in the patient's particular position would want to know.... [this precedent] 'marks the rejection of the paternalistic approach to determining how much information should be given to patients'."[21]

Legally, physicians must disclose "material risks," which include impairment of the physician caused by any use of drugs, disease, or alcohol that increase the risk of an operation—such risks must be disclosed to the patient. In the past, most deliberations regarding informed consent have focused on whether or not the informed consent adequately described the risks inherent in the surgical procedure itself and have not focused on the risks associated with the procedure being done in the hands of that particular health care provider at that time. Surgeons are understandably resistant to attempts to change the standard of informed consent from the published risks associated with various procedures to surgeon-specific and site-specific risks, for fear that it would open up a Pandora's box, including the issue of violating the privacy rights of a surgeon to protect information about his or her own medical history.[22] Evidence is accumulating, however, that many factors, including prior experience of the surgeon, whether the hospital has a high or low volume of similar cases, and the availability of electronic medical records, affect the risk of operative complications and adverse events during hospitalization.[21] It is within this context that we must view the premise that is the subject of today's debate, namely, that sleep-deprived surgeons should not be allowed to operate without the patient's consent.

Given the principle of autonomy and the patient-centered standard of disclosure, physicians have a duty to disclose to the patient any condition of the treating physician that an ordinary reasonable person in the patient's particular position would likely consider a material risk (i.e., would likely consider to be significant) and therefore want to know. [...] The key question is whether an ordinary reasonable person in the patient's particular position would likely consider extended duration work hours and consequent sleep deficiency to be a material risk and whether the patient would therefore want to know if his or her surgeon had been working for 24, 48, or 72 hours straight before undertaking an elective surgical procedure.

Several national polls have indicated what patients want to know. For example, one poll asked about the subjects' response if they learned that the doctor who is about to perform their surgery has been on duty for 24 consecutive hours.[23] Respondents reported that they would be very likely (65%) or somewhat likely (21%) to feel anxious about their safety; moreover, 60% of respondents reported that they would assume that it was very unlikely (31%) or somewhat unlikely (29%) that the surgical procedure would go well. Thus, 6 of 7 Americans would likely consider the status of a surgeon who has been on duty for 24 consecutive hours to be a material risk, and 6 of 10 believe that this would likely adversely affect the outcome of their surgery. Therefore, it is the surgeon's duty to disclose that condition and seek the patient's consent to operate in that condition before proceeding with the operation. Furthermore, respondents reported that they would be very likely (45%) or somewhat likely (25%) to ask for a different surgeon if they learned that the doctor who was about to perform their surgery had been on duty for 24 hours. So, 70% of Americans indicate that knowing that a surgeon who was about to perform their surgery had been on duty for 24 consecutive hours would influence their medical care decisions: it is the surgeon's duty to disclose that condition and seek the patient's consent to operate in that condition before proceeding with the operation.

The Boards of Directors of the Sleep Research Society and the National Sleep Foundation endorsed model legislation in 2005 that would establish "a requirement for physicians who have been awake for more than 22 of the prior 24 hours to inform their patients of the extent and potential safety impact of their sleep deprivation and to obtain consent from such patients before providing clinical care or performing any medical or surgical procedures." Given the extensive evidence that various aspects of neurobehavioral performance, including judgment regarding one's impairment, are degraded to a degree that is, on average, comparable to a blood alcohol concentration of 0.05–0.10 g/dL when persons are awake for 24 hours,[24] and that the average physician-in-training is impaired by an amount equivalent to a blood alcohol concentration of 0.05 g/dL when working frequent extended duration shifts, patients have a right to be informed if their physician has been on duty for 24 hours or more and the right to decide whether to take the risk of receiving care from that provider.

Con

Carlos A. Pellegrini, MD

Should a surgeon who has been awake for 22 of the previous 24 hours not be allowed to operate without the patient's written informed consent? My position is that informed consent is not the right solution.

The rationale for obtaining informed consent from this patient under the circumstances described above is as follows: The operation performed by a surgeon who has not slept for 22 hours imposes a higher risk. The patient has a right to know that there is an increased risk of complications (patient's autonomy). The patient's knowledge of an increased risk will result in actions that mitigate the risk.

Let us examine each of these three assumptions.

DOES AN OPERATION PERFORMED BY A SURGEON WHO HAS NOT SLEPT FOR 22 HOURS IMPOSE A HIGHER RISK?

The issue of sleep deprivation and fatigue and its effects on medical care came to a head in the 1980s after the death of Libby Zion, a patient who had been admitted to a New York hospital and was treated by a resident who eventually claimed that fatigue caused by lack of sleep had impaired his decision-making abilities. [...]

This case fueled interest in the impact of sleep deprivation leading to a considerable number of studies. Those studies can be divided into two general types: those conducted in laboratories under controlled situations, and those conducted by physicians (surgeons in our case) examining the effect of different work patterns on the outcomes of operations. The majority of the studies performed in controlled situations showed that vigilance, decision-making, and other attributes are affected progressively by acute sleep deprivation of the type under consideration in our case. A few experimental and controlled studies, however, have shown that while sleep deprivation manifested itself in sleepiness scales and increased overall cognitive workload, the subjects were able to perform technical tasks and to learn new tasks after nearly 24 hours of sleep deprivation—something also pertinent to our discussion.[25]

Conversely, studies that measured the relationship of sleep deprivation to outcomes of surgery have had varying results. On one extreme is the observation of Rothschild and colleagues[26] that in a subset of surgeons who had had less than 6 hours of "sleep opportunity" before an elective case (measured between the end of an emergency case while on call and the initiation of an elective case), the complication rate rose from 3.4% to 6.2% when compared with cases the surgeons had performed when they had not been on call or operated during the night. Of interest, however, is that, even in this study, when all cases and all surgeons are considered, there were no significant differences in the outcomes of elective operations whether the surgeon had or had not been operating the night before the elective case. The authors themselves acknowledge that they did not know whether or not the surgeons had slept the entire night before the "control" cases when they were not on call, and that there were potential confounders created by the retrospective nature of the study. On the other extreme are the findings of a more recent paper by Chu and colleagues[27] in which the researchers evaluated the effects of sleep deprivation on the outcome of more than 4,000 consecutive cardiac surgical procedures and found no difference at all in the results with sleep deprivation of the kind we are discussing today. In between these two extremes there are other studies that have focused on the effect of reduction of resident work hours and workload of surgeons, and so forth, with varying results and many of these studies showing no effect on the outcome of patients.

At the end of the day, well-controlled studies are impossible to do, and many studies that have looked at physicians' working hours and compared them to outcomes have failed to show an association. It is clear that while controlled studies show a progressive deterioration in our ability to do certain tasks, the failures of the studies to demonstrate influence on the outcome may be related to the fact that those involved use a number of fatigue mitigation techniques (such as physical fitness, periods of short naps, use of coffee, and others), to actually mitigate tiredness. The same has been true for the studies that have examined the effects of the implementation (in 2003) of an 80-hour work week for residents and mandatory periods of rest.[28] Examination of patient outcomes has shown varying results, and the largest cohort examined comprising all admissions to the VA failed to show any difference between the before and after 80-hour eras.

The argument above is not intended to defy logic; acute and chronic sleep deprivation by logic should impact on the surgeon's performance. However, the [clinical] studies have shown that there is no clear, measurable, reproducible relationship between the number of hours a surgeon has been working and the outcomes of an elective procedure.

THE PATIENT HAS THE RIGHT TO KNOW—BUT WHAT?

There is no question that the patient has a right to know everything that may affect the outcome of a procedure that he or she is about to undergo. However, mandating that the surgeon disclose to the patient the amount of sleep that the surgeon had over the preceding 24 hours without a clear measurable effect on the patient's outcome is not indicated. Furthermore, doing so just before an operation, at the time of maximum vulnerability on the part of the patient, is inhumane. Even further, if surgeons believe that they are tired and may not be offering the patient the best operation, surgeons' ethics would insist that the surgeons excuse themselves from doing it. Therefore, asking a surgeon to discuss with the patient the potential for sleep deprivation to affect outcome (assuming the surgeon believed that to be true) at the same time that we ask the surgeon to behave professionally (and therefore abstain from doing the operation) makes no sense to me.

It is not only that this becomes impractical, but if surgeons were to be obligated to disclose whether they were on call and did not sleep, should they also disclose whether they were able to sleep well? Whether they were awake part of the night at home? Whether there are issues of health among family members that kept a surgeon awake or worried? And what about financial worries, marital problems, and so many other issues that are known to affect the ability of humans to concentrate. How far is this disclosure supposed to go?[29]

I understand that it is "convenient" to take something as objective as having been on call versus not having been on call or having performed an operation the night before versus not having performed an operation the night before as elements that can be easily determined and easily measured and put them in the consent. But why do that in the face of a lack of demonstration of a clear effect on outcomes? And if it was clear that it affected outcomes, wouldn't it then be an obligation of the system to protect the patient and the surgeon by prohibiting the performance of the operation? Why would informing the patient be the best solution in this case? What if the patient agrees? Can a system—assuming the information was clear on the effect of complications—accept the patient's wish? [...]

MITIGATING THE RISK

I believe there are many ways to mitigate the potential risks associated with excessive workloads, night call, and sleep deprivation. First, the solutions start with the surgeon. Appealing to professionalism and arming the surgeons with enough information about the effects of sleep deprivation and fatigue would result in the development of strategies by the surgeon. I am not talking about the "last line of defense," namely, the surgeon noting that he or she is fatigued and deciding not to do an operation. I am talking about the adequate planning of the surgeon's life in terms of overall fitness, hours worked, how to accommodate the unpredictability of surgery, and how to best position himself or herself for work. Informed consent is the ultimate expression of professionalism between a surgeon and a patient. Everything that the surgeon believes [...] may bear on the outcome should be discussed with the patient in the most transparent fashion well before the operation is decided upon. A mechanical disclosure of duty hours, while the patient is awaiting surgery, while asking that the patient sign a "specially designed form" as has been proposed, is the antithesis of informed consent and places the patient in an unfathomable position, choosing between a surgeon who is trusted and a totally new person who may not be known to the patient or the family.

The second layer that I see as a solution is the immediate environment in which surgeons performs their work. Groups of surgical divisions or sections in the academic world and surgical partners in private practice in the outside world should be looking out for one another, and they should make their rules as to whether or not elective procedures are allowed to be performed after a night on call. In those cases, local rules for groups and for teams may have much more relevance. For example, if the calls are normally ones that are extremely demanding, then there should be no room for surgeons to schedule elective cases the next day. Conversely, in situations where the call may not be very demanding and where most of the time the surgeon can obtain a good night's sleep, then the scheduling of elective cases maybe more permissive.

Developing high-performing teams, emphasis is placed within a team on the need to have persons that are fit for duty. In this environment, persons are familiar with the concept of "mutual support," situational awareness, and mutual monitoring, and the ability of any member of the team to "stop the line" just before or even during the operation represents another layer of protection and mitigates the risk.

The fourth element is the institution itself—and here is where I believe the bulk of the responsibility ultimately will lie. Yes, it will require giving up part of the autonomy that surgeons have had over the years, but ultimately, making use of modern technology, the institution should assure by its rules (eventually applied through the teams) that everyone is "fit for duty."

Systems must change to respond to current knowledge in terms of cognitive workloads and the effect of fatigue on performance. When discussing safety in medicine, we frequently turn to aviation, an industry known for its devotion to safety. Most recently, the Federal Aviation Administration introduced regulations further addressing pilot fatigue. It did so in a multi-faceted way that takes into consideration specific factors that affect performance.[30] Extending our comparison of the informed consent, perhaps those who defend that theory would consider it appropriate for the crew to disclose to passengers the number of hours worked, the number of sectors flown, and the degree to which they may be sleep deprived. Instead, the system simply sets rules that precludes crews from flying those planes. Our rules should mandate that hospitals develop system changes to protect patients and surgeons alike that are not based on informed consent but on internal rules founded in the type of work that a given hospital carries on. Every surgeon should take fatigue management courses, and the systems should incorporate fatigue mitigation techniques that are known to work. [. . .]

Thus, the idea of obtaining informed consent is, in my opinion, an easy way out. It deflects a responsibility to patients that should be shared by the system, the team, and the surgeons; and it asks the patients to provide, with their signatures, permission to proceed to do something that may not be in their best interest. I believe it is the surgeon, and ultimately the system, who must rise to this occasion and accept the responsibility for the delivery of the best possible surgical care.

Concluding Remarks
Robert M. Sade, MD

Czeisler [. . .] and Pellegrini agree on several points: lack of sleep compromises neurobehavioral performance, and the ethical and legal standards for informed consent require that surgeons disclose to patients all material issues that can affect the outcome of a planned operation. Their main disagreements focus on the nature of the material risks posed by a surgeon's sleep deprivation and who should bear the burden of deciding whether an operation should go forward.

A critical issue in this debate is the real-world question of whether and to what degree attending surgeons' lack of sleep affects the outcomes of their surgical procedures. Czeisler cites a single study of practicing surgeons—his group's recent paper found that complications after procedures were higher when surgeons were on call the night before than when they were not. Their study had several serious flaws; most important was absence of any data on the surgeons' actual time of sleep when on or off call—being on call does not necessarily mean lack of sleep, nor does off call necessarily mean a full night's rest. In response, Pellegrini cites several other studies that have shown no difference in surgical outcomes performed by sleep-deprived versus well-rested surgeons.

None of the available studies has been well controlled. Such studies are needed, but it seems unlikely that we will ever have a randomized controlled trial evaluating the effects on surgical outcomes of various degrees of practicing surgeons' sleep deprivation. In the absence of reliable data, what should be done in the interest of patient safety? That question lies at the heart of this debate.

In the face of uncertainty about the presence or degree of elevated risk to patients, we might wonder whether it is premature to mandate a consent process that is likely to confuse and frighten patients immediately before an operation, a time when they are not well situated to receive new information and make a thoughtful, deliberate decision. Perhaps the weight of making decisions about surgical procedures in the face of the surgeon's suboptimal sleep would best be borne by the institution and the surgical team, as well as by the surgeon. Mandated disclosure and written consent of the patient seem too blunt an instrument to advance the goal of patient safety. The mitigation strategies outlined by Pellegrini might better serve the interests of patients without violating their autonomy and informational needs.

What will policy makers do with the facts, assertions, and beliefs presented in this debate, in this era of increasing regulation of the health care system? The policy of mandated work hours for physicians-in-training has been solidly entrenched for several years—such regulation may lie on the road ahead for practicing surgeons as well.

References

1. Section 405.4. Medical staff. New York Comp Codes R & Reg. Title 10 § 405 (1989). http://w3.health.state.ny.us/dbspace/nycrr10.nsf/11fb5c7998a73bcc852565a1004 e9f87/bc8961f6b14230318525677e00726457?opendocument. Accessed September 4, 2012.
2. Accreditation Council for Graduate Medical Education. The ACGME's approach to limit resident duty hours 12 months after implementation: a summary of achievements. Chicago: Accreditation Council for Graduate Medical Education. http:// www.acgme.org/acwebsite/dutyHours/dh_dutyhoursummary2003-04.pdf. Accessed September 4, 2012.
3. Nurok M, Czeisler CA, Lehmann LS. Sleep deprivation, elective surgical procedures, and informed consent. *N Engl J Med.* 2010;363:2577–9.
4. Pellegrini CA, Britt LD, Hoyt DB. Sleep deprivation and elective surgery. *N Engl J Med.* 2010;363:2578–9.
5. Friedman RC, Bigger JT, Kornfield DS. The intern and sleep loss. *N Engl J Med.* 1971;285:201–3.
6. Patrick GTW, Gilbert JA. Studies from the Psychological Laboratory of the University of Iowa. *Psychol Rev.* 1896;III: 468–83.
7. Barger LK, Cade BE, Ayas NT, et al. Extended work shifts and the risk of motor vehicle crashes among interns. *N Engl J Med.* 2005;352:125–34.
8. Czeisler CA. The Gordon Wilson Lecture: Work hours, sleep and patient safety in residency training. *Trans Am Clin Climatol Assoc.* 2006;117:159–89.

9. Czeisler CA, Buxton OM. The human circadian timing system and sleep-wake regulation. In: Kryger MH, Roth T, Dement WC, eds. *Principles and Practices of Sleep Medicine*. St Louis, MO: Elsevier Saunders; 2010:402–19.

10. Czeisler CA, Gooley JJ. Sleep and circadian rhythms in humans. *Cold Spring Harb Symp Quant Biol*. 2007;72:579–97.

11. Venkatraman V, Chuah YM, Huettel SA, Chee MW. Sleep deprivation elevates expectation of gains and attenuates response to losses following risky decisions. *Sleep*. 2007;30: 603–9.

12. Roehrs T, Burduvali E, Bonahoom A, Drake C, Roth T. Ethanol and sleep loss: a "dose" comparison of impairing effects. *Sleep*. 2003;26:981–5.

13. Lim J, Dinges DF. Sleep deprivation and vigilant attention. *Ann NY Acad Sci*. 2008;1129:305–22.

14. Anderson C, Horne JA. Sleepiness enhances distraction during a monotonous task. *Sleep*. 2006;29:573–6.

15. Wertz AT, Ronda JM, Czeisler CA, Wright KP. Effects of sleep inertia on cognition. *JAMA*. 2006;295:163–4.

16. Lockley SW, Cronin JW, Evans BE, et al. Effect of reducing interns' weekly work hours on sleep and attentional failures. *N Engl J Med*. 2004;351:1829–37.

17. Ayas NT, Barger LK, Cade BE, et al. Extended work duration and the risk of self-reported percutaneous injuries in interns. *JAMA*. 2006;296:1055–62.

18. Arnedt JT, Owens J, Crouch M, Stahl J, Carskadon MA. Neurobehavioral performance of residents after heavy night call vs. after alcohol ingestion. *JAMA*. 2005;294:1025–33.

19. Rothschild JM, Keohane CA, Rogers S, et al. Risks of complications by attending physicians after performing nighttime procedures. *JAMA*. 2009;302:1565–1572.

20. Sox HC, ed. Medical professionalism in the new millennium: a physician charter. *Ann Intern Med*. 2002;136:243–6.

21. Veerapen RJ. Informed consent: physician inexperience is a material risk for patients. *J Law Med Ethics*. 2007;35:478–85.

22. Heinz C. How much is enough? Patients' right-to-know v privacy rights of health-care providers. *Law Govern*. 2004;7: 1–21.

23. National Sleep Foundation. 2002 "Sleep in America" poll. Washington, DC: National Sleep Foundation. http://www.sleepfoundation.org/sites/default/files/2002sleepinamericapoll.pdf. Accessed September 19, 2012.

24. Falleti MG, Maruff P, Collie A, Darby DG, McStephen M. Qualitative similarities in cognitive impairment associated with 24 hours of sustained wakefulness and a blood alcohol concentration of 0.05%. *J Sleep Res*. 2003;12:265–74.

25. Tomasko JM, Pauli EM, Kunselman AR, Haluck RS. Sleep deprivation increases cognitive workload during simulated surgical tasks. *Am J Surg*. 2012;203:37–43.

26. Rothschild JM, Keohane CA, Rogers S, et al. Risks of complications by attending physicians after performing night-time procedures. *JAMA*. 2009;302:1565–72.

27. Chu MW, Stitt LW, Fox SA, et al. Prospective evaluation of consultant surgeon sleep deprivation and outcomes in more than 4000 consecutive cardiac surgical procedures. *Arch Surg*. 2011;146:1080–5.

28. Hegar MV, Truitt MS, Mangram AJ, Dunn E. Resident fatigue in 2010: where is the beef? *Am J Surg*. 2011;202:727–32.

29. Keune JD, Kodner IJ, Healy GB. Disclosing sleep: an ethical challenge. *Bull Am Coll Surg.* 2011;96:20–1.
30. Federal Aviation Administration. Fact sheet—Pilot fatigue rule comparison. Washington, DC: Federal Aviation Administration. http://wwwnew.faa.gov/news/fact_sheets/news_story.cfm?newsid=13273&omnirss=fact_sheetsaoc&cid=103_f_s. Accessed September 19, 2012.

8

Are Thoracic Surgeons Ethically Obligated to Serve as Expert Witnesses for the Plaintiff?

Donald C. Watson, Jr., Francis Robicsek,
and Robert M. Sade[*]

Introduction
Robert M. Sade, MD

Medical negligence lawsuits have been growing in both number and size of awards to plaintiffs for many years. In the last few years, however, the effect on physicians, especially surgeons, has become noxious, and record numbers of surgeons are choosing early retirement or abandoning medicine to work in other fields. Tort reform is high on the agenda of nearly every medical association and specialty society.

The villain of this piece is generally believed to be trial lawyers, who profit greatly from huge awards in malpractice cases, often far beyond their injured clients' share of the bounty. The anger of many if not most physicians is directed at the plaintiff's bar, to the extent that they refuse to testify for the plaintiff in any malpractice suit, especially when the defendant is a member of their own specialty.

Yet, there may be problems with this viscerally held position. In providing legal testimony, a physician's primary ethical obligation is to tell the truth as he sees it without bias that favors one side or the other. That may make irrelevant the side of a lawsuit for which a physician testifies. There are many other considerations of course, but there is an underlying vexing question: if a thoracic surgeon regularly testifies in medical negligence lawsuits, does he have an ethical obligation to serve as expert witness for plaintiffs as well as defendants?

---

[*]Watson DC Jr, Robicsek F, Sade RM. Are thoracic surgeons ethically obligated to serve as expert witnesses for the plaintiff? *Ann Thorac Surg.* 2004;78:1137–41. Copyright Society of Thoracic Surgeons, republished here with permission.

This question was debated at the 50th Annual Meeting of the Southern Thoracic Surgical Association by two of our most esteemed colleagues, both former presidents of the Association and both possessing special expertise in legal issues: Donald Watson and Francis Robicsek. They present their adversarial positions after the presentation of this case, which served to focus the debate.

CASE

Doctor Loyall is a cardiothoracic surgeon with a large experience and excellent results in aortic surgery. He has been sued several times by patients who had complications of surgery, usually paraplegia, but also false aneurysms and other problems. He has lost a case only once when, contrary to the merits of the case, a jury was emotionally swayed by the appearance of the plaintiff, an attractive young woman whose right leg was amputated because of a complication after aortic surgery.

Doctor Loyall testifies in negligence cases two to three times a year in defense of other surgeons who have been sued, usually for complications of aortic surgery. He receives a telephone call from an attorney in another state. He hears the story of a 55-year-old man who is now paraplegic after removal of a descending thoracic aortic aneurysm extending into the distal aortic arch. The operation in question was done with a clamp-and-sew technique, with a cross-clamp time of 67 minutes. It was done by a thoracic surgeon who has been in practice for 5 years, after finishing his training at a program that is now on probation for inadequate operative experiences for their trainees. The surgeon is not yet board certified.

It then becomes clear to Dr. Loyall that the lawyer represents the plaintiff. He has a personal policy of never testifying for plaintiffs, so he ends the conversation, declining to be involved, despite the strong likelihood of substandard judgment or technique or both.

Was Dr. Loyall wrong in refusing to testify for the plaintiff in this case, on the grounds that physicians have an ethical obligation to testify for plaintiffs as well as for defendants in medical liability cases?

Pro
Donald C. Watson, Jr, MD

The principle question is important: are thoracic surgeons ethically obligated to serve as expert witnesses for the plaintiff? Two ethical arguments follow showing that absent other disqualifying factors, thoracic surgeons are obligated to serve as expert witnesses for the plaintiff or the defense. That of course assumes that the surgeon is able to offer testimony and that the merits of the case justify such testimony. Doctor Loyall was wrong in refusing on only ethical grounds to testify for the plaintiff.

Ethics discussions help us decide the bases upon which we pursue the things we value and the ultimate criteria for what we do. However, they serve only as advisory. The specifics of each situation vary. Conclusions are often subjective and almost always involve judgment. Differences in opinion between competent people can and do exist on many important ethical issues. We must be respectful of and take into consideration others' points of view. These ethical considerations, as suggested by Pellegrino,[1] are also undergoing a metamorphosis. The ethical framework of medicine is changing.

Two cautions should be acknowledged. We must beware of politically correct actions that have shaky ethical foundations. Armey suggests, "Politics sooner or later makes a fool of everyone."[2] In the long run, actions supported by sound ethical principles should prevail. Additionally, although used in a different context, a political activist suggested, "If we don't stand for something, we may fall for anything." Thoracic surgeons must stand for moral principles and use professional standards or we are likely to fall for the antithesis.

Two concepts of "ethical" are expanded upon. The first involves moral, that is, right behavior standards. The second demands conforming to accepted professional standards of conduct. All other criteria being met, each line of reasoning forms an independent ethical justification for the position that thoracic surgeons are obligated to serve as expert witnesses for the plaintiff or the defense.

A brief summary of five foundations of ethical thought, in idealized societies, is in order.[3] [...] Plato described the common good in a society of individuals. Opining that one's own good is firmly linked to the good of the community, he concluded that individuals are ethically bound by the pursuit of common values and goals. Subsequently Aristotle expressed the fairness and justice approach by noting that equals should be treated equally. In our judicial system, the plaintiff and the defendant are equals, thus requiring equal treatment for the plaintiff and the defendant. As this notion was later pursued in ethics discussions, favoritism and discrimination were considered unjust and wrong. Additionally, the virtue approach maintains the existence of certain ideals toward which we should all strive. Relevant virtues include compassion, generosity, integrity, fairness, self-control, and prudence. Then, in the 18th century Kant suggested a rights approach focusing on an individual's right to choose. When living in a community, the individual's rights include truth, privacy, freedom from harm, and what is promised by a consenting individual. Finally, the utilitarian approach, a 19th century conception of Bentham and Mill, suggested that actions are ethical only when they provide the greatest balance of good over evil.

Four medical moral principles of behavior have evolved with these foundations in ethics. The Hippocratic Oath suggests that we do no harm and help others, principles of nonmaleficence and beneficence. Patient autonomy, the third principle, has recently risen in importance but is not germane to the question posed. The fourth principle of justice insists that we do the right thing for patients and be fair in those actions. Justice is, more often than not, the most difficult to resolve.

These foundational principles of ethics and medicine, that is, right behavior standards, force us to ask what implications naturally follow when applying them to the question posed? These implications are that Dr. Loyall was (1) not serving the common good, (2) treating equals unequally, (3) failing to reach for virtuous goals, (4) ignoring the rights of individuals to truth and freedom from harm, (5) failing to tip the societal balance of good over evil, (6) failing to help future patients, (7) potentially allowing harm to future patients, and (8) failing to provide expert information available for the best possible evaluation of what was just. It is reasonable to conclude that by refusing, on only ethical grounds, to testify for the plaintiff, Dr. Loyall was wrong.

A second independent concept of ethical actions demands conformity to accepted professional standards of conduct. [...] Our profession has standards and is guided by major organizations with established principles of behavior. As a matter of ethical behavior, thoracic surgeons are obligated to comply with them in their actions. The American Medical Association (AMA) suggests that as citizens and professionals, physicians have an ethical obligation to assist in the administration of justice.[4] The American College of Surgeons (ACS) Code of Conduct[5,6] suggests that surgeons, in part, must accept responsibilities to serve as effective advocates for patients' needs, to provide the highest quality of surgical care, and to participate in self regulation by setting, maintaining, and enforcing practice standards. By refusing on purely ethical grounds to testify, Dr. Loyall was wrong by not fulfilling this ethical obligation to conform to accepted standards of physician conduct. Doctor Loyall would not be assisting in the administration of justice, would not accept responsibilities to advocate for patients, and would not help to calibrate and improve the quality of surgical care, or setting, maintaining, and enforcing standards of practice.

In general, when considering two ethical alternatives it is helpful to ask five questions namely, which alternative (1) best respects the moral rights of those affected, (2) leads to the best overall consequence, (3) treats, in process, the parties equally, (4) advances the common good, and (5) develops moral virtues? In balance, greater good over evil is achieved when physician experts provide the best possible information and advice to a system adjudicating a dispute. Physicians are ethically obligated to testify for the plaintiff or the defendant depending on their ability and the merits of the case. We must stand for moral principles of behavior. Professional standards define those principles.

A few caveats are in order. First, this issue is emotionally charged. Emotional reactions about colleagues testifying against colleagues are intense. Thoracic surgeons are not exempt from these most human reactions. This response often interferes with our collective ability to objectively engage the question posed.

Second, many other important issues are related to this ethics question, distracting us from the principle at hand. These distractions include but are not limited to disordered, even chaotic, medical-legal systems, qualifications of experts, legal requirements of experts, adversarial nature of legal proceedings, differences between medical truth and legal truth, specific case circumstances, and practicality of testifying. [...]

Third, in our daily actions, we must consider practical consequences. Politically correct actions, which may be in opposition to moral obligations, allow us to get along within our community and to survive with less stress. The penalty for violating a strictly moral obligation is primarily personal. The penalty for adhering to a moral principle, in violation of loyalty, can be steep. Some surgeons, in all subspecialties, have stood on moral principle only to have their lives adversely affected because the community viewed that moral stance as not loyal.

Fourth, if one is to testify, one should adhere to established standards. The ACS[5] and the Society of Thoracic Surgeons (STS)[7] have described qualifications and standards of behavior for expert witnesses. [...] The ACS and STS suggest there is an obligation to testify when appropriate. [...] The AMA also suggests that expert witnesses, irrespective of being called by either the plaintiff or the defense, must not become advocates and must remain nonpartisan.[8]

In conclusion, based on fundamental ethical principles for behavior of individuals living within a community and professional code of conduct standards, Dr. Loyall was wrong in refusing on purely ethical grounds to testify as an expert witness for the plaintiff. The reality of medical-legal proceedings in our society, however, presents a number of confounding issues making adherence to this ideal practice difficult.

Con
Francis Robicsek, MD, PhD

Society has its way of dealing with important issues. One way is to make them laws. The treating physician is a "factual" witness who has a legal obligation to testify to the treatment his patient received. In contrast, just as an uninvolved physician does not have any legal obligation to accept an unknown patient, a medical expert may testify voluntarily, albeit paid. While he is supposed to render an unbiased opinion in our peculiar medico-legal system, his involvement is called upon only if it promotes the invoking party. If it does not, his testimony will neither be given nor heard.

Whenever a physician is asked to render an expert opinion, he may legally, as well as ethically, decide not to get involved. He may feel unprepared and unwilling to be interrogated for hours, have his credentials questioned, his family life scrutinized, and his character assassinated by an overzealous attorney.

Or he may be a conscientious objector who believes that our tort system is wrong and does not help the injured; it does not punish the negligent but often hurts the innocent physician and provides a windfall for the attorney. He may think the only way to change it is not to participate, but he might be willing to assist a colleague innocently accused and does not consider it his duty to get involved in procedures against fellow physicians.

Or he can say the "public trust," which goes with his medical license, obliges him to try to make the best of the system, to cooperate with it, and make choices on a daily basis.

Any of the above may be fitting to one's own ethical choice and should be respected. It is not unethical. What is unethical is for someone to render inappropriate testimony for any reason, for any party. That is today's main ethical problem and the reason why some physicians are reluctant to testify. They simply do not want to be identified with the readily available group of dubious witnesses who fill our courtrooms with pseudoscience and are willing to testify "for or against" depending upon who pays their fee.

To believe that obliging our profession to testify may clean up the situation is naïve. While some attorneys indeed seek an honest reliable opinion, others are looking for a witness who says what they want to hear. They will go from one potential witness to the other until one is found who is either naïve or loose enough to serve their purpose.

The Trial Bar wants us to actively support the tort system by providing a readily available list of witnesses. Our answer is this: we are ready if you are ready! Give us a process that fairly and speedily compensates the injured patient, punishes the negligent physician, protects from frivolous, costly litigation—and they will not find a more cooperative partner than we are. We are ready to sit down tomorrow to discuss no-fault insurance, review panels, mandatory mediation, free, impartial witnesses to the court—whatever.

There is indeed a problem with medical experts—not with those who do not testify, but with some of those who do. While some of them, be it motivation by either economic or by intent, do provide a fair and honest testimony, others are less than truthful. For our professional organizations to open the floodgates of "readily available" witnesses without any quality control of their testimony would be highly counterproductive. Before we accept the concept that it is everybody's ethical duty to testify, and we provide a list of experts obliged to testify, we should fulfill our already existing ethical duty to clean up expert testifying. Ten years ago I recommended to the Council of the STS that medical expert testimony should be reorganized as a professional activity and thus subject to peer review, and that a grievance process should be made available to both parties. By this mechanism, improper testimony can be readily exposed and false witnesses censored and hence removed from the system.

This process has now been applied by the American Association of Neurological Surgeons (AANS), which found that one of their members provided "inappropriate and unprofessional" testimony and they suspended his membership.[9] The member countersued. The case in which the American Medical Association, the American College of Surgeons, and the Illinois State Medical Society filed a joint "friend of the court" brief supporting the AANS was reviewed by the Seventh Circuit US Court of Appeals and decided in favor of the AANS. The US Supreme Court declined to review the case.[10] However, the event was labeled by some trial lawyers as an "unacceptable intrusion and egregious assault by an overly anxious, embittered group of physicians who are willing to do anything to pressure their colleagues not to testify."

Until we make significant strides in this regard, or even thereafter, medical experts testifying should remain an issue of personal conscience. I may have testified in the case in question, either for the defendant or the plaintiff, depending upon additional information, but I do not castigate those who exercised their First Amendment right by keeping their mouth shut. My feelings are best expressed by the words of Dr. Mark Gorney[11] published in the Bulletin of the American College of Surgeons: "The moment of truth is at hand when you must elect all circumstances considered whether to act as an expert witness against a colleague. Only you, in the loneliness of your mind, can decide which road to follow, because in one direction the circumstances may be overwhelming for it, whereas in the other, something inside is saying, 'There but for the grace of God go I.'"

Concluding Remarks
Robert M. Sade, MD

Few topics stoke a surgeon's fire as much as malpractice litigation. Watson and Robicsek have presented starkly contrasting views of how Dr. Loyall should have responded to the plaintiff's attorney who was soliciting his opinion. The essayists agree on the central ethical imperatives of medical testimony: all testimony should be truthful, as the surgeon understands the truth, and the witness should have expertise in the area under litigation. After that, their points of view and reasoning sharply diverge. [...]

The case itself removes most of the issues that usually complicate medical-legal discussions. Disdain for the tort system is not, for Dr. Loyall, a barrier to testifying because he regularly testifies in lawsuits. His qualifications as an expert witness in this case are not in doubt. The adversarial environment of negligence lawsuits and the wide chasm between medical (scientific) and legal (authoritative) standards of truth have not bothered him in the past, as he has not rejected testifying as an expert. We are left with a single reason for his consistent refusal to testify for plaintiffs and their attorneys, based in emotion: he was once deeply stung by the arbitrary injustice of the medical-legal judicial system. There are undoubtedly additional questions of fact related to the patient's injury in the case at hand, but Dr. Loyall has summarily dismissed them as irrelevant. The central question—whether Dr. Loyall was wrong in refusing to testify for the plaintiff—is stark.

Watson's conclusion that Dr. Loyall was wrong not to testify is based on a nexus of ethical reasoning that stretches across several centuries of ethical thought that would now fall under the rubric of professionalism. Robicsek's finding that Dr. Loyall did nothing wrong is based on the narrow grounds of the right of every American to speak or to remain silent. At issue here is the nature of professional ethics: are the professional decisions and actions of physicians bound only by the laws governing society in general or do physicians bear additional legitimate extralegal obligations (that is, ethical obligations) by virtue of the special circumstances inherent in the patient-physician relationship?

Ethics and law are closely related, overlapping to some extent, but essentially separate. To say, as Watson does, that Dr. Loyall has an ethical obligation to testify for the plaintiff if the facts justify such testimony is not to say that he should be hauled into court unwillingly or lose his medical license if he refuses to testify. He has a legal right not to testify, just as Robicsek says. But if Watson's view of professional ethics is correct, then Dr. Loyall was nevertheless wrong in refusing to testify.

Robicsek's commitment to a legalistic view of Dr. Loyall's obligation to testify does not require that he reject professional ethics as Watson has described it. He could have it both ways, asserting both the right not to testify and the importance of professional ethics, by arguing, as some have, that legal testimony is not part of professional practice so should not be subject to the usual ethical standards of the practice of medicine, to peer review, or to oversight by medical licensing boards. He did not make that argument, however, so we cannot be certain where he stands, but I suspect that he is as deeply committed to professional ethics as any of us.

Our essayists have persuasively argued distinct visions of professional decision making. Each of us is likely to face similar decisions in the future, unless there is an early resolution of the malpractice crisis, which seems unlikely. If and when that time comes, our decision to say yes or no will embody the particular view of professionalism we have embraced.

References

1. Pellegrino ED. The metamorphosis of medical ethics. *JAMA*. 1993;269:1158–62.
2. Armey D. *Armey's axioms*. Hoboken, NJ: John Wiley & Sons; 2003.
3. Markkula Center for Applied Ethics. Thinking ethically: a framework for moral decision making. Santa Clara, CA: Santa Clara University. http://www.scu.edu/ethics/practicing/decision/thinking.html. Accessed October 24, 2003.
4. American Medical Association. E-9.07 Medical testimony. Chicago: American Medical Association. http://www.ama-assn.org/ama/pub/category/8539.html. Accessed October 18, 2003.
5. Gruen RL, Arya J, Cosgrove EM, et al. Professionalism in surgery. *J Am Coll Surg*. 2003;197:605–10.
6. Spencer FC, Guice KS. The expert medical witness: concerns, limits, and remedies. *Bull Am Coll Surg*. 2000;85:22–5.
7. Society of Thoracic Surgeons Board of Directors. Statement on the physician expert witness. *STS News*. 2003;9:6–7.
8. American Medical Association. Board of Trustees Report 5-A-98. Chicago: American Medical Association. http://www.thruthinjustice.org/amareport.htm. Accessed October 18, 2003.
9. Rice B. Malpractice experts: the penalty for bearing false witness. *Med Econ*. 2002;15:36–9.
10. Hollowell EE, Zaremski MJ, Wecht CH. Expert testimony in medical malpractice cases—new hazards. Paper presented at the annual meeting of the American Academy of Forensic Sciences, February 21, 2003, Chicago.
11. Gorney M. Expert witnesses caught in a moral dilemma. *Bull Am Coll Surg*. 2003;88:11–14.

SECTION 3

Relationships with Patients— Autonomy and Consent

Robert M. Sade

A physician shall, while caring for a patient, regard responsibility to the patient as paramount.

—Council on Ethical and Judicial Affairs, American Medical Association, Code of Medical Ethics

Questions of how physicians should relate to patients lie at the core of medical ethics. In the practice of medicine, the first responsibility of physicians is to the patients they treat. Out of respect for patients' right of self-determination, physicians must transmit to patients sufficient information about their illnesses to allow them to understand what is happening to them and to be able to make reasonable decisions about their health care. Patients must be respected as persons, and their medical needs must receive timely attention. All information about the patient's life and medical condition must be held in strict confidence, and the patient's privacy must be respected.

Because the practice of surgery usually involves physical invasion of the body, the process of informed consent is especially important in the relationship between surgeons and patients. The fundamentals of informed consent—its precondition and conditions—are fairly straightforward and well known to surgical residents and practicing surgeons. The precondition must be met before the consent process can continue: The patient must have the capacity to make decisions. If the patient lacks capacity, then a proxy (an agent appointed by the patient) or surrogate (a person authorized by law to make decisions on the patient's behalf) makes decisions in place of and for the patient. The basic conditions of informed consent are disclosure and consent. Patients must be given information about their illness and reasonable treatment alternatives, transmitted in a form that they can understand in sufficient detail to make a reasoned decision. Finally, patients must authorize execution of diagnostic tests or treatments.[1]

The process of informed consent occurs every day, so it seems familiar and straightforward. Yet the process is more complex than it seems because of the intricate interplay between the details of the illness, the range of possible interventions, the surgeon's beliefs about what is medically best, and the patient's capacity to understand the information and come to a decision. How much information should be conveyed? What methods of presentation optimize the patient's understanding? How can one ensure that the patient actually understands the information? How can one measure the depth of understanding? How should the surgeon respond if the patient doesn't want to listen to explanations and asks the surgeon to do whatever the surgeon thinks is best? When if ever can a procedure be carried out without the patient's consent? What can be done if a patient is competent and rational but still refuses treatment of a life-threatening condition? How much decision-making authority do surrogate decision-makers have, especially if the surgeon disagrees with their choices? These are just a few items on the long list of complicated questions that pertain to informed consent. Excellent discussions of the ethics of informed consent are available for medicine in general[2] and for surgery in particular.[3]

Given these complexities, it is not surprising that serious conflicts can arise within the patient–surgeon relationship, many of which are difficult to resolve. Several such conflicts and controversies have been debated in Ethics Forum sessions.

Chapters

Chapter 9 addresses one of the fundamental principles of patient care, the requirement for the physician to respect the patient's autonomy.[4] The idea of autonomy has many implications; for example, in cases of disagreement between physician and patient, the patient's choice is ultimately decisive. An extensive body of law and ethical deliberation has indicated that a patient has the right to determine what happens to his own body. If the patient lacks decision-making capacity, a proxy or surrogate makes decisions in his stead. When a patient is anesthetized, he clearly no longer has the capacity to make decisions, but his previous instructions during the informed-consent process or in the form of an advance directive continue to control what happens to his body. A particularly difficult situation is that of the Jehovah's Witness, whose religious beliefs prohibit the use of blood transfusions, even when required to save the patient's life. Are there circumstances under which a patient's refusal of life-saving transfusions can be overridden by a surrogate?

The case in **chapter 10** describes a situation that reverses the conflict in the previous case.[5] The patient has a limited prognosis due to lung cancer. After lobectomy, he has a complicated postoperative course leading to multisystem failure. The surgeon believes the patient has a reasonable chance of good-quality survival and insists on moving forward with dialysis for renal failure. The patient's wife, his surrogate decision-maker, demands that dialysis not be instituted on grounds that her husband would not have wanted it. The surgeon is faced with a decision: doing what the patient's wife wants or overriding her decision by seeking a court order to continue treatment.

Disclosure of medical errors to patients and their families has been a major area of contention ever since the 1999 report of the Institute of Medicine, *To Err is Human: Building a Safer Health System*, which brought the problem of hospital deaths due to medical errors to the public consciousness. In the vignette that focuses the debate in **chapter 11**, a surgeon mistakenly ligates a branch pulmonary artery during an intended pulmonary lobectomy, necessitating an extension of the operation to include the entire lung. Ultimately this complication leads to the patient's death.[6] Does the surgeon have an ethical obligation to inform the patient and his family about the mistake he made, or do the potential dire consequences of disclosure to himself justify concealing the truth?

A different problem regarding disclosure of a surgical error occurs when the error is not the surgeon's but is the mistake of another surgeon who operated on the patient previously. **Chapter 12** introduces the case of a patient who has a bronchopleural fistula subsequent to a pneumonectomy ten days previously.[7] The first surgeon failed to do a lymph node biopsy that would have aborted the procedure that led to the pneumonectomy. The second surgeon approaches the first surgeon, describes the error that was made, and suggests that the first surgeon talk to the patient about it. Concerned about litigation, the first surgeon refuses. Is the second surgeon obligated to tell the patient about the error?

In providing information to patients regarding a current illness, physicians must disclose alternative courses that are consistent with good medical judgment. Occasionally, however, a patient may ask for treatment that is outside acceptable medical standards for what the patient believes is good reason. In **chapter 13**, a young man with Marfan syndrome has an aortic aneurysm that is not yet ripe for operation, but intervention is nearly inevitable within a relatively few years.[8] He is about to lose insurance coverage and asks the surgeon to go ahead with the operation, even though the aneurysm is not large enough to justify intervention by strictly medical criteria. Is it reasonable for the surgeon to do what the patient wants, or should he steadfastly remain within the limits of standard surgical practice?

Much of the disease burden in this country—as much as 50% by some estimates—is caused by lifestyle choices made by the patient, such as drinking too much alcohol, eating too much food, driving too fast, or engaging in otherwise dangerous activities. Some self-inflicted diseases can lead to expensive interventions, raising the question of the extent to which surgeons are obligated to provide such operations after the patient repeatedly fails to refrain from self-damaging behavior. **Chapter 14** presents the vignette of a patient who abuses cocaine intravenously, undergoes aortic-valve replacement for native-valve endocarditis, and subsequently develops prosthetic-valve endocarditis after he relapses to intravenous cocaine abuse.[9] What is the surgeon's obligation to replace the infected prosthesis after repeated episodes of drug abuse?

References

1. Faden RR, Beauchamp TL, Nancy M. P. King NMP. *A History and Theory of Informed Consent.* New York: Oxford University Press; 1986.
2. Miller F, Wertheimer A. *The Ethics of Consent: Theory and Practice.* New York: Oxford University Press; 2010.
3. Jones JW, McCullough LB, Richman BW. Informed consent and disclosure. In: *The Ethics of Surgical Practice.* New York: Oxford University Press; 2008:12–51.
4. Naunheim K, Bridges C, Sade RM. A Jehovah's Witness patient who faces imminent exsanguination should be transfused. *Ann Thorac Surg.* 2011;92(5):1559–64.
5. D'Amico TA, Krasna MJ, Sade RM. No heroic measures—how soon is too soon to stop? *Ann Thorac Surg.* 2009;87:11–18.
6. Mavroudis C, Mavroudis CD, Naunheim K, Sade R. Should surgical errors always be disclosed to the patient? *Ann Thorac Surg.* 2005;80(2):399–408.
7. Moffatt-Bruce S, Denlinger C, Sade RM. Another surgeon's error: must you tell the patient? *Ann Thorac Surg.* 2014;98(2):396–401.
8. Estrera AL, Ikonomidis S, Ikonomidis JS, Sade RM. Impending loss of insurance coverage is an indication to proceed with complex, expensive surgery. *Ann Thorac Surg.* 2010;89(6):1709–16.
9. DiMaio JM, Salerno TA, Bernstein R, Araujo K, Ricci M, Sade RM. Ethical obligation of surgeons to non-compliant patients: can a surgeon refuse to operate on an intravenous drug-abusing patient with recurrent aortic valve prosthesis infection? *Ann Thorac Surg.* 2009;88(1):1–8.

9

Should a Jehovah's Witness Patient Who Faces Imminent Exsanguination Be Transfused?

Keith S. Naunheim, Charles R. Bridges,
and Robert M. Sade*

Introduction
Robert M. Sade, MD

The right of every person to reject unwanted medical therapies, whether or not the choice is consistent with good clinical practice or medical judgment, is well established in ethics and law. The right to reject treatment can be exercised directly by the patient or indirectly by the patient's surrogate or proxy decision maker. Generally speaking, first-person directives take precedence over surrogate/proxy decisions; that is, a valid directive by a patient, such as a living will or an organ donor card, cannot ordinarily be overridden by a surrogate/proxy unless the patient has given that person specific authority to do so.

A Jehovah's Witness signature on a Jehovah's Witness card refusing blood transfusion and on the operative permission form repeating her refusal ordinarily allows no wiggle room: the surgeon is obligated to honor her refusal, even in the face of life-threatening hemorrhage. But what if her Jehovah's Witness husband demands that her life be saved with blood transfusions, claiming that she is currently incapacitated and unable to change her mind about transfusion, which he, as the person who knows her best and the one she has designated as her health care agent, is certain she would do if she were able to do so. Drs Keith Naunheim and Charles Bridges reach differing conclusions about what is the right thing to do under such circumstances.

---

*Naunheim K, Bridges C, Sade RM. A Jehovah's Witness patient who faces imminent exsanguination should be transfused. *Ann Thorac Surg.* 2011;92(5):1559–64. Copyright Society of Thoracic Surgeons, republished here with permission.

CASE

A 59-year-old Jehovah's Witness with severe rheumatic mitral stenosis and insufficiency, Josephine Rutherford, has an advance directive naming her husband, Frank, who is also a Jehovah's Witness, as her health care agent. She has a preprinted Jehovah's Witness card that she signed 2 years previously, refusing blood transfusions. On the operative permission form, she signs the clause refusing transfusion and her husband signs as witness.

She undergoes mitral valve replacement, and unexpectedly suffers the rare complication of posterior perforation of the left ventricle with exsanguinating hemorrhage. The surgeon, Dr. Percy Thomas, tells the family she is going to die without transfusions. Her Jehovah's Witness husband states that his wife does not have the opportunity to change her mind, and, as her health care agent, he must make the decision for her. He is sure she would change her mind if she knew death from blood loss is now a certainty—she has often expressed to him how much she has to live for. The patient's two adult children, a 25-year-old pregnant daughter (who is a Jehovah's Witness) and 29-year-old son support the request to give the patient the blood she needs to survive.

Dr Thomas urgently calls the hospital attorney, who tells him that the state's Uniform Health Care Decisions Act (UHCDA) provides protections that allow for a strong case to be made for legal immunity from civil or criminal liability, no matter what decision the surgeon makes.[1] He should make his determination, the attorney says, on ethical grounds. What should the surgeon do?

Pro
Keith S. Naunheim, MD

This Jehovah's Witness patient should be transfused. The problems surrounding transfusion in Jehovah's Witness patients are some of the most controversial ethical issues faced in medicine. The Jehovah's Witness religion was initially instituted under the name the Watchtower Bible and Tract Society founded in 1884 by Charles Taze Russell in Western Pennsylvania. In 1931, the Watchtower Bible and Tract Society was reincorporated by a society of international Bible students, and the name of the religion was changed to Jehovah's Witnesses. The religion is based primarily on the "end of the world" prophecy as interpreted from Bible readings. Teachings from this religion specify that Jehovah's Witnesses are the only "true" Christians, and that only such true believers will be saved at the time of Armageddon and the second coming of Christ. At that time, all those who are not true believers will be destroyed. Mr Russell first suggested Armageddon would occur in 1914 but it had not yet arrived at the time of his death in 1916. His successor, Joseph Franklin Rutherford, rewrote the doctrine and subsequently predicted Armageddon would occur in 1918, 1920, and 1925. The doctrine of this religion also specifies that only the Jehovah's Witness leadership can provide a true interpretation of the Bible, and this must be followed strictly by all believers; individualism is strongly discouraged. Also, any members of the religion who openly criticize the leadership or their teachings are considered to be apostates and disloyal to God and thus subject to penalties such as excommunication and expulsion from the community. This latter punishment suggests the apostate will be shunned, not only by the society as a whole, but by family members as well.

The Jehovah's Witness leadership has held many controversial views regarding medical issues, views that have gradually evolved over the last few decades. There was a time in which the Jehovah's Witness leadership considered the American Medical Association to be representatives of Satan and "tricksters" who tried to mislead the population into inappropriate medicines and surgical procedures. There had been prohibitions against the utilization of aluminum cookware, which was reported to cause cancer and insanity. Vaccinations were characterized as "pus cocktails," and organ transplantation was equated with "cannibalism." Over the last several decades, these latter two treatment modalities have become accepted by the Jehovah's Witness leadership and are now "matters of conscience" for all of the Jehovah's Witness membership.

The prohibition for utilization of blood was first announced in 1945, and has been based on at least three citations from the Bible: (1) Genesis 9:4 "But you must not eat meat that has its life blood still in it." (2) Leviticus 17:2 "None of you may eat blood, nor may any foreigner residing among you eat blood." (3) Acts 15:29 "You are to abstain from food sacrificed to idols, from blood, from the meat of strangled animals and from sexual immorality."

The transfusion of blood products is interpreted by the Jehovah's Witness leadership as equivalent of "eating blood" because the patient receiving a transfusion is the one who consumes the blood product. Even this prohibition has evolved somewhat over the past 2 decades. Originally, all forms of blood products were banned, including specific clotting factors (as administered to hemophiliacs), immunoglobulin, and even albumin. Consumption of any these or the more standard types of transfusions (whole blood, packed red blood cells, platelets, or fresh frozen plasma, whether heterologous or autologous) were thought to warrant excommunication from the religion and eternal damnation at the time of judgment. However, at present, the Jehovah's Witness leadership believes that albumin, immunoglobulin, and specific clotting factors can be administered if the individual practitioner's conscience allows.

Many critics have attacked the transfusion prohibition as being "an irrational belief" and thus an inappropriate foundation for making any medical decision regarding receiving blood products. However, Jehovah's Witness religious dogma does not appear any more "irrational" than the belief of many other religions. [...] Arguing against the transfusion prohibition on the basis of "irrational beliefs" appears somewhat hypocritical for any practitioner of religion whose basic tenets require faith, for example, the blind belief in a non-provable entity or practice.

I believe there are three important issues pertaining to the administration of blood in Mrs Rutherford's case and questions that must be answered: (1) Was the consent voluntary or was it given under duress? (2) Did the patient fully grasp the gravity and scope of the operation? (3) Can the family supersede the decision of the patient?

WAS THE CONSENT GIVEN UNDER DURESS?

With regard to voluntary consent, the patient did sign the consent outlining the prohibition of transfusion and also carried a card in her wallet documenting same. The question of duress, however, is a more subtle one. There can be a little doubt that the religious practices of Jehovah's Witnesses can be considered somewhat coercive. The prospect of being expelled from one's community and even from one's family can be frightening; such a concept will exert great emotional pressure upon the patient making decisions regarding blood products. In many instances, a pastor or church member will accompany the patient and his or her family to make certain that "the whole truth" is revealed to the patient and the physician involved does not "mislead" or "trick" them into accepting transfusions. There have even been instances in which hospital employees who are Jehovah's Witness practitioners have reported on other Jehovah's Witnesses who have agreed to receive transfusions, thus condemning them to harsh punishment within their community. Is this type of peer pressure not duress? Can one confidently assume that the consent was entirely voluntary? At the very least, some doubt exists regarding the voluntary nature of such consent.

DID THE PATIENT GRASP THE GRAVITY AND SCOPE OF THE OPERATION?

A complete informed consent includes a thorough discussion of the procedure. That entails an outlining of the nature of the intervention, all reasonable alternatives to the treatment, and recommendations as well as the risks and potential benefits of the procedure. The complication outlined in the above clinical scenario (posterior perforation of the left ventricle) is both exceedingly rare and remarkably complex. It is very difficult to believe that the patient actually could comprehend that a complication with a less than 1% incidence could eventually endanger her to the point where her survival chances were less than 50/50 even with the benefit of transfusion. [...] Many patients cannot recount what they were told even within the hour after the informed consent process. Because of this, I believe the best guide regarding the level of comprehension for this patient would come from the family. Indeed, both the husband and the daughters stated that the patient did not fully grasp the ramifications of her transfusion decision and insisted that, had she truly understood the possibilities, she would want to be transfused. I, for one, would not suggest my judgment regarding the patient's state of mind was more accurate than that of the family with whom she lived. The family's insistence that she did not understand in this case is critical; thus, I cannot be certain that her consent was fully informed considering their attestation to the contrary.

CAN THE FAMILY'S DECISION REGARDING TRANSFUSION SUPERSEDE THE PREVIOUS DECISION OF THE PATIENT?

In 1993, the National Conference of Commissioners on Uniform State Laws drafted and approved the UHCDA. This act has been ratified by several states and defines the specific powers of health care agents during the time of incapacity on the part of a patient. It was in effect at the time of this clinical scenario. The act specifically states that an appointed "surrogate shall make the decision in accordance with the surrogate's determination of the patient's best interest." In this case, the husband and daughters [sic] all agreed that transfusion was in the patient's best interest, and the hospital attorney confirmed that such a decision was arguably legal and appropriate. Thus, under the dictates of this act, it is wholly appropriate for the family's decision to supersede that of the patient.

In summary, there is nothing clean and certain about the ethical issue within the scenario. The basic ethical values that are usually referred to in such clinical situations include the following: autonomy—the patient has the right to refuse or accept offered treatments; beneficence—a practitioner should act in the best interest of the patient; nonmaleficence—"first do no harm" (*primum non nocere*); justice—fair and equal distribution of treatment and health care resources; dignity—the patient and the doctor both have the right to dignity; and truthfulness—patients must be informed regarding all options and ramifications.

While it is sad, it is also true that in difficult situations such as the clinical scenario above, not all the ethical values can be fulfilled simultaneously. Transfusing the patient to save her life fulfills the value of beneficence while at the same time potentially violating the value of autonomy. However, the decision by the husband and daughter [sic] on behalf of the incapacitated patient certainly fulfills the legal definition of appropriate practice and, in my opinion, fulfills the ethical value of autonomy as well. I believe that, in this case, transfusion of this Jehovah's Witness patient is both justifiable and correct.

Con
Charles R. Bridges, MD, ScD

This Jehovah's Witness patient should not be transfused. The Jehovah's Witness faith has grown remarkably since its inception in 1869, now including more than 7 million followers in 236 countries.[2] The Watchtower Society is the governing body of the Jehovah's Witnesses, and in 1945, this body introduced a ban on accepting blood transfusions. As a result, Jehovah's Witnesses nearly universally refuse to receive blood products. In fact, most are quite dogmatic about the fact that they would rather die than receive a transfusion.[3] Their refusal to accept blood products is based on a literal interpretation of the passages in the Old Testament that forbid them to do so. In fact, even the option of preoperative autodonation and banking of blood for perioperative use is excluded as once the blood has been disconnected from the body's circulation, it is no longer acceptable. These restrictions notwithstanding, innovative blood conservation techniques[4] including meticulous surgical technique, use of miniature heart-lung circuits, retrograde and antegrade autologous priming, autologous normovolumic hemodilution, and use of an in-line cell saving device for red cell salvage during cardiopulmonary bypass, can be utilized with excellent results even in complex cardiac surgical procedures in these patients.[5] Moreover, the Watchtower Society has left the decision to accept fractions of the primary components (i.e., cryoprecipitate, albumin) to the individual Jehovah's Witness, while forbidding the acceptance of the "primary components" of blood, defined as red blood cells, white blood cells, platelets, and plasma.[6] Some would argue that the Jehovah's Witness refusal to accept blood products represents a form of irrational religious zealotry. However, unlike many other arguably less than scientifically rational religious beliefs, the most recent data suggest overwhelmingly that blood transfusions are associated with an increase in mortality and morbidity that is a direct consequence of the transfusions themselves and not due to uncorrected confounding issues. This point is best illustrated by the observation that there is a direct relationship between the age of the blood transfused and its negative impact on mortality and other complications, hence implicating the blood rather than the condition of the patient receiving it.[7] Thus, rather than representing irrational religious zeal, it is perhaps more appropriate to describe the Jehovah's Witness's aversion to blood transfusions as emblematic of divine scientific insight!

INFORMED CONSENT TO SURGERY

In 1914, Judge Benjamin Cardozo wrote a landmark opinion in the case Schloendorff v The Society of New York Hospital, which legally defined simple consent and changed the history of American medical ethics. Cardozo wrote: "Every human being of adult years and sound mind has a right to determine what shall be done with his body; and a surgeon who performs an operation without his patient's consent commits an assault, for which he is liable in damages ... except in cases of emergency, where the patient is unconscious, and where it is necessary to operate before consent can be obtained."[8]

Clearly, in this case, although the patient is indeed unconscious, it was the surgeon's duty to discuss the precise scenario presented, namely, intraoperative life-threatening hemorrhage, with the patient and the patient's family before the procedure. One might argue that, for a minor surgical procedure, it would not be necessary to discuss life-threatening bleeding but for a cardiac surgical case, it should always be discussed as a possibility.

Furthermore, it is the surgeon's duty to provide sufficient information to the patient and the patient's family in advance of the case so that the patient can anticipate how he or she would be expected to react to situations that are likely to occur. Thus, although ventricular perforation is itself a rare complication of mitral valve replacement, potentially life-threatening bleeding is not an uncommon occurrence during cardiac surgery. Failure to discuss this scenario is a failure to provide adequate information for true informed consent. Moreover, it is the surgeon's duty to accept the patient's religious beliefs, values, and morals, independent of whether the surgeon finds these beliefs to be rational.

COGNITIVE UNDERSTANDING

The surgeon's duty is to help the patient to develop "cognitive understanding" of the procedure. Cognitive understanding requires that patients appreciate their present condition, the procedure proposed, and that their decisions will have consequences. These consequences are best understood as a series of probabilities attached to a group of potential outcomes, each of which may be associated with either an improvement or a worsening of the patient's condition and possibly even in the patient's demise. Only when fully apprised of these probabilities and outcomes, each a function of the patient's decision, can the patient make an informed decision. It is the surgeon's charge to correct any misunderstanding the patient may have, to improve their fund of knowledge, and to help them to understand both the nature and the consequences of the options available to them. Throughout this process, the surgeon must respect the patient's autonomy.

PREVENTIVE ETHICS

This case represents a failure of "preventive ethics." Here, it is the surgeon's responsibility to ascertain that the patient fully understands her condition and the probable impact of her refusal to accept blood products on the expected outcome. Because some Jehovah's Witnesses fear that they will be shunned by their community if they were to accept blood products, the surgeon must explore whether the patient's understanding has been clouded by emotional factors, anxiety, financial obligations, and the like. Only if such factors can be excluded or managed through counseling can informed consent be obtained. Having established true evaluative understanding, the surgeon should acknowledge value conflicts that exist and develop a management plan (including all likely eventualities) and make sure the plan is in accord with the patient's values and beliefs. These are the tenets of preventive ethics. Adequate preventive ethics in this case would have obviated the need to address this issue of life-threatening hemorrhage after the surgery had commenced. It arguably should have been discussed before the procedure to prevent the ethical dilemma. The surgeon's first response to refusal of blood transfusion should have been to review with the patient her understanding of the condition and its benefits and risks.

SUMMARY

In the case presented, the surrogate decision makers for Josephine Rutherford (the patient's husband and two daughters [sic]) have been asked to provide "substituted judgment" for the patient since she is unconscious. In this case, the surrogates believe that the patient would want to be transfused if she knew that she would otherwise die. However, Dr Thomas has every right and indeed a duty to ignore the wishes of these surrogates if he has a reasonable degree of certainty that the surrogates are mistaken, regardless of their views. In this case, there should be a reasonable degree of certainty that the patient would not want to be transfused, given that she has both signed a card refusing transfusions 2 years ago and again signed a consent form before the procedure refusing transfusions. There should be no doubt. As alluded to above, the principles of preventive ethics and cognitive understanding imply that in the context of true informed consent the surgeon should already know exactly what the patient would want under these circumstances. However, in the absence of such absolute knowledge, given the patient's written refusal to accept blood products, given that bleeding is common during cardiac surgery, and given that consent for cardiac surgery necessarily implies that the patient understands that death is a possibility, the principles of transitive logic (eg, if A implies B, and B implies C, and C implies D, then A implies D) dictate that the patient must have known that her refusal to accept blood products might lead to her death. Therefore, in keeping with her written expressed wishes, the patient must be allowed to die without a transfusion.

Concluding Remarks
Robert M. Sade, MD

For the purpose of this debate, we accept the hospital attorney's opinion that the UHCDA provides immunity from civil or criminal liability to the surgeon, whether he chooses to transfuse or not to transfuse. [...] So Dr Thomas's decision should be made on ethical grounds, that is, what is the right thing to do: transfuse in an attempt to save the patient's life, or withhold transfusion and allow the patient to die? Both essayists present their cases clearly and logically. Both base their analyses on the principle of respect for autonomy. The nature of autonomy has been understood in many different ways, but generally, most analysts accept the minimal components of an autonomous decision as a choice that is made intentionally, with understanding of the relevant information, and with freedom from controlling influences.[9]

Intentionality is generally taken to be binary, whereas understanding and voluntariness can be matters of degree. For example, a professor of biology and an illiterate grade school dropout lie at opposite ends of a spectrum of ability to comprehend medical information. Similarly, a range of influences can have greater or lesser impact on a patient's decision-making freedom—persuasion, manipulation, and coercion are different kinds of influences. Persuasion is not a controlling influence if a physician's balanced presentation of facts and honest reasoning moves a patient to a choice recommended by the physician, but could be controlling if the physician's balanced and honest discussion produces an emotional reaction that drives the patient's decision. Manipulation impels a patient toward a certain choice when the physician presents information in a biased manner, misrepresents facts, or withholds information; manipulation is always a controlling influence that compromises autonomous decision making. Coercion—the use of force or the threat of force or harm—also undermines autonomy.

Protecting autonomous decision making is the primary purpose of informed consent. The process of informed consent requires the presence of several elements that signal the centrality of respect for autonomy. These elements are generally understood to be competence, disclosure of relevant information, understanding of that information, voluntariness of decision making, and consent that both chooses an option and authorizes the chosen procedure.[10] [...]

The patient's husband, who is also her health care agent, asserts that the patient would have changed her mind and accepted transfusions if she had known that death were imminent. The most commonly used standard by which agents make decisions for a patient is substituted judgment: in the absence of a relevant and specific advance directive, the agent must choose the option that the patient would have chosen had she not lacked decision-making capacity. But in this case, Mrs Rutherford has made a first-person decision not to have blood transfusions, a decision that generally cannot be overridden by others. There are situations, however, in which overriding a first-person directive may be justified. In clinical settings, as the severity of risk of harm to the patient increases, there is a parallel increase in justification for overriding an advance directive.[11] The dilemma in this case is the clash between the patient's clear directive and the most severe of risks, death by exsanguination. To her husband and children, overriding Mrs Rutherford's directive does not undermine her true beliefs and values, rather, it respects and restores her autonomy, a position that Dr Thomas could find plausible.

Under the circumstances of this case, there seems to be no clearly right or wrong answer. The precise nature of autonomy and of its protector, the process of informed consent, has not been decisively resolved in the biomedical ethics literature, and the courts still find difficult cases at the edges of settled law. Both Naunheim and Bridges have made cogent arguments in support of their positions. Under the UHCDA, they both seem to have made a legally defensible case and, in my view, they both have presented positions that are reasonable and ethically acceptable.

I close with a caveat: the UHCDA was adopted by only a few states, and the statutes and case law governing informed consent in the remaining states display great variation. A surgeon who faces a similar case would be on ethically defensible grounds to choose either to provide or to withhold transfusion, but legally, would be prudent to consult the health care institution's legal staff before reaching any conclusion about the most appropriate course of action.

References

1. Uniform Health Care Decisions Act. National Conference of Commissioners of Uniform State Laws. Chicago: Uniform Law Commission; 1993. http://www.law.upenn.edu/bll/archives/ulc/fnact99/1990s/uhcda93.pdf. Accessed April 15, 2011.
2. About Jehovah's Witnesses. Brooklyn, NY: Jehovah's Witnesses; 2010. http://www.watchtower.org/e/statistics/worldwide_report.htm. Accessed July 11, 2011.
3. Hughes DB, Ullery BW, Barie PS. The contemporary approach to the care of Jehovah's Witnesses. *J Trauma*. 2008;65:237–47.
4. Sniecinski R, Levy JH. What is blood and what is not? Caring for the Jehovah's Witness patient undergoing cardiac surgery. *Anesth Analg*. 2007;104:753–4.
5. Ferraris VA, Ferraris SP, Saha SP, et al. Perioperative blood transfusion and blood conservation in cardiac surgery. *Ann Thorac Surg*. 2007;83:27–86.

6. Dandolu BR, Parmet J, Isidro A, et al. Reoperative cardiac surgery in Jehovah's Witness patients with patent internal thoracic artery grafts: how far can we push the envelope? *Heart Surg Forum.* 2008;11:E32–3.

7. Koch CG, Li L, Sessler DI, et al. Duration of red-cell storage and complications after cardiac surgery. *N Engl J Med.* 2008;358:1229–41.

8. Jones JW, McCullough LB, Richman BW. A comprehensive primer of surgical informed consent. *Surg Clin North Am.* 2007;87:903–18.

9. Beauchamp TL, Childress JF. Respect for autonomy. In: *Principles of Biomedical Ethics,* 6th ed. New York: Oxford University Press; 2009:99–149.

10. Meisel A, Roth L. What we know and do not know about informed consent. *JAMA.* 1981;246:2473–77.

11. Kleinig J. *Paternalism.* Totowa, NJ: Rowman and Allanheld; 1983:76.

10

No Heroic Measures

HOW SOON IS TOO SOON TO STOP?

Thomas A. D'Amico, Mark J. Krasna, Diane M. Krasna, and Robert M. Sade*

Introduction
Robert M. Sade, MD

As cardiothoracic surgeons, we face many difficult problems in our professional lives, and base most decisions on clinical judgment developed and honed during many years of training and experience. Some decisions, however, are based on more than weighing scientific evidence and outcome probabilities, and they require value judgments on such matters as the desirability of alternative outcomes. Among the most difficult judgments we make are those that conflict with the views of the patient or the patient's proxy (i.e., agent appointed in advance by the patient) or surrogate (i.e., agent authorized by law) decision maker. [...] The case below illustrates just such a difficult surgeon–family conflict and it is the focus of the debate that follows.

THE CASE OF THE RESOLUTE WIFE

John Cooper is a 40-year-old restaurant owner, who has a wife and two children, 20 and 22 years old. He is a 45-pack/year smoker and complains of chest pain, located in the right chest wall. A chest roentgenogram shows a mass in the right upper lung field. Diagnostic workup discloses squamous cell carcinoma of the lung, stage IIB (T3N0M0), invading the chest wall. His surgeon,

---

*D'Amico TA, Krasna MJ, Sade RM. No heroic measures—how soon is too soon to stop? *Ann Thorac Surg.* 2009;87:11–8. Copyright Society of Thoracic Surgeons, republished here with permission.

Dr. William Ashley, performs a difficult right upper lobectomy with chest wall resection. The pathology report confirms the histology and stage of the cancer; the margins of the surgical specimen have no residual tumor and the lymph nodes contain no malignant cells.

The patient does well initially, but on postoperative day (POD) 2, [...] a chest roentgenogram shows pneumonia. Increasing distress requires reintubation and transfer back to the cardiothoracic intensive care unit. On POD 4, the chest roentgenogram shows early signs of a bilateral fluffy infiltrate [...]. By POD 6, it is clear that the patient has adult respiratory distress syndrome. Dr. Ashley has excellent rapport with the family, which seems to be cohesive and is devoted to their husband and father, respectively. The surgeon informs the family of the patient's steadily worsening prognosis.

By POD 8, the lung problem is worse and signs of renal failure have appeared. Dr. Ashley spends considerable time with the patient's wife explaining her husband's clinical condition, including the likelihood that he will soon require hemodialysis. For the first time, she mentions that she and her husband have talked about the use of "heroic measures" if one of them should develop a serious or terminal illness from which full recovery was unlikely, and he did not want such measures. The patient's wife determines that dialysis should not be used.

Dr. Ashley explains that the patient's chance of recovery is not high, but is not zero, and dialysis might successfully manage his renal failure, allowing his lungs time to recover. The patient's wife is unconvinced. The surgeon suggests that they wait over the weekend, and see what happens, as the decision can be delayed for a few days. The patient's wife agrees; she is also willing to talk with the hospital ethics committee. Committee members meet with her several times over the weekend.

On POD 11, the need for dialysis is imminent; the potassium level now is 5.9 mg/dL and rising. Managing the adult respiratory distress syndrome is still difficult, but it has not become worse over the weekend, and no cardiotonic drugs have been required. Dr. Ashley discusses the situation again with the patient's wife, also with the ethics committee representatives present. The surgeon again expresses his belief that it is in the patient's best interest not to withhold dialysis. He has a reasonable chance of surviving his pulmonary and renal problems (with the surgeon's guess of perhaps a 20% probability of leaving the hospital alive with a good quality of life) and a fairly good chance of surviving his cancer (published data suggest a 50% chance of being alive in 5 years). Moreover, in this day and age, dialysis and artificial ventilation cannot be considered heroic treatment. The ethics committee scrupulously carries out its role as educator and mediator. In the end, the patient's wife still insists on withholding dialysis.

Dr. Ashley now sees two options. He can follow the decision of the patient's wife and allow his patient, with a potentially treatable organ failure, to die soon from progressive renal failure. Alternatively, the other option based on the grounds of doing what is in the patient's best interest, he can ask the hospital attorney to seek a court order to continue treatment. He wants to do the right thing for his patient, but he is not sure which course is best. He decides to ask two of his colleagues for their thoughts.

Pro
Thomas A. D'Amico, MD

[...] The need for physicians, patients, and families to confront the issues of withdrawal of support and medical futility, as highlighted in this hypothetical case, is important and unfortunately familiar to cardiac and thoracic surgeons. Decisions regarding the use, withdrawal, or withholding of life-sustaining care are usually not difficult to make. When there is uncertainty about prognosis and the rights of others to make decisions for the patient, medical, ethical, and potentially medical/legal controversies may be difficult to manage.

Although conflicts have arisen in several reported cases in which a patient was competent to make a decision about end-of-life care,[1] conflicts regarding withdrawal of support more commonly occur when the patient lacks the capacity to express his or her wishes regarding a specific decision.[2] One study demonstrated that physicians and families are responsible for the majority of the decisions about life support in intensive care units, because fewer than 5% of patients are able to communicate with clinicians at the time the decision is made.[3] Conflicts commonly arise when a physician recognizes medical futility and the family does not.[4] Less commonly, the family expresses the desire to withhold or withdraw support, against the physician's judgment, as in this case. In addition, this case is complicated by the lack of a living will or written advance directive, and the issue of a surrogate's right to decision making is an element of the conflict.

The intended peripheral role of law when end-of-life dilemmas arise is often forgotten in debates such as this. The law prohibits active killing, and clear advance directives must be followed if they have been properly executed. But within these bounds, end-of-life questions are almost always resolved privately, by patients, their physicians, and their family members, working with nurses, social workers, and members of the clergy. Within wide boundaries, we must honor the wishes clearly stated by the patients. This commitment not only safeguards the liberty and dignity of the patient, but it also protects against family strife when a patient's intentions are clear.

Regarding the primary question posed by this scenario of whether Dr. Ashley should ask the hospital attorney to seek a court order to continue treatment, the only possible answer is no. First, based on precedents, it is unlikely to be successful. Second, there are other options. This summary, however, does not do justice to the difficult decision-making process entailed in this case and others like it. To fully address the complex issues that define this case, Dr. Ashley must answer the following questions: What are the chances of the patient surviving this critical illness with a reasonable quality of life outside the hospital? What measures must be taken to accomplish his recovery? How much suffering will further care impose on the patient's wife and his family? What resources would be expended in that care? In the absence of a written advance directive, how can the patient's wishes best be expressed? If the patient's wife is not justified in being allowed to make this decision to withdraw support, what decisions would she be capable of making? I will address these questions sequentially.

What are the chances of the patient surviving this critical illness with a reasonable quality of life outside the hospital? Evaluation of prognosis requires assessing age, cancer stage, severity of illness, presence of organ dysfunction, reversibility of ongoing processes, and chance of cognitive function beyond the intensive care unit.

At 40 years of age, the patient is relatively young, which improves his chance of recovery and also supports an aggressive strategy. [...] As he battles postoperative pneumonia, sepsis, adult respiratory distress syndrome, high ventilatory support, and renal failure imminently requiring dialysis, the severity of illness is best described as high, and the possibility of complete recovery as relatively low. [...]

What measures must be taken to accomplish his recovery? Further efforts to achieve recovery would include acute and possibly chronic dialysis, tracheostomy, and prolonged ventilatory support, gastrostomy, and rehabilitation. [...] Although all of these measures are offered routinely in the intensive care unit, are they reasonable to apply to a man with a poor prognosis if he would be likely to decline if he was capable?

How much suffering will further care impose on the patient and his family? Although the suffering imposed on the patient difficult to assess, the suffering imposed on the patient's wife would likely be high. It certainly seems that she has given the decision to withhold dialysis careful consideration. She has involved her husband's surgeon and the hospital ethics committee for advice, and she has stated specifically that she and her husband had discussed this difficult decision, and that he would refuse further care. Thus, one would conclude that the imposition of further (unwanted) care would be traumatic and injurious to the family.

What resources would be expended in that care? Although a surgeon's primary responsibility is to optimize the outcome of the patient's care, it is irresponsible to ignore the issues of cost and resource utilization. [...] In this case, resource expenditure could be justified if consent for its use (i.e., specifically dialysis) were to be obtained.

In the absence of a written advance directive, how can the patient's wishes best be expressed? [...] [The surgeon must] address the issues of critical illness and the patient's wishes regarding decisions in the informed consent process. Although this issue is not specified in the hypothetical scenario, one can only assume that either the topic was not discussed or that the patient's wife is correctly representing her husband's wishes, because Dr. Ashley does not dispute the point. Thus, in the absence of a written advance directive, decision-making for a patient at the end-of-life is made by the next of kin, or the patient's wife. She articulates that she and her husband have addressed this issue previously, and there is no reason to doubt her. Therefore, decisions regarding consent for further care are clearly hers to make.

If the patient's wife [...] is capable and empowered to make decisions consenting to the care to the current stage of care, she is equally capable and empowered to make decisions declining care (assuming effective communication with Dr. Ashley).

RECOMMENDATIONS

In considering these questions, one can make the following recommendations for Dr. Ashley:

1. Do not take the case to court, but consider other options.
2. Talk to the entire family about what the patient would want in this situation. [...] Remember that family members often do not understand information regarding diagnosis, prognosis, or treatment, and physicians often miss important opportunities to allow patients and family members to discuss their personal values and goals of therapy.[5]
3. Delay urgent dialysis with other clinical alternatives to allow further dialogue. Hyperkalemia could be temporarily managed with calcium, glucose, and insulin. [...] [T]he option of peritoneal dialysis could be discussed as well.
4. Propose a negotiated approach in regard to reaching specific clinical goals and using these goals in the decision making in regard to continuing or withdrawing care. One option would be to set a goal for a specific time limit for dialysis, to allow recovery of the lungs and the kidneys.

It would not be wrong to proceed with dialysis if the family supported it. If further support is withheld, that decision could not be criticized if the family believes that it represents the patient's wishes. If the family refuses, it would be inappropriate to insist on dialysis based on what is known now about the patient's preferences and his chance of survival.

CONCLUSION

Surgeons should strive to understand clearly the ethical and legal issues involved in end-of-life care, including the function of an advance directive, healthcare power of attorney, individual state medical futility acts, and American Medical Association policy on these issues.[6] Unfortunately, only 20% to 30% of adults are estimated to have advance directives, and in 35% of those, the directives cannot be found when needed. Utilize consults from ethics committees or palliative care services to improve end-of-life care. Address impending issues before a decision must be made urgently or emergently. Negotiate decisions based on clear, easily understandable goals and milestones. The overarching goal of courts, clinicians, and others with a say in end-of-life disputes should be to pursue private, family-based decisions within the wide limits set by law. Practice medicine in the hospital, not the courtroom [...].

Con

Mark J. Krasna, MD, and Diane M. Krasna, CRNA

[...] We strongly believe that unless treatment causes unneeded pain or suffering to no avail, it is incumbent on a physician to act in the patient's best interest to provide care and treatment with every resource available. We believe this is a moral and ethical obligation based on the principles of beneficence and nonmaleficence (i.e., being of benefit to the patient and doing no harm). Hippocrates suggested three major goals of medicine: "cure, relief of suffering, and refusal to treat those who are overmastered by their diseases."[7] Some might use these words to advocate stopping treatment, but we will explain the smokescreen that has been inappropriately promoted and continues to be advocated by those who argue for cessation of all curative treatment with very loose boundaries. We also hope to demonstrate how to distinguish between futile, "heroic" care and what is realistic, supportive care during an acute postoperative crisis. Good communication with patients and their families preoperatively and postoperatively is imperative. An operative consent covering postoperative situations and giving the surgeon the latitude necessary to act in the patient's best interest is needed. We must educate patients, their families, and collaborative healthcare workers to fully understand the difference between medically appropriate, supportive care, and end-of-life palliative care.

CONSENT

Informed consent is a central legal and ethical concept for this discussion. Legally speaking, consent is explicit or implied. The patient entered into an explicit contract with Dr. Ashley when he came to his office and consented to surgery. The patient expressed his desire for surgery, fully knowing its possible life-threatening complications and potential long postoperative course. Dr. Ashley assured the patient of his commitment to steer him through all of that just previously mentioned as his surgeon, to the best of his ability, as per the operative permit and Dr. Ashley's explanations before surgery.

The World Medical Association Declaration on the Rights of the Patient states: "The patient has the right to self-determination, to make free decisions regarding himself/herself. The physician will inform the patient of the consequences of his/her decisions. A mentally competent adult patient has the right to give or withhold consent to any diagnostic procedure or therapy. The patient has the right to the information necessary to make his/her decisions."[8] Good communication between physician and patient is essential for truly informed consent. This involves explaining complex diagnoses, treatments, and prognoses in simple language, ensuring the patient's grasp of the information, answering questions, and explaining advantages and disadvantages of the options. [...]

ADVANCE DIRECTIVES

While we are told that the patient gave an oral advance directive, we do not believe that it "holds water" postoperatively. [...] A clear distinction must be made between patients facing unexpected, futile, long-term care and the current scenario; what is being proposed by Dr. Ashley in this case is appropriate, supportive care with a reasonably hopeful outcome. Professional responsibility of a physician to do no harm also implies the moral authority to judge the benefits of medical interventions. Arrogance aside, who knows better than the physician, from his experience with similar cases and scenarios as to what can work and what should be tried.

We are told that the proposed treatment plan for dialysis has been explained to the patient's wife and she had refused on the grounds that she and her husband had "talked" about the use of "heroic measures" if one of them should develop a terminal illness from which recovery was unlikely. Dr. Ashley repeatedly expresses his feelings that it is in the patient's best interest for the wife not to withhold dialysis; today, dialysis and mechanical ventilation cannot be considered "heroic treatment."

ETHICS COMMITTEE

The ethics committee educates and mediates, but in the end the patient's wife still insists on withholding dialysis. Dr. Ashley is left with two options: (1) allow the patient's wife to decide to let his patient with potentially treatable organ failure to die unnecessarily soon from progressive renal failure, or (2) on the grounds of doing what is in the patient's best interest and what the doctor has been contractually engaged to do, he must ask the hospital attorney to seek a court order to continue treatment.

Here we will emphasize Dr. Ashley's obligation both morally and ethically to act on his patient's best interests. We will look at the implementation of the ethics committees, their limitations, and possible risks of coercion, unintended or intended, and the appropriateness or inappropriateness of empowering a body of perhaps less medically knowledgeable people to advocate for the patient.

It is incumbent on physicians operating on advanced lung cancer to have excellent communication skills. They must explain the difficulties anticipated and sometimes dreaded, and the steps that will be taken to correct postoperative complications and actually prepare an explicit, informed consent stipulating postoperative treatments that would or could be interpreted or misinterpreted as heroic, life saving, and possibly misconstrued as futile. Legally, consent may be given orally or in writing. Consent is implied when the patient indicates a willingness to undergo a procedure or treatment by his behavior. For treatments that entail risk or discomfort, it is preferable to obtain explicit written consent. Situations in which the patient voluntarily gives decision-making authority to a physician or third party are exceptions to the requirement for informed consent. This is implied with postoperative complications, and the surgeon is expected to do what is in the patient's best interest. Does the informed consent supersede the advance directive? After thoracic procedures, the consent generally includes management of perioperative complications, such as bleeding that requires emergency surgery. [...]

EDUCATION AND COMMUNICATION

The patient's wife has limited medical knowledge at best; the ethics committee in a perfect world would have profound understanding of the postoperative care available and be able to articulate and convince the patient's wife that the surgeon's recommendation is appropriate and in the patient's best interest. Too often, ethics committees are empowered to sign off on care or assume that they need to consider allocation of finite institutional resources and miss the conflict that the patient is being used as a means to the family's or hospital's ends.

A discussion on withholding and withdrawing life-sustaining therapy and the surrogate's role and commitment to supporting the patient's rights and best interests is detailed in the official statement of The American Thoracic Society adopted by their board of directors in March 1991. It supports the decision "to continue life-sustaining treatment when the patient no longer has decision-making capacity, based on the knowledge of the patient's preferences, values, and goals, and their commitment to supporting the patient's rights and best interests."[9] The surrogate should make the same decisions about the patient's care as the patient would have made if capable of doing so, concerning the use of life-sustaining therapy [. . .]. [The policy] goes on to detail circumstances when a surrogate can't make a decision, and it outlines a reasonable process for a patient's physician and other healthcare providers to make decisions for the patient based on what is determined to be "in the patient's best interest." This process should be as reasonable and objective as possible, weighing the benefits for starting or continuing a certain life-sustaining therapy against its burdens on the patient. If the benefits of the therapy exceed the burden, the therapy should be administered. [. . .]

FUTILE CARE

The word "futile" is derived from Latin roots meaning, "that which easily pours out, is ineffective, or useless." It is also defined as frivolous or lacking serious purpose, and implies a decision about outcome probability that we do not have, ignoring the wide range of treatments for a given diagnosis.[10] The ethical principles of beneficence and nonmaleficence underlie and define treatment goals, so the purpose of a life-sustaining intervention should be restoration or maintenance of a patient's well being, not mere prolongation of biological life. On this basis, a life-sustaining intervention may be withheld or withdrawn from a patient without the consent of the patient or surrogate if the intervention is judged by the physician to be futile. A life-sustaining intervention is considered futile if reasoning and experience indicate that the intervention would be highly unlikely to result in meaningful survival for that patient.[11] Here, meaningful survival specifically refers to a quality and duration of survival that would have value to that patient as an individual. [. . .]

Predictive models such as the APACHE III systems are useful in large populations, but they are not intended to predict an individual's risk of death. There are no precise measurements to predict an individual's outcome with comparable precision. Physician experience and intuition often serve the patient's best interest.[12]

CONCLUSION

If the patient's wife cannot be convinced by a step-by-step plan for appropriate life-supporting measures intended to improve the patient's outcome, it is incumbent on Dr. Ashley to seek a court order to continue treatment. This would not have been necessary if the doctor had adopted our current practice in which we discuss suspending specific aspects of any existing advance directive for a defined period of time during the preoperative informed consent conversation with the patient and those closest to him. Then we record the joint decision in the medical record.

The patient and physician and the physician and family relationships are most likely to be optimal with excellent communication from the outset with compassionate conversations, acknowledgment of an advance directive, agreement to suspend it for a specified time, and education about the meaning of specific scenarios in the context of postoperative complications and their management. [...] Working well together would hopefully eliminate the need for judicial involvement to achieve what everyone's goal should be (i.e., serving the patient's best interest).

Concluding Remarks
Robert M. Sade, MD

D'Amico and Krasna and Krasna provide an illuminating discussion, presenting discordant perspectives on this difficult problem. Two issues lie at the core of the quandary facing Dr. Ashley: (1) the distinction between the substituted judgment and best interest standards when making decisions for incapacitated patients and (2) the extent of decision-making authority of proxies (i.e., agents appointed by the patient) and surrogates (i.e., agents designated by law or the judicial system).

THE STANDARD FOR SURROGATE DECISION MAKING

Most state law and most commentators on medical ethics prioritize substituted judgment over best interest. This priority of the substituted judgment standard is plainly stated in Maryland law (where Dr. Krasna practices):

> Any person authorized to make health care decisions for another under this section shall base those decisions on the wishes of the patient, and if the wishes of the patient are unknown or unclear, on the patient's best interest.[13] The ethical distinction between substituted judgment and best interest is clearly described and the priority of substituted judgment is supported by the American Medical Association's Code of Medical Ethics [...].[14]

Both discussants fail to identify this distinction. D'Amico does not mention the best interest standard at all, even though circumstances in this case arguably might justify application of this standard. Krasna and Krasna state or imply that the surgeon's primary concern must be the patient's best interest (in a narrowly construed medical sense), but that position is contrary to both law and widely accepted medical ethics.

PROXY OR SURROGATE AUTHORITY TO MAKE DECISIONS

The authority vested in proxies and surrogates, according to both ethics and law, to make decisions on behalf of patients is stated clearly in the American

Medical Association Code: "Physicians should recognize the proxy or surrogate as an extension of the patient, entitled to the same respect as the competent patient." Those who would override a surrogate's decision should ask themselves whether they would come to the same conclusion if the patient had made the same decision. [...]

In both ethics and law, surrogate decision makers have essentially the same authority as the patient would have, if capable. Therefore, the central dilemma in this case is not whether the family believes that withholding dialysis represents the patient's wishes, as D'Amico believes, nor whether providing dialysis is in the patient's best interest, as Krasna and Krasna assert. The critical question is the validity of the patient's wife's decision and belief that her husband's oral directive included the withholding of dialysis (i.e., whether her decision truly reflects the choice that her husband would have made if he were capable of making this decision). No evidence suggests that the patient's wife has ulterior motives in her decision-making or that she is primarily serving her own interests rather than those of her husband; she is, for all intents and purposes, a competent, trustworthy surrogate decision maker.

In the end, we find that we cannot tell Dr. Ashley what is the right thing for him to do, because he failed to give his colleagues, Drs. D'Amico and Krasna, a critical piece of information. The patient's wife judges that her husband would have considered dialysis "heroic" and would not want to continue treatment. To resolve the question of the right thing to do, Dr. Ashley must first put aside his personal beliefs about the meaning of "heroic," about what course is medically indicated, and about the desirability of the quantity and quality of life in case of survival. Then he must decide, after weighing all the information at his disposal, whether the patient's wife has correctly judged that her husband would have refused dialysis. If the preponderance of evidence indicates that her judgment is accurate, the surgeon is ethically bound to honor her substituted judgment and withhold dialysis. If the evidence indicates that her judgment is mistaken, he is justified in seeking a court order to continue treatment and initiate dialysis.

At the end of the road, when all avenues for agreement have been explored and disagreement persists, the decisive factor is what the patient chooses. When the patient is incapable of choosing at the time of decision, the proxy or surrogate's choice is decisive *if* it accurately reflects what the patient would have wanted. Fortunately, we do not often have to disentangle the skein that lies beneath that "if."

References

1. Reynolds SR, Cooper AB, McKneally M. Withdrawing life-sustaining treatment: ethical considerations. *Thorac Surg Clin.* 2005;15:469–80.

2. Burns JP, Truog RD. Futility: a concept in evolution. *Chest.* 2007;132:1987–93.

3. Way J, Back AL, Curtis JR. Withdrawing life support and resolution of conflict with families. *BMJ.* 2002;325:1342–5.

4. Lautrette A, Darmon M, Megarbane B, Joly LM, et al. A communication strategy and brochure for relatives of patients dying in the ICU. *N Engl J Med.* 2007;356:469–78.

5. Tulsky JA. Beyond advance directives: importance of communication skills at the end of life. *JAMA.* 2005;294:359–65.

6. Truog RD, Mitchell C. Futility: from hospital policies to state laws. *Am J Bioeth.* 2006;6:19–21.

7. Fine RL, Mayo TW. Resolution of futility by due process: early experience with the Texas advance directives. *Ann Intern Med.* 2003;138:743–6.

8. Cotler MP, Gregory DR. Futility: is definition the problem? Part I. *Camb Q Healthc Ethics.* 1993;2:219–24.

9. American Thoracic Society. Withholding and withdrawing life-sustaining therapy. *Am Rev Respir Dis.* 1991;144:726–31.

10. Truog RD. Tackling medical futility in Texas. *N Engl J Med.* 2007;357: 1–3.

11. World Medical Association Declaration on the Rights of the Patient, revised at the 171st Council Session, Santiago, Chile, October 2005: http://www.wma.net/e/policy/14.htm.

12. Knaus WA, Wagner DP, Draper EA, et al. The APACHE III prognostic system: risk prediction of hospital mortality for critically ill hospitalized adults. *Chest.* 1991;100:1619–36.

13. Code of Maryland. Health–General, Title 5, Subtitle 6. Section 5-605 (c)(1) http://mlis.state.md.us/asp/web_statutes.asp?ghg&5-605. Accessed June 2, 2008.

14. Council on Ethical and Judicial Affairs. E-8.801 Surrogate decision-making. American Medical Association, Code of Medical Ethics: current opinions with annotations, 2006–2007 ed. Chicago: American Medical Association. http://www.ama-assn.org/apps/pf_new/pf_online?f_n.browse&doc.policy.les/HnE/E-8.081.

11

Should Surgical Errors Always Be Disclosed to the Patient?

Constantine Mavroudis, Constantine D. Mavroudis,
Keith S. Naunheim, and Robert M. Sade*

Introduction
Robert M. Sade, MD

Mistakes made in the care of patients, especially in the hospital setting, have drawn a great deal of attention since the 1999 report of the Institute of Medicine (IOM), To Err is Human: Building a Safer Health System.[1] The IOM famously cited an estimate of 44,000 to 98,000 deaths a year due to medical errors [...]. The highly intense, complex care required by most cardiothoracic surgical patients might logically seem to provide rich substrate for the occurrence of mistakes. They undoubtedly occur, and surgeons, beginning early in the last century, have created a culture of openly admitting and discussing their mistakes during routine morbidity and mortality conferences.

Open discussion of mistakes, however, has been mostly confined to those weekly conferences; full disclosure to patients has not been as universally practiced. Much of the ethics literature suggests that the best way to handle health care errors is to disclose them fully to patients. This policy is advised in the face of rising incidence and award levels of negligence lawsuits against physicians. Does a policy of disclosure make sense? If we follow such a policy, are we taking the high road or the road to self-destruction? Are we being saints or are we being martyrs? [...]

---

*Mavroudis C, Mavroudis CD, Naunheim K, Sade R. Should surgical errors always be disclosed to the patient? *Ann Thorac Surg.* 2005;80(2):399–408. Copyright Society of Thoracic Surgeons, republished here with permission.

To focus the discussion, a case was presented in which a surgical error was committed under circumstances that allowed the surgeon the opportunity safely to conceal it.

CASE

Mr. Sirius Lunger is 51 years old and has a history of smoking (80 pack-years), emphysema, and recent onset of hemoptysis. He is found to have a mass in his right upper lobe, and Dr Waffle, a thoracic surgeon, does a bronchoscopy, which reveals a mass in the right upper lobe bronchus. The biopsy demonstrates squamous cell carcinoma. Doctor Waffle schedules Mr. Lunger to undergo right upper lobectomy, but tells the patient and his family (wife and three teenage children) that he may need to remove more than just the lower lobe, which he will decide when he visually inspects the cancer.

During the operation, Dr Waffle, assisted by an operating room nurse, identifies the pulmonary vessels in the hilum, then ligates and divides the anterior trunk to the upper lobe and a second upper lobe branch. As he completes the dissection and is preparing to ligate the pulmonary veins, he realizes that he has inadvertently ligated and divided both the anterior trunk and the ongoing pulmonary artery in the fissure; he has no other choice than to remove the right lung, despite the risks entailed by the patient's chronic lung disease. He completes the dissection of the right pulmonary veins, ligates them, and finally dissects, divides, and oversews the right mainstem bronchus, completing a right pneumonectomy.

Postoperatively, Dr Waffle is uncertain what to tell the patient and his family. He believes that openness and full disclosure is generally the right thing to do, and that, if Mr. Lunger does not do well, a lawsuit is less likely if he tells the whole story. He realizes, however, that he has already mentioned to the patient and his family the possibility of a more extensive operation than lobectomy, and he was the only one in the operating room who knew of the misplaced ligature. He also believes that if disclosure of his mistake leads to lengthy malpractice litigation, which is a distinct possibility, it would be a major distraction from his practice and very bad publicity for himself, his partners, and his hospital. A jury would be likely to have great sympathy for Mr. Lunger's young family, and this could well lead to an unjustified, emotionally based adverse verdict and financial ruin for his own family. Doctor Waffle tells the patient and the family that the more extensive resection was required, and does not mention inadvertent arterial ligation.

Because of the chronic lung disease in the remaining lung, Mr. Lunger cannot be removed from ventilator support, and ten days later, he develops antibiotic-resistant pneumonia. Three days later, still on the ventilator, he dies of respiratory insufficiency. Doctor Waffle, as is his usual practice, expresses his sympathy to the family, sends a note of condolence, and attends the funeral, all of which is much appreciated by the family.

Should Dr Waffle have disclosed his technical error?

Pro
Constantine Mavroudis, MD, and Constantine D. Mavroudis

Truth telling in medicine, as in the case in question, isn't always as straightforward as it sounds. Disclosing an error to a patient is never easy and may have important adverse consequences for the doctor. It is not enough to simply state "that truth is always the best policy"; it is important to explore why this might be so.

So, what did Dr Waffle actually do? He performed a comprehensive diagnostic assessment of Mr. Lunger. He conducted an informed consent interview with Mr. Lunger and his family, which included the possibility that he might have to perform a pneumonectomy if it were found that the tumor spread to adjacent parts of the lung. During the operation, Dr Waffle experienced unknown circumstances that led to errors in judgment-technique. This resulted in an unwanted pneumonectomy instead of the planned lobectomy. Mr. Lunger died from pulmonary insufficiency, which may or may not have been prevented, regardless of the extent of pulmonary resection.

What happened to Dr Waffle, who is a board-certified thoracic surgeon with excellent credentials? A root-cause analysis would have to consider the following questions. Were there anatomic anomalies such as distortion of the pulmonary artery due to the tumor that could have been overlooked or unappreciated? Was an informed assistant (senior resident or colleague) in the room during the operation? Were there environmental distractions that were not controlled (eg, loud talking, music playing, excess operating room traffic)? Did Dr Waffle suffer a lapse in concentration due to some psychological or organic reason? The fact still remains that whatever the possible personal or system causes, the complication occurred.

If Dr Waffle (1) decides not to disclose the incident to the patient and family, (2) chooses to hide the incident from his colleagues, and (3) succeeds in his deception, he will have only to deal with his conscience [...]. If, on the other hand, Dr Waffle decides to disclose all the facts to the patient and family and offers an apology, he still faces the reality of a litigious society with unjust laws that treats medical errors in a tort system where there is a milieu of punishment and financial devastation. There is, therefore, significant conflict between ethical considerations (do the right thing) and self-preservation (protect one's self).

HISTORICAL PHILOSOPHICAL CONSIDERATIONS

Aristotle did not live in a time of medical litigation and we can only speculate what his thoughts would be concerning this modern day societal problem. His Nicomachean Ethics were based on the moral virtues of courage, temperance, prudence, and justice.[2] [...] Aristotle would argue that Dr Waffle and Mr. Lunger entered into an agreement, based on the moral virtue of justice. Doctor Waffle would treat Mr. Lunger in the same manner that he would want to be treated had he, in fact, been the patient. It would follow that Dr Waffle would be duty bound to disclose the truth in all aspects of care with Mr. Lunger based on this situation.

One would assume that Plato would agree with this scenario, except that Plato suggested that lying in certain circumstances is not immoral.[3] For instance, lying or intentional deception to one's enemy would not be immoral. Furthermore, intentional deception, when done in the patient's best interests, is considered by him to be morally justified. [...]

Kant's moral theory is considered by some to be the foundation of modern bioethics.[4] His basic tenet is the primacy of autonomy and dignity of the individual ("the principle of humanity"). For Kant, morality can exist only by virtue of our autonomy as rational beings. The moral worth of an action is not related to the beneficial outcome that it may bring, but whether it is done from a sense of duty or obligation. Kant's moral law or "categorical imperative" states, "Act only on that maxim through which you can, at the same time, will that it should become a universal law of values." Every act has to stand on its moral virtue and be judged as if it were to become a universal law of nature. Kant could not condone lying for any reason because to do so violates the principle of the "categorical imperative." [...]

The English school of Utilitarianism based its moral theory on the "utility" or outcome of an act rather than its motive. To act morally was to act in such a way that the amount of benefit or pleasure achieved was maximized and the harm or "pain" minimized—the "greatest good for the greatest number." [...]

At first sight, it may be hard to imagine that much pleasure will be achieved by Dr Waffle telling his patient that he has made a serious error. However, consideration of Dr Waffle's pain takes a far too narrow view of Utilitarianism, which is a doctrine not of personal expediency but a consideration of the greater societal good. [...]

MODERN TRENDS

[...] So what should Dr Waffle do? The proper course of action for this ill-fated surgeon is to do the following: (1) disclose the entire incident as it occurred in a straight-forward fashion, indicating that it was an error, (2) try to give the best explanation possible as to why this happened, (3) tell the family what steps that he is taking to prevent such an occurrence from happening again, and (4) apologize. This line of thinking has been reported by multiple authors recently and has been supported by classic ethical thought.

Mazor and associates conducted a questionnaire survey, involving 1,500 members of a New England-based health maintenance organization, which yielded a 66% response rate.[5] [...] The results showed that full disclosure yielded better patient satisfaction, an enhanced trust between patient and physician, and a positive emotional response. [...]

Osmon and associates studied the reporting of medical errors in an intensive care unit experience.[6] They concluded that medical errors are common among patients in the intensive care unit and that an error can result in the need for additional life-sustaining treatments, which can contribute to patient death. They urged the development of a nonpunitive reporting system, which could maximize the chance for analysis and improved patient care. Krizek reviewed the ethical issues of adverse events and identified five types of medical errors (judgmental, technical, expectations, systems, and mechanical).[7] [...] He urged that we eliminate the culture of blame, insist on truth telling with full disclosure, and use these opportunities to improve all aspects of patient care. [...]

Gallagher and associates tested the patients' and physicians' attitudes on reporting medical errors in focus groups.[8] Both groups had unmet needs following medical error events. Patients wanted full disclosure and an apology. Physicians agreed with disclosure but wanted "to choose their words carefully." Moreover, physicians worried that an apology could create legal liability which, in some states, it can. Krizek states, "delivering truth in an artful fashion does not have to be a lie," by which he meant that he would find the correct words to be kind and thoughtful to his patient while disclosing the medical error. However, this raises the slippery slope argument that truths told in an "artful fashion" could shade into intentional deception.

The distinction between lying and intentional deception is discussed by Jackson [...].[9] Jackson notes, "Doctors and nurses, like everyone else, have a prima facie duty not to lie—but again, like everyone else, they are not duty bound to avoid intentional deception, lying apart; except where it would involve a breach of trust." [...] The "breach of trust" phrase is central to Dr Waffle's dilemma and illustrates the difference between intentional deception to hide an error to fulfill Dr Waffle's interests and intentional deception to hide the diagnosis of a fatal disease where the doctor is presumably trying to serve the patient's interests (however misguidedly) rather than his own. It would appear that even in Jackson's approach, Dr Waffle must disclose the error in a forthright manner in order to avoid violating the breach of trust covenant.

Disclosing a medical error, especially when the physician feels personally responsible, requires a great deal of moral courage. However, as most physicians come to recognize, the practice of medicine itself requires courage, including the courage to honestly face and endure one's mistakes. [...] Surgical training aims to instill in its future practitioners the habit of choosing the right thing to do so good results will be achieved, even under pressure. The right thing includes an acknowledgement of error and a commitment to excellence. To commit an error may be blameworthy; to lie about it is cowardly.

In the end, it is Kantian ethical theory that best supports full disclosure of medical errors in a forthright and clear manner. A physician must respect the patient's dignity and act with beneficence, sympathy, conscience, and without arrogance. He is duty bound to maintain the interests of his patients and his profession over his own. [...] The expected virtues of competence and compassion of the physician, together with the expected virtues of gratitude and compliance of the patient, will energize the process for an Aristotelian just end.[10]

Con
Keith S. Naunheim, MD

My opponent has utilized Kantian philosophy, Aristotelian logic, and Platonean ethics as the foundation for his argument. As intelligent and enlightened as these philosophers were, the principles they espoused do not necessarily provide adequate guidance for the 21st century thoracic surgery practitioner. [...]

First, I think it is important that we make some assumptions regarding this vignette. Those assumptions would include that the practitioner involved, Dr Waffle, was a well-trained and competent thoracic surgeon. Further, I would make the assumption that on the day of the surgery he was unimpaired by drugs or alcohol. Finally, it seems appropriate to believe that the resulting injury was entirely unintentional and that the surgeon did the very best job he could on that given day. If these assumptions are agreed upon then I feel strongly that nondisclosure is an acceptable and preferable option.

There is an underlying ethical paradox in the practice of medicine in the 21st century. Despite the fact that medical mistakes are inevitable, the standard for medical practice has evolved to the point at which only perfection is acceptable. This appears to be the opinion of the lay press as well as politicians and the population at large. It is also true that this belief is inculcated into physicians and surgeons throughout their medical school and residency. During training, we are taught that human life is sacred and nothing less than perfection is acceptable when performing diagnosis and treatment. This goal, while laudable, is entirely unrealistic and ignores the preponderance of literature that demonstrates that human error is a fact of life.

The "science" of human error, which has been extensively studied within business and industry, is not taught during medical training. Rather, students of medicine have been led to believe that error is avoidable and thus any mistake is "wrong." Commonly, errors are treated as a failure of character. Perhaps the best example of this may be the morbidity and mortality conferences attended by most thoracic surgeons during their training. The overwhelming attitude was "how can there be an error without negligence?" By endorsing this attitude, we have become our own worst enemies. Mistakes in medical care are inevitable and this is now becoming widely recognized. [...]

One of the most important things to determine in this patient's scenario is the assignation of "blame." One question that must certainly be asked is whether the operative actions and the resulting mortality were indeed a cause and effect? During training, surgeons are taught that they are responsible for everything that happens to a patient and it logically follows that the surgeon will be responsible for any errors or bad results that occur. While the logic appears sound the conclusion is absurd. Surgeons do not have the power to control all outcomes. In the present case, the patient had serious underlying chronic obstructive pulmonary disease. Such patients are at an increased risk for postoperative pneumonia and ventilator dependence, as occurred in this patient. Although the performance of a pneumonectomy in lieu of a lobectomy may have increased the risk of respiratory insufficiency and pneumonia, it is impossible to determine that those complications would not have arisen even in the face of a simple lobectomy.

Surgery is a risky business and during the process of informed consent Dr. Waffle certainly communicated that to the patient and his family. The patient accepted the risk for potential complications, including harm, which might come due to a difficult or problematic dissection as occurred. [...]

There are many ethical theories that might be applied to this particular clinical situation including Aristotelian ethics, ethical egoism, ethical relativism, deontology, and utilitarianism among others. The vast majority of thoracic surgeons are not experts in the ethical realm but most, I believe, can easily grasp the theory of consequentialism. [...] Consequentialism suggests that one ought to do that act which realizes the best overall net consequences when one considers both the harm and the benefit to all those involved.

In the scenario outlined, one must therefore consider the harm and the benefit to the patient and his family. In addition, however, it is appropriate to consider the harm and potential benefit to the surgeon. The decision that is made regarding disclosure should be the best one with regard to the overall net consequences to both the patient and his family as well as to the physician. It is often suggested that benefits and harms to the patient may carry greater weight than those to the physician.

Thus, reasons to disclose the intraoperative misstep would include any significant benefit to the patient and his family as well as any benefit to the doctor that comes secondary to disclosure. Reasons not to disclose would be those things that cause patient or family harm as well as harm to the surgeon involved.

Theoretically, in many clinical situations acknowledging or disclosing such a mistake may benefit patients in several ways. [. . .] [T]he only "patient benefit" or goal that might be fulfilled is the potential for "fair" compensation via litigation. Somehow the words "fair" and "litigation" just don't seem to belong in the same sentence in the 21st century medicolegal world.

There are yet other reasons that could potentially support the decision to disclose. These would be classified as "doctor benefit" and would include the fact that acknowledging a mistake may benefit the doctor in some situations. [. . .] It has been suggested that disclosure can potentially decrease the chance of a lawsuit. [. . .] There is but a single study that suggests disclosure may decrease the risk of a lawsuit but other literature and common sense suggest otherwise.[11]

[. . .] Witman and associates performed a survey of patient attitude towards medical mistakes in the outpatient setting.[12] [. . .] Based on their findings, the arguments that disclosure can help avoid legal action seems naively optimistic and the likelihood of lawsuit avoidance highly improbable.

[. . .] In consequentialism, one must also consider the reasons why the physician should not disclose the error. The rationale for this approach would include issues of "patients/family harm" and "physician harm." In general, acknowledging mistakes could potentially harm patients in a couple of ways. First, it might inhibit present or future patient/doctor relationships or patient family relationships. Secondly, it could incite greater anger or emotional distress in a patient who has been harmed or in the family of a patient who has been harmed. Of these two, only the latter would possibly come into play. The present and/or future patient/doctor relationship, as has been stated above, has no real role since the patient has expired and the relationship has disappeared. However, there is certainly a chance that there could be greater anger, anxiety, and emotional distress on the part of the family if they were informed that surgical error may or may not have played a role in the death of their loved one.

"Physician harm" must also be considered in consequentialism when considering reasons not to disclose. The doctor could be harmed by inducing anxiety and severe emotional distress during and after disclosure. In addition, he runs the potential for the loss of respect, patient referrals, hospital privileges, and perhaps even contracts. Thus, there is a significant potential economic loss and almost certitude with regard to an increase in malpractice premiums. None of these potential harms to the doctor is obviated by the death of the patient and thus these must be considered when one thinks of valid reasons not to disclose. [. . .]

In summary, the issue can be looked at from a number of perspectives. From the medical perspective, no matter what the surgeon chooses to do, the patient will not "undie." One cannot help the expired patient and there is no medical reason to disclose. From an emotional standpoint, the family will not grieve "better" and the surgeon is not likely to find a great deal of consolation following an act of contrition. The patient/doctor relationship, cited often as a reason to disclose, really does not come into play as the patient has expired. With regard to physician guilt, it is unlikely that unburdening one's soul in and of itself would be beneficial. [...] Finally, it gets down, as it often does, to a question of money. Most surgeons I know would be happy if appropriate compensation could be provided to patients and/or their families without resorting to the legal system. The current tort system is adversarial in nature and it has been demonstrated that monetary awards really bear little correlation to the damage done. Looking to the current medical tort system for economic justice would be like asking a used car dealer for "fair price." [...]

Like all physicians, we strive to provide fair and ethical treatment for all patients. But fairness and ethics should be a two-way street. Over the last decade, American medicine has been assaulted from many directions. Not only has society as a whole not stepped up to defend our profession, rather they are instigating and driving many of the negative changes. [...] The Platonean idea of virtue was meant to apply to the entire society, not just individuals. Requiring surgeons to be more virtuous than society as a whole, while idealistic, is neither fair nor reasonable.

In the above clinical scenario, the surgeon has no duty to disclose the intraoperative occurrences. The patient had a significant underlying disease and may very well have died no matter what occurred at the time of surgery. Disclosure would provide no significant good or benefit other than subjecting the surgeon to the likelihood of a bitter contentious and ultimately unfair malpractice suit. A disclosure would serve no real principle of justice or fairness. Just because one is a virtuous physician does not mean one must become a martyr.

Concluding Remarks
Robert M. Sade, MD

In analyzing Dr. Waffle's error in the operating room, Mavroudis reviews a range of philosophical ethical systems, from the ancient era, through the Enlightenment, to contemporary times. By combining Aristotelian teleological and Kantian deontological approaches, he reaches the conclusion that Dr. Waffle should disclose everything about the error to the patient and the patient's family. Naunheim utilizes a different philosophic system, consequentialism, to reach the opposite conclusion: Dr. Waffle should keep the potentially damaging information to himself. Naunheim reaches this conclusion after weighing the benefits and harms (pleasure and pain to a Utilitarian) that will occur to both the patient and the surgeon, depending on disclosure or nondisclosure.

While ethicists have relied on a wide range of philosophic reasoning in constructing ethical systems, the codes of behavior used by physicians for centuries have been based on certain principles that have found broad support within the medical profession. The most fundamental principle, found in virtually every contemporary code, is essentially this: "A physician shall, while caring for a patient, regard responsibility to the patient as paramount."[13] All surgeons accept this principle and are guided by it every day. Yet, while the patient's best interests are the most important considerations, they are not the only ones. Physicians also have obligations to others: family, colleagues, hospitals, and wider communities. Physicians are not required to place themselves in harm's way to such an extent that their ability to continue to care for current and future patients is seriously jeopardized or their personal lives are gravely threatened. [...]

It is important for physicians, when faced with great uncertainty in threatening situations, to avoid acting on emotional reactions, such as anger toward society for failing to protect physicians adequately, outrage at trial attorneys for making life miserable for unfortunate physicians who come within their sights, or fear of patients who present real or apparent threats. Physicians faced with threatening situations should be guided by cool reason grounded in the principles of medical ethics. This means that they should give great weight to patients' interests, allowing their own interests to override those of their patients only when the threat of harm is grave and the jeopardy it imposes is serious.

Making the right decision requires that physicians assess as accurately and objectively as possible the real threat to their own interests and to their ability to care for patients in the future. Availability of more complete data that document actual risks to physicians arising from full disclosure of surgical errors to patients will help us to make better-informed decisions. Our deliberations should also include objective assessment of personal observations and experiences in similar situations.

Various philosophical traditions, as presented by our debaters, have not produced a definitive answer to the question of how Dr. Waffle should respond to his dilemma. In all probability, there is no single answer that would apply to all physicians in all situations. Broadly accepted principles of medical ethics can provide a helpful guideline; however, when deliberating on the many factors to be considered, the heaviest weight should be placed on doing what is best for the patient—in this case, disclosure of the facts and the trust such openness generates. At the end of the day, however, we must rely on judgments based on dispassionate interpretation of the inconclusive data that are available, in the context of personal observations, to determine just how much Dr. Waffle—and we, when our times come—should tell the patient.

References

1. Institute of Medicine. *To Err is Human: Building a Safer Health System.* Washington, DC: National Academy Press; 2000.
2. Aristotle. *The Nichomachean Ethics,* Book III. Ross, D (trans). London: Oxford University Press; 1954.
3. Plato. *Republic,* II:382. Jowett, B (trans). In: *The Dialogues of Plato,* Vol. 1. New York: Random House; 1937.
4. Bernstein M, Brown B. Doctors' duty to disclose error: a deontological or Kantian ethical analysis. *Can J Neurol Sci.* 2004;31:169–74.
5. Mazor KM, Simon SR, Yood RA, et al. Health plan members' views about disclosure of medical errors. *Ann Intern Med.* 2004;140:409–18.
6. Osmon S, Harris CB, Dunagan WC, Prentice D, Fraser VJ, Kollef MH. Reporting of medical errors: an intensive care unit experience. *Crit Care Med.* 2004;32:727–33.
7. Krizek TJ. Surgical error: ethical issues of adverse events. *Arch Surg.* 2000;135:1359–66.
8. Gallagher TH, Waterman AD, Ebers AG, Fraser VJ, Levinson W. Patients' and physicians' attitudes regarding the disclosure of medical errors. *JAMA.* 2003; 289:1001–7.
9. Jackson J. Telling the truth. *J Med Ethics.* 1991;17:5–9.
10. Mavroudis C. Presidential address: a partnership in courage. *Ann Thorac Surg.* 2003;75:1366–71.
11. Kachalia A, Shojania KG, Hofer TP, et al. Does full disclosure of medical errors affect malpractice liability? The jury is still out. *Jt Comm J Qual Saf.* 2003;29:503–11.
12. Witman AB, Park DM, Hardin SB. How do patients want physicians to handle mistakes? *Arch Intern Med.* 1996;156: 2565–9.
13. Council on Ethical and Judicial Affairs. Code of Medical Ethics: current opinions with annotations, 2004–2005 ed. Chicago: American Medical Association; 2004:xiv.

12

Another Surgeon's Error

MUST YOU TELL THE PATIENT?

Susan D. Moffatt-Bruce, Chadrick E. Denlinger, and Robert M. Sade*

Introduction

Robert M. Sade, MD

The question of whether physicians should report medical errors to patients and their families has been the subject of much commentary ever since the 1999 report of the Institute of Medicine, To Err is Human: Building a Safer Health System, which brought the problem of hospital deaths due to medical errors to public attention.[1] A general consensus has been reached among bioethicists and within the medical profession: physicians have an ethical obligation to patients to disclose errors made during their health care. Much less clear is a closely related but quite different problem: is a physician obligated to disclose errors made by others when those others will not personally disclose them? [. . .]

THE CASE OF THE MISSING BIOPSY

A 72-year-old man is referred to Dr. Paul Jones with the new diagnosis of bronchopleural fistula. He under went right pneumonectomy 10 days previously, performed by Dr. John Lapps, a cardiothoracic surgeon in another part of the state, after having under gone induction chemoradiation therapy for stage IIIA non-small cell lung cancer, clinically staged. This procedure

* Moffatt-Bruce S, Denlinger C, Sade RM. Another surgeon's error: must you tell the patient? *Ann Thorac Surg.* 2014;98(2):396–401. Copyright Society of Thoracic Surgeons, republished here with permission.

was complicated by hemorrhage. The final pathology report disclosed multi-station mediastinal lymph node disease.

A review of the operative note reveals that no frozen sections were sent. Dr. Jones is surprised that Dr. Lapps did not obtain a biopsy specimen of the mediastinal lymph nodes by a less invasive procedure than thoracotomy, or at least after thoracotomy but before pneumonectomy. If the patient had been his originally, he, like most thoracic surgeons, would have biopsied the nodes, and the patient would not have undergone pneumonectomy. Dr. Jones intends to describe to the patient and his family what he believes needs to be done now. Before he talks with the patient and his family, however, he contacts Dr. Lapps, describes the error Dr. Lapps made in not obtaining a lymph node biopsy specimen, and encourages him to report this to the patient. Worried about a possible lawsuit, Dr. Lapps refuses to do so. Dr. Jones will answer honestly any questions the patient and his family might ask, but wonders if he should tell them about Dr. Lapps' omission.

Pro
Susan D. Moffatt-Bruce, MD, PhD

Dr. Jones must tell the patient and his family about Dr. Lapps' omission. Several ethical principles support this stance. Before taking a pro or con stance, however, a preface must be made. This is a very challenging and perhaps not unfamiliar scenario. With patient care becoming more complex and care teams being more diverse, this is likely to become a sadly familiar situation. Having said that, I will outline ethical principles, as well as expand on, what the benefits are in dispelling myths about care that may not be true and unveiling the reality of the clinical scenario presented here: Dr. Lapps' omission likely did not meet the standard of care. Lastly, I will review what tactics and teaching must be part of the surgeon's armamentarium to properly care for the patient and render this a very professional disclosure.

The ethical principles that support Dr. Jones telling the patient and his family that Dr. Lapps should have biopsied the mediastinal lymph nodes, thereby obviating the need for a pneumonectomy, include (1) the surgeon's professional obligation; (2) the surgeon's integrity; (3) the patient's right to informed care and to be fully engaged in his care; and (4) the patient's right to informed consent regarding further care he will require.

The American Medical Association Code of Medical Ethics helps render clarity to the surgeon's professional obligation to tell the family that Dr. Lapps has made an error in judgment in completing the pneumonectomy. The Code states, "Situations occasionally occur in which a patient experiences significant medical complications that may have resulted from the physician's mistake or judgment. In these situations, the physician is ethically required to inform the patient of all the facts necessary to ensure understanding of what has occurred."[2]

Furthermore, the American College of Physicians Ethics Manual states "Physicians should disclose to patients information about procedural or judgment errors made during care, as long as such information is material to the patient's well-being. Errors do not necessarily imply negligent or unethical behavior, but failure to disclose them may."[3] This statement leaves no ambiguity that surgeons, and in particular, Dr. Jones, are obligated and it is their professional duty to disclose an error of another surgeon once it has been discovered. Professional self-regulation requires sharing and acting on information collectively and should become our professional norm.

So, the professional codes of conduct under which we should ethically work support the disclosure of Dr. Lapps' error by Dr. Jones. Where does the patient's care and expectations come into this debate? Every patient is entitled to what is truly informed care. That is to say, patients are entitled to honest information. When asked, Dr. Jones must be truthful and answer to the best of his ability about what transpired to render such to the patient under his care. He may choose to not use words like "error" and "mistake" but rather choose more productive and less judgmental words such as "clinical opinion" and "divergence from." If he is not asked, Dr. Jones is still obliged to render an appropriate disclosure as it pertains to the patient's clinical care. Patients and families should not have the burden of trying to discover "what happened" or how it should happen that, in this instance now, the patient is facing additional care by another surgeon.

Financial burden to the patient should be relieved. Often patients and families will need help after such a serious error that is now going to prolong their care, and they will have difficulty accessing compensation without information about what really happened. Family must be kept informed along with the patient about the long-term care plan. The patient had initially consented to 5 to 7 days of hospitalization time, and now his care has likely turned into a prolonged stay. In addition, the patient may have been moved from his local environment and is now in an unfamiliar city with the family incurring additional costs. The patient's needs are very real, and as professionals, we are expected to put the needs of the patient and the family above our own. Honest and expeditious disclosure will serve to move beyond blame to advocacy for the patient.

The patient is entitled to informed consent. This will be a particularly important component of this patient's care because Dr. Lapps' omission has now required further intervention and care by Dr. Jones. For the patient and his family to give informed consent for additional therapy or surgical intervention, they must understand the clinical course thus far. This has the potential to be important for the patient as well as the surgeon and their own relationship, particularly if an additional operation is fraught with the potential for further complications or prolonged care. To be truly informed, a patient has to understand what care rendered to them resulted in the current state of their disease.

Although surgeons may be ethically obligated to disclose errors, pressures from society and the medical profession itself make it very difficult for physicians and surgeons to rush to disclose in a timely and professional manner. In one recent study, only approximately one-third of patients who had some experience with a medical error said that a health professional involved in the incident disclosed the error or apologized.[4]

Most physicians have trained in a culture that supports "shame-and-blame" approaches to medical errors. Shame, fears about blame, and worries about legal liability also play a role in the underreporting of medical errors. Most physicians have trained—and some continue to train—in poor working conditions that include heavy workloads, inadequate supervision, and poor communication. All those factors contribute to medical mistakes, which are often very difficult to take responsibility for. A balance must be found between "non-blame" and appropriate accountability.

In theory, there are many benefits to a timely and appropriate disclosure. There are data [. . .] supporting that good, open, and honest communication improved patient satisfaction and, ultimately, outcomes. Improved surgeon-patient relationships and, ultimately, improved patient and family satisfaction results from open communication and honesty.[5] Although the research suggests that good communication about adverse events may reduce litigation and malpractice payouts, I must concede that data are lacking from studies to indicate how to disclose other's errors while minimizing the risk that a patient will initiate a claim.

There is also the well-being of the surgeon to consider after an error has been made. One study, for example, demonstrated that when house staff could no longer deny or discount a mistake, they were plagued by profound doubts and guilt. For many, "the case was never closed," even when they finished their training.[6] [. . .] Gallagher and colleagues recently published a very timely article in the New England Journal of Medicine whereby the tactics and teaching required to meet the patient's needs were explored in depth.[7] The authors speak to the concept of "explore, do not ignore" when a colleague's possible error has occurred. The clinician's first obligation is to obtain the facts; inaccurate or speculative information is damaging.

Only Dr. Lapps will know exactly what happened during the care or operation. To engage with the surgeon to give him the opportunity to correct assumptions and join the disclosure process is the first step. This should ideally be a very professional surgeon-to-surgeon discussion so that it is productive rather than disruptive. Approaching Dr. Lapps with curiosity rather than accusation will be much better received. The goal is to engage the practitioner to help determine how to disclose an error, if together you decide there has indeed been one, as well as determine if there are others to which the disclosure must be made (i.e., institution, The Joint Commission). In fact, Gallagher and colleagues give us guidance on how best to proceed with the disclosure, in that sometimes additional people should be present, including medical directors or department chairs. If Dr. Lapps were to decline the invitation, then disclosure must proceed, and when asked, Dr Jones is obliged to always tell the truth. [...]

Lastly, coaching and support for the surgeon who has to disclose an error of his own or another needs to be provided. This is never an easy or pleasant process but one that will turn the focus to patient-centered care as opposed to surgeon-centered protection. The earlier we start this training and setting expectations around appropriate accountability, apology, and disclosure the better; medical school is the ideal initial forum.

In conclusion, Dr. Jones is obligated to discuss the potential error with Dr. Lapps, thereby verifying the facts and determining whether an error was made or not. Dr Jones then must provide the surgeon the opportunity to disclose the error to the patient and family and to truly be part of the accountability process. Ultimately, the patient and family must be informed because it is a shared professional responsibility, of all surgeons, to provide transparent disclosure of errors that impact patient outcomes.

Con

Chadrick E. Denlinger, MD

Several recent statements provide guidance related to the disclosure of medical errors by physicians to the patients for whom they have been providing care. It is fair to conclude that a consensus has been reached regarding our ethical duty to inform patients of our own medical errors. In addition to being the ethically acceptable practice, disclosing ones' own errors is critical for preserving trust between patients and physicians.

Arguments supporting nondisclosure because of concerns for provoking anxiety or confusion have largely been discredited. Therefore, most agree that medical errors should be disclosed to the patient by the physicians involved as soon as reasonably possible given their overall medical situation.

The situation of Dr. Jones disclosing an error involving Dr. Lapps, who practices at a different institution, is significantly different. Encountering medical errors involving other physicians is extremely common. In fact, a recent survey of practicing clinicians found that more than two-thirds of physicians had encountered a peer's medical error within the prior 6 months, although 90% of them had received little or no prior training on how to manage this situation.[8] Given the frequency in which analogous situations occur, it is instructive to think of our own situations and ask ourselves "how did

I respond?" rather than to ask hypothetically "how would I respond?" As we reflect on prior situations, we should realize that our prior actions were guided by our own ethical code and sense of justice.

Several years ago, I accepted a patient from another hospital and I quickly realized that the patient had, in my opinion, been mismanaged at the previous institution. As I treated the patient, I focused on the current situation and what treatments were necessary. We did not discuss the prior care at another hospital. Eventually the patient recovered and returned to a normal lifestyle, but this only came after an initial prolonged hospitalization and numerous subsequent admissions for minor procedures and a few significant operations. Over the course of the following year, the patient and family began asking questions related to my opinion of what had occurred at the prior hospital and I answered openly and honestly.

In preparation for the discussion involving Drs. Jones and Lapps, I conducted my own survey of 20 different colleagues scattered throughout the United States as well as several individuals at my own institution. Those surveyed were provided a succinct review of the case and were asked, "should I have discussed with the patient regarding the previous care?" Those surveyed were asked that in addition to treating the patients, should I have:

A. told the family that I agreed with the prior management;
B. offered no opinion regarding the prior management, but answer honestly if asked; or,
C. proactively told the family that I thought the prior management was inappropriate.

Everyone surveyed responded that that I should have answered questions honestly when asked, but that I should not have proactively informed the patient or family that the prior management was inappropriate.

The topic of disclosing medical errors involving a different physician has recently been addressed in other publications. The authors acknowledge that existing guidelines emphasize the importance of disclosing errors pertaining to our own practice, but they offer little guidance on disclosing mistakes involving others. This lack of guidance heightens the clinician's uncertainty about what to do.[7] There are three primary challenges with disclosing another's mistakes. Most importantly, it is often difficult to determine exactly what happened when a physician was not directly involved in the event in question.

Second, it is difficult to understand what conversations occurred between the physician(s) involved and the patient regarding the risks and benefits of various treatment options. Furthermore, there is likely some uncertainty regarding the degree of patient involvement in selecting a given treatment pathway.

Finally, opinions differ about what constitutes a medical error. Potential errors exist on a spectrum ranging from "not what I would have done" but within the standard of care to blatant errors suggesting medical incompetence. These three issues contribute the lack of clarity of the appropriate response when we encounter a peer's medical error.

Several examples in the literature illustrate the difficulty with determining what defines a medical error. In 1991, the Harvard Medical Practice Study investigated the number of adverse outcomes and deaths that occurred as the result of negligent medical errors.[9] For the purposes of that study, more than 30,000 medical records from New York state were randomly selected and screened by nurses to identify patients with adverse outcomes. The screeners identified nearly 8,000 patient records as showing evidence of adverse outcomes.

Two physicians then independently reviewed each of these records. The vast majority of the reviewers were board-certified surgeons or board-certified internists. Each reviewer received specific training for the purpose of the study to educate him or her about what constituted an adverse outcome and what constituted medical negligence. The inter observer reliability of identifying adverse outcomes was good, with a k value of 0.61. Conversely, the physicians' opinions regarding negligence were far less reliable, with a k value of only 0.24.

The authors acknowledge that judgments regarding the causes of adverse outcomes or negligent care are difficult and sometimes inaccurate. The fact that physicians had difficulty determining whether or not a standard of care had been met was really not surprising given the complexity of medical care. A second similar study involved pairs of anesthesiologists independently reviewing the appropriateness of care in more than 100 actual malpractice claims.[10] The 2 reviewers agreed on the appropriateness of care in 62% of the cases. Each reviewer thought the care was appropriate in 27%, and they both thought the care was inappropriate in 32%. Interestingly, the 2 reviewers disagreed on whether or not the care was appropriate in 38% of cases (k = 0.37).

These two studies highlight the fact that physician medical record reviewers who receive specific training that prepares them to properly identify negligent or inappropriate care have a substantial degree of disagreement. If this is true, it is unacceptable for each of us to assume that we are capable of correctly judging the appropriateness of care provided by other previously treating physicians and to inform patients of our opinion.

Given the degree of disagreement between expert reviewers, consideration should be given to when the disclosures should end. In the current case, if Dr. Jones informs the patient that Dr. Lapps has provided negligent care, what are the ethical responsibilities of subsequent physicians taking care of the patient? Almost certainly, the patient will be transferred to an intensive care unit where care will be provided, in part, by intensivists. If one adopts the policy that we are all responsible to disclose medical errors involving other physicians, then we should also be responsible to share our opinion regarding reviews of care rendered other physicians. Therefore, the intensivist would be responsible to inform the patient of his or her opinion of Dr. Lapps' care and would also be responsible for providing an opinion about the appropriateness of comments made to the family by Dr. Jones regarding Dr. Lapps' care. This scenario would continue when the patient leaves the hospital and the primary physician involved in his care is the primary care physician.

Physicians have strong opinions about how they would like their colleagues to disclose information when their own care is thought to be negligent. A recent survey presented physicians with clinical vignettes where adverse outcomes occurred.[8] [...] Regardless of the severity of the outcome, approximately two-thirds of all respondents indicated that they would report their opinion to the original physician rather than report their opinion to the patient when they were the one observing the error. However, when the respondent was the physician responsible for the error, 93% of the respondents expected their peers to report the error to them.

When encountering medical errors involving other physicians, the most appropriate response is to speak directly with those involved. This may clarify the rationale behind decisions that were made and will expound the discussion that occurred with the patient before rendering treatment. After this discussion, the 2 physicians may agree that no Harmful error had occurred and therefore nothing needs to be disclosed. Alternatively, the physicians may agree that there was an error and they agree upon who should disclose the error to the patient and when this should occur. A third scenario is that the 2 physicians disagree either on whether an error occurred or they disagree on how the information should be disclosed to the patient. Under these circumstances, institutional guidance should be sought given the frequent disagreements even among expert reviewers related to the appropriateness of previous care.

In conclusion, Dr. Jones should not tell the patient that he believes Dr. Lapps made a medical error for several reasons: Medical errors involving other physicians must be first discussed with the physicians involved to fully understand the decisions that were made. Second, there is frequent lack of agreement regarding the appropriateness of care Previously provided. Entangling a patient and their family in the midst of differing medical opinions would likely increase their anxiety beyond the stress already felt because of the illness itself. Therefore, only a collaborative approach to accountability can fully meet the needs of patients after harmful medical errors have occurred and the physician involved is no longer taking care of the patient.

Concluding Remarks
Robert M. Sade, MD

Both essayists make persuasive arguments to support their positions. A few of their arguments are less than convincing, however. Moffatt-Bruce, for example, claims that her citations of sections of the American Medical

Association Code of Medical Ethics and the American College of Physicians Ethics Manual support the disclosure of Dr. Lapps's error by Dr. Jones. The American Medical Association Code does not support disclosure of another physician's error; it refers to a physician disclosing his own mistake.[2] The American College of Physicians Manual is more ambiguous than she asserts; it does not mention reporting errors of others.[3] Elsewhere, however, in support of her position, the American College of Physicians is much clearer about the obligation of a physician to report another physician's error: "The patient has both an ethical and a legal right to the information [about another clinician's mistake]".[11]

Denlinger wants us to believe that a great deal of uncertainty surrounds the question of whether or not an error occurred, which is assumed by Moffatt-Bruce to be a fact. In the Jones-Lapps scenario, however, Dr. Jones talks with Dr. Lapps, and it is clear that Dr. Lapps's refusal to disclose the omission of a lymph node biopsy is not based on denial that an error occurred but is based on fear of a lawsuit.

Moffatt-Bruce and Denlinger share many points of agreement. They both agree that Dr. Jones must discuss the omission of the biopsy with Dr. Lapps and that the 2 surgeons should jointly determine whether or not an error was made. They agree that Dr. Lapps should be offered an opportunity to disclose the omission to the patient and that a collaborative approach to resolution of the issue is needed.

Their major disagreement is on the final step of the process, after Dr. Lapps refuses to participate in disclosure of the omission. Moffatt-Bruce speaks of a "shared professional responsibility" to ensure disclosure of what happened to the patient, which is ethically necessary. Denlinger similarly speaks of a "collaborative approach to accountability" but stops at that point, leaving open the question of whether disclosure of the omission is obligatory.

Discussion of physicians' responsibility to report their own mistakes to patients is extensive in the medical and the bioethics literature, but little commentary can be found about disclosure of errors made by other clinicians. The best exploration of this subject is the recent report of Gallagher and coworkers,[7] which was cited by both essayists. The article provides a closely reasoned analysis of how to deal with errors made by other clinicians. The general conclusion is that patients and their families should be informed of errors or deviations from standard practice, as a matter of openness, honesty, and trust. The authors consider several different relationships between a clinician who makes an error and another clinician who discovers the error. One of those relationships involves a physician who discovers an error made by a physician at another institution, mirroring our scenario. In the situation of Drs. Jones and Lapps, the strategy they describe suggests that when Dr. Lapps refuses to participate in disclosing the misadventure to his former patient, Dr. Jones should seek assistance from the senior leadership at his own institution in deciding how to proceed, and in the best of circumstances, should be advised by a "disclosure coach" to ensure a well-considered, carefully planned discussion with the patient and his family—what Gallagher and colleagues describe as "skillfully executed disclosure conversations."

Our essayists disagree about whether reporting the error to the patient and his family is ethically obligatory. They agree on one critical issue, however: when a possible error is reported to the patient, it must be done with careful attention to the words and manner of communication to minimize adverse emotional responses by the patient and the family and to avoid burdening them unnecessarily.

References

1. Institute of Medicine. To err is human: building a safer health system. Washington, DC: National Academy Press; 2000.
2. AMA Council on Ethical and Judicial Affairs. Opinion 8.12, Patient information. Code of Medical Ethics: current opinions with annotations. 2012–2013 ed. Chicago: American Medical Association; 2012:290.
3. American College of Physicians. American College of Physicians ethics manual. Fourth ed. *Ann Intern Med.* 1998;128:576–94.
4. Blendon R, DesRoches C, Brodie M, et al. View of practicing physicians and the public on medical errors. *N Engl J Med* 2002;347:1933–40.
5. Kachalia A, Kaufman SR, Boothman R, et al. Liability claims and costs before and after implementation of a medical error disclosure program. *Ann Intern Med.* 2010;153:213–21.
6. Kachalia A. Improving patient safety through transparency. *N Engl J Med.* 2013;369:1677–9.
7. Gallagher TH, Mello MM, Levinson W, et al. Talking with patients about other clinicians' errors. *N Engl J Med.* 2013;369: 1752–7.
8. Asghari F, Fotouhi A, Jafarian A. Doctors' views of attitudes toward peer medical error. *Qual Saf Health Care.* 2009;18: 209–12.
9. Brennan TA, Leape LL, Laird NM, et al. Incidence of adverse events and negligence in hospitalized patients. *N Engl J Med.* 1991;324:370–6.
10. Posner KL, Caplan RA, Cheney FW. Variation in expert opinion in medical malpractice review. *Anesthesiol.* 1996;85:1049–54.
11. Fato M, Herrin VE. Must you disclose mistakes made by other physicians? *ACP Internist* 2003 (November). http://www.acpinternist.org/archives/2003/11/mistakes.htm. Accessed February 25, 2014.

13

Impending Loss of Insurance Coverage Is an Indication to Proceed with Complex, Expensive Surgery

Anthony L. Estrera, Sharon Ikonomidis,
John S. Ikonomidis, and Robert M. Sade*

Introduction
Robert M. Sade, MD

[...] The first principle of medical ethics relates to physicians' fidelity to patients: "A physician shall, while caring for a patient, regard responsibility to the patient as paramount."[1] The principle of beneficence tells us that we should do what is best for the patient, but what do we mean by the phrase "best for the patient"? Do we mean what is medically best, a determination that is within the domain of the physician's expertise, or do we mean what the patient believes is best? Usually, the patient gets to choose among available therapeutic alternatives, but some alternatives that are desired by a patient may not be available. For example, a patient who asks for a prescription for antibiotics in order to prevent the sniffles that just appeared from turning into a full-blown upper respiratory infection actually is requesting an irrational therapy. The physician should not provide the desired prescription but instead should provide an explanation of why it is not indicated.

Similarly, when a patient faces loss of health insurance coverage, a cardiothoracic surgeon could find himself flirting with the boundaries of ethical behavior. We describe below a patient with a known surgical disease who asks a cardiothoracic surgeon to repair the problem because he will soon lose

*Estrera AL, Ikonomidis S, Ikonomidis JS, Sade RM. Impending loss of insurance coverage is an indication to proceed with complex, expensive surgery. *Ann Thorac Surg*. 2010;89(6):1709–16. Copyright Society of Thoracic Surgeons, republished here with permission.

his health insurance coverage. The problem is that standard indications for surgery are not yet present, which raises the question of whether the surgeon should operate as the patient requested, on financial grounds. The surgeon wants to do what is best for the patient, but is the patient asking for something the surgeon should not provide?

THE CASE OF THE PREMATURE OPERATION

William Hochman, a 22-year-old college senior, will graduate in a few months. His health needs have always been covered by his father's health insurance policy, which is a benefit of his work as a janitor in a local apartment building. The insurance has reimbursed most of the expenses associated with the diagnostic testing that led to the diagnosis of Marfan syndrome a few years ago. When his last computed tomographic scan and echocardiogram showed slowly expanding diameter of his ascending aorta and a leaking aortic valve, William asked his internist to refer him to a surgeon who has a great deal of experience with aortic surgery.

The surgeon, Dr. Karl Geschickt, has now reviewed William's history, examined him, and thoroughly inspected his computed tomographic scans and echocardiograms. The surgeon tells William what he already knows: his ascending aorta has expanded from 3.6 cm two years ago to 4.0 on last week's scan, and his echocardiograms demonstrate mild aortic regurgitation. He definitely does not need an operation now, but at this rate of progression, an operation almost certainly will be needed within a few years.

William explains that, as an art history major, he expects to have a hard time finding a full time job when he graduates, and on the day of his graduation from college, he will no longer be eligible for coverage under his father's policy, and neither he nor his parents can afford to buy an individual health insurance policy. He tells the surgeon that he understands the nature of his disease and the future need for aortic surgery, but because of his insurance and financial situation, he needs to have the inevitable operation now rather than in a few years. Should Dr. Geschickt accommodate this young man's need? Should he operate now?

Pro
Anthony L. Estrera, MD

We all know the ethical principles that guide our clinical decisions: autonomy, beneficence, nonmaleficence (do no harm), and justice.[2] In carrying out our medical duties, we as clinicians identify maladies and plan treatments in order to improve the patient's well being. At the same time, the treatment applied must minimize the risk for complications and death for the patient, otherwise the treatment should not be undertaken. Prior to doing so, we establish a contractual agreement or informed consent with the patient for this service.

The decision to perform the procedure will generally depend on two factors: the medical indications for the procedure and patient preferences. Albert Jonsen and colleagues[3] define medical indications as the "data about the patient's physical and psychological condition that suggest diagnostic and therapeutic activities aimed at realizing the overall goals of medicine: prevention, cure, and care of illness and injury." Thus, "medical" facts justify the diagnostic and therapeutic interventions. Two critical questions regarding the "medical facts" are the following:

1. How are the medical facts determined?
2. Can the medical facts be affected by factors not traditionally considered medical?

Advocates of unrestricted advocacy, such as ethicists Albert Jonsen and Eric Cassell, suggest that these contextual factors should not be considered when determining clinical decisions. Cassell[4] maintains that "the sick are sick not because of human agency and intent but overwhelmingly because of the actions of fate." Jonsen and colleagues also note that factors external to the patient-physician relationship should never be decisive over patient welfare. In essence, supporters of unrestricted advocacy believe that only medical facts should determine clinical care.

In contrast, proponents of restricted advocacy note that considerations of justice do furnish a moral basis for individual action, because principles of professional ethics derive from roles specified by just institutions. Ethicist Norman Daniels, a proponent of restricted advocacy, points out that "dispensing with justice is not an option, because justice inheres in our very conception of the professional's moral role."[5] In essence, contextual factors do influence our decisional capacity.

I believe that medical recommendations are based on clinical judgments, but these judgments may be influenced by contextual factors such as economics. Our choices as physicians do have economic consequences on our patients and will ultimately influence ours and the patients' decisions. What happens if one does not consider, at least in part, economic factors in the clinical decision?

Generally, we have assumed that "medical" facts were what we traditionally accepted as the physiological, pathological, and psychological events related to the patient. Although this is what we were taught in medical school, the "medical" facts are not the only factors that contribute to the patient's wellbeing. I submit to you that just as important, and critical to the patient's well-being, are the social and economic issues immediately at hand.

It is often impossible for us to be completely empathetic with our patients, especially this patient, Mr Hochman, who has Marfan syndrome. It is likely he has learned as much as he could regarding his condition and realizes that although his aorta is not enlarged enough to indicate surgery (so he is told), his aortic root has enlarged from 3.6 cm to 4.0 cm. Knowing that his aorta has enlarged must be an overwhelming concern for him. In addition, he has also learned that having his abnormally enlarged aortic root places him at risk for rupture and early death. Although Dr. Geschickt cannot tell him with any certainty what these risks are, he is informed that future surgery will be needed within a few years. He further realizes that even if his aorta does not rupture, he may still suffer an aortic dissection and that if this occurs, his long-term prognosis worsens. He further realizes that the rest of his aorta may be at risk for further aneurysmal degeneration and that he will most likely require further interventions to replace the remainder of his aorta. He lives in fear. How can one say that this fear does not affect his well-being?

Medical "indications" are driven by the "fear" of the unknown. There is no way we can predict the future, but as clinicians we attempt to do this every day. It is the anticipation of what may happen in the future that often dictates what we do in the present. This is the nature of our profession. [...]

In thoracic surgery, a solitary pulmonary nodule (SPN) in a 50-year-old patient has up to a 50% chance of harboring a malignancy.[6] A patient who smokes is sent to your office with a new SPN, with results of a needle biopsy, and positron emission tomography/computed tomographic scans that are negative for malignancy. The patient asks you to resect the SPN. Would you? Again the emotion of fear (of cancer) drives your decision.

For this same patient, it is December 21, 2009. You have seen him and offer him surgery (you are an expert in thoracoscopic techniques) and he understands the potential need for a thoracoscopic lobectomy—a complex, expensive procedure—on January 4, 2010. But ... He asked you to perform the procedure as soon as possible; i.e., before the end of the year. This is because he has already paid his deductible ($250), and his out-of-pocket expenses ($1,250) for the year have been covered; if the procedure is performed before the new year he will not incur any added expenses. Would you accommodate him? How does this differ from impending loss of insurance coverage? Economic issues do influence our decisions and thus should be considered when deciding to operate. Impending loss of insurance coverage may be of great importance to some patients. [...]

Lack of health insurance might kill up to 45,000 Americans per year. Wilper and colleagues[7] analyzed 9,000 surveys from 1986 to 1994, then followed through 2000 and identified that the uninsured had a 40% higher risk of death than those with health insurance. Extrapolated to 2005 census data, this accounted for 44,789 deaths. The authors speculated that these deaths occurred because uninsured patients did not seek medical attention for fear of not being able to pay for it.

In another study, Himmelstein and his colleagues[8] found that 62.1% of all bankruptcies in the US have a medical cause, which had risen 50% since 2001. Because of the fear of death, and the fear of bankruptcy (economic devastation), impending loss of health insurance becomes very important and cannot be ignored when deciding to perform surgery.

In summary, the moral argument that impending loss of insurance coverage is an indication to proceed with complex, expensive surgery is valid, and is consistent with these principles of medical ethics:

1. Beneficence: Loss of insurance coverage as one of the indications for surgery will provide a benefit for Mr Hochman and eliminate the risk for proximal aortic dissection and rupture.
2. Nonmaleficence: In the hands of a skilled surgeon (Dr. Geschickt), the procedures can be performed safely.
3. Justice: Performing surgery prior to loss of insurance is fair because the patient (or his father) has already paid for surgical benefits.
4. Autonomy: In my opinion this is the most important principle in this case, and it is exercised by both Dr. Geschickt and Mr Hochman.

Thus, impending loss of insurance coverage is an indication to proceed with complex, expensive surgery.

Con

Sharon Ikonomidis, MS, PhD, John S. Ikonomidis, MD, PhD

> *"The delivery of medical care is to do as much nothing as possible."*
> — *Samuel Shem, The House of God, 1978*

The ethical dilemma presented in the case of William Hochman is whether or not the patient should be offered preemptive (and costly) cardiovascular surgery while he has medical insurance coverage, to avoid future possibility of needing surgery and not being able to pay for it, even though the surgeon deems the operation to be not medically indicated.

We argue that a patient should not receive preemptive cardiovascular surgery that is not medically indicated because such an act would violate basic tenets essential to the appropriate practice of medicine. Brett succinctly states the issue in this way: "It is important to recognize that the structure and regulation of medical practice in the United States clearly reflect a broad social mandate for clinicians to exercise independent professional judgment and to resist the patient's requests for harmful or non-beneficial interventions."[9] Accordingly, the proper role of the surgeon is to do what is best, both from a medical and moral point of view, for the health of the patient. This is based on the fundamental principle of beneficence or nonmaleficence as repeated in our medical oaths which express promises made by the medical profession to the members of societies in which they practice. The principles of beneficence and nonmaleficence date back to the Hippocratic oath (4th century BC) and resurface in the American Medical Association Code of Medical Ethics (1847 to 2010), the American College of Surgeons Fellowship Pledge (1913), and the World Medical Association's Declarations of Geneva (1947) and Helsinki (1964), to name a few.[10]

The cardiac surgeon, upon consideration of the patient's suitability for surgery, must determine the risk-to-benefit ratio of the procedure. Surgery is not medically indicated if it is determined that the risk(s) of undergoing surgery outweighs the potential benefits of such treatment for the patient's health. Thus, to recommend or proceed with such surgery would constitute a violation of the commitment to nonmaleficence. Surely it is always safer (and thus of optimal nonmaleficence) to not perform surgery that is not absolutely necessary!

The obligation of the cardiac surgeon to promote the patient's cardiac health is paramount over non-health related considerations. When a requested procedure is unacceptable by current standards, as in Mr Hochman's case, non-health related considerations become entirely irrelevant. In addition, we maintain that it is inappropriate for someone whose expertise lies in a specific clinical application to make value judgments about another's economic condition; especially when such judgments impact the physical health of that person. The poor economic state-of-affairs which exists in this country does indeed affect individuals' access to health care. However, this is a social problem to be addressed by society as a whole; the burden should not lie on the shoulders of individual physicians to fix our socioeconomic problems whether they affect access to health care or not. Such considerations are secondary at best and are not strictly speaking within the scope of the individual surgeon's duties.

The risk-to-benefit ratio factored into a decision of whether or not to proceed with surgery is arguably the most relevant piece of information the patient will receive from the surgeon in terms of making this choice. If the risks clearly outweigh the potential benefits of having a major operation when it is not indicated, as they do in this case, it is doubtful that the patient would choose to proceed. The surgeon may deflate the importance of this information by giving serious weight to (irrelevant) nonmedical risks or benefits, but doing so constitutes a violation of the fundamental (Kantian) duty of respect for persons because the patient's autonomous decision-making capacity has been biased by irrelevant information. For Kant[11], autonomous persons are "ends in themselves" who determine their own futures and thus are never to be treated merely as means to the ends of others. Respect for autonomy is a very important ethical principle, perhaps the most important in the surgeon-patient relationship. We honor it by not accepting as germane and important irrelevant facts that bias the patient's decision-making process.

[...] In the present case, with an ascending aortic diameter of 4.0 cm, the patient in question does not satisfy the "accepted" criteria for surgical aneurysm repair. The probability that this patient's ascending aorta will ever reach 5.0 cm in diameter is unknown but likely is less than 100%. As such, the possibility exists that the patient is an "anomaly" and does not experience sufficient additional aortic dilatation so as to require surgery. Also, it is currently unknown exactly how long it would take for the aneurysm to reach 5.0 cm in diameter and (or) what the patient's risk of dissection would be over this time period. Moreover, during this indeterminate period of time, new advances in medical therapy may become available which could reduce or halt the tendency toward aneurysm formation and hence prevent the requirement for surgical intervention. [...]

Also, who can say with certainty that the patient will not be able to afford surgery after his medical insurance has expired? The patient may win the lottery or receive an inheritance or have a friend or family member who offers to pay the costs. Though perhaps unlikely, the point is that the decision to have surgery should not be based on future uncertainties (whether medical or financial) but rather must be based on what is presently known to be medically indicated.

Another major ethical concern arising from this case, in which the patient receives preemptive surgery due to present affordability and future financial uncertainty, is one of social justice. Here we are concerned specifically with a principle of distributive justice defined as "a matter of the comparative treatment of individuals' characteristic of modern democratic theory."[12] Justice is providing access to treatment for all patients who need it (or for whom surgery is medically indicated). Injustice is sometimes providing access to treatment for patients on the basis of need (or for whom surgery is medically indicated) and sometimes providing access to treatment for patients on the basis of something other than need (or for whom surgery is not medically indicated). We contend that allowing for the impending loss of insurance coverage to be an indication for surgery poses a clear injustice as it allows for a qualification for surgery that is not applied equally across the patient population. [...]

In terms of health care distribution within the broader social community, if cardiac surgeries that are not medically indicated are allowed (like cosmetic surgeries), then cardiac surgery allocation becomes morally problematic because a system would be created in which society's members who need surgery but cannot afford it are bumped by those who can afford (albeit temporarily in this case) but do not really need it! If the primary goal of medical practice is to heal the sick then surely the allocation of life-saving medical resources to those who do not require them is an unjust form of distribution, not to mention a financial waste.

Consider the converse possible outcome in which the patient undergoes surgery and does not fare well. Choosing to operate on patients when not medically indicated may place the surgeon on very unstable ground from a medico-legal standpoint where the law chooses to define this operation as failing to meet an appropriate standard of care. If the patient (even though he requested the surgery in the first place) or the family decides to sue for medical malpractice it is likely that, in a court of law, "expert" witnesses, presumably experienced thoracic aortic surgeons, will not agree with the decision to proceed with a nonmedically indicated operation based on pending loss of insurance.

What this would mean for our medical insurance companies is also important. There is the possibility that insurance rates would escalate drastically if cardiac surgeons make a practice of operating on patients who request surgeries before their insurance policy terms expire. This would present a social injustice to those who have worked hard for years to pay for decent medical coverage but have been fortunate enough not to have needed major surgery and hence the coverage to pay for it. Why should their rates go up? Preemptive surgery may end up costing society more with respect to medical insurance premiums. Conversely, from the standpoint of physician reimbursement, while it is clear that expanding the scope of operative indications to patients proven to not require surgery has the potential to benefit the surgeon financially, the long-term consequences may be dire. It is highly likely that this practice will be detected and could lead to charge of fraud with the potential for loss of the right to care for patients altogether. It is also possible that the payor, upon review of the case, may deny payment on the basis of breech of the standard of care. Because many institutions submit billings on behalf of the surgeon, the institution, in addition to the surgeon, may assume culpability for fraudulent billing practices should an audit be conducted.

CONCLUSION

Although fiscal matters must dictate much of how the medical system functions, it is not in accordance with our medical ethical principles that such matters dominate decisions at the cardiac surgeon-patient level. In the case considered herein, concern for Mr. Hochman's present ability to pay for his operation must not precede or occlude concerns for his cardiovascular health. Patients should not receive cardiovascular surgery that is not medically indicated. We conclude, then, that impending loss of insurance coverage does not serve as an indication to proceed with cardiovascular surgery.

Concluding Remarks
Robert M. Sade, MD

THE ARGUMENTS

The Belmont Report of 1979[13] [...] identified three ethical principles relevant to research: respect for persons (respect for autonomy), beneficence, and justice. In the same year, Tom Beauchamp and James Childress[14] split off from beneficence a fourth principle, nonmaleficence. These four principles, often referred to as the Georgetown Mantra, are commonly used in ethical analysis. Both discussions of the William Hochman case are based on these principles, but they reach very different conclusions. [...]

One of the difficulties of using a prescriptive analysis of ethical issues, such as the Beauchamp-Childress formulation, is illustrated by the discussions above; the defining terms are open to many different interpretations, sometimes diametrically opposed. Nevertheless, such discussions provide a useful starting place for analysis. The opposing authors disagree on the points noted above, but they agree on at least two issues: standard indications for operating on Mr. Hochman are not present at this time, and nonmedical factors should generally be considered in treatment deliberations. [...]

The disagreement between the two positions can be attributed in part to language, namely, the meaning or usage of terms such as benefit, unnecessary surgery, and standard of care. The ambiguity of those terms allows divergent usages, leading to critical questions. Whose valuation of benefits versus risk counts? If the indications for operation are outside current standards, should non-medical factors be excluded? Is an operation that does not meet standard indications unnecessary, and are unnecessary operations automatically unsafe? We might also ask how the risks borne by the surgeon and society at large should be weighed in the deliberations.

WHOSE VALUATION OF BENEFITS VERSUS RISK COUNTS?

A widely accepted method of making decisions in medicine is "shared decision making." Different interpretations of how this method should work have been described; in general, it means that the physician and the patient exchange information and reach agreement on the best treatment option. The physician supplies information based on his expertise and the patient supplies information about his values and preferences. Applying this model to the current case, Mr. Hochman's values and preferences seem clear—he wants the operation—and if Dr. Geschickt agrees with the patient, he will do it. If Dr. Geschickt disagrees with the patient, believing instead that an operation at this time would be wrong, he can, as Ikonomidis and Ikonomidis suggest, try to persuade the patient to abandon the idea of an operation now. If the patient is persuaded, there is agreement and no operation is done.

If, however, the patient is not persuaded and still wants the operation, Dr. Geschickt has the option of agreeing to operate or of refusing. If he chooses the first option, they agree, but if he chooses the second, the patient is left with two choices: not having the operation or finding another surgeon. Both the patient and the physician are autonomous individuals and, while they seek consensus, which is usually achieved, agreement might not be possible. The surgeon might be correct in his belief that the risk-benefit balance weighs more heavily on the side of risk, but the patient might be willing to take that risk because the benefit, in this case, avoiding the need for paying out-of-pocket for surgery in the future, carries much more weight for him than for the surgeon. If Dr. Geschickt refuses to do the surgery, he does so on the basis of his own value system, not the patient's; that is, he exercises his own professional autonomy.

IF THE INDICATIONS FOR OPERATION ARE NONSTANDARD, SHOULD NONMEDICAL FACTORS BE EXCLUDED?

Estrera and Ikonomidis and Ikonomidis agree that non-medical factors such as the patient's preferences should be weighed when there is more than one acceptable surgical option, but they disagree when the surgery being requested is "not absolutely necessary." Estrera still weighs those factors, but Ikonomidis and Ikonomidis discount them entirely on grounds of safety: "Surely it is always safer (and thus the optimal nonmaleficence) to *not* perform surgery that is not absolutely necessary!"

An enduring difficulty with this position has been the meaning of the words "necessary" and "unnecessary." [...] There seems to be no solid ground for asserting that an operation indicated by parameters outside standard limits is ipso facto unnecessary. Underlying the question of whether Mr. Hochman's operation should be considered unnecessary is the question of whose values weigh more heavily, the patient's personal values or the physician's medical standards. Unnecessary to whom and by what measure? This question circles back to the discussion of shared decision making, leaving us with the quandary of adjudicating firmly held opposing view of physician and patient. [...]

HOW SHOULD THE RISKS BORNE BY THE SURGEON AND SOCIETY AT LARGE BE WEIGHED?

My discussion thus far has focused on the risks and benefits confronting the patient, but at least two other parties have a stake in this decision to operate or not: the surgeon and society at large. Doing this operation exposes Dr. Geschickt to certain potential harms, according to Ikonomidis and Ikonomidis. If the procedure is determined to be below the standard of care, he could face a charge of fraud by the insurance company when he submits his bill. If the operation results in serious complications, unlikely though this is, he could face a lawsuit for malpractice. Society could be harmed by violations of social justice through unjust allocation of resources if the rich can satisfy their desires for unneeded procedures and preempt the use of those resources by patients who are less well off, according to Ikonomidis and Ikonomidis. [...]

CONCLUSION

The persistently indeterminate meanings of several terms (e.g., unnecessary surgery, benefit, standard of care) leave us with no clear solution to Dr. Geschickt's dilemma [...]. We can advise him to follow the primary principle of medical ethics, do what is best for the patient, but that would be begging the question, for what is best for the patient is precisely the disputed issue. [...]

The informed consent that is so familiar to us is not a signed piece of paper, as many residents seem to believe, but is a process grounded in two ethical principles: respect for the patient as an independent moral agent and beneficent guidance of the patient toward choices that are right for him. As surgeons, we also are moral agents, guided by our own values, knowledge, and professional judgment in dealing with our patients. Out of respect for one another, neither patient nor physician should attempt to impose unwanted options on the other. That is why Dr. Geschickt could rightfully choose either of the two options that are open to him and also why he should listen to the advice of both Estrera and Ikonomidis and Ikonomidis before making his decision.

References

1. Council on Ethical and Judicial Affairs, American Medical Association. Principles of medical ethics, VIII. Code of Medical Ethics: current opinions with annotations, 2008–2009 ed. Chicago: American Medical Association; 2008:xv.
2. Beauchamp TL, Childress JF. *Principles of Biomedical Ethics*. 5th ed. New York: Oxford University Press; 2001.
3. Jonsen A, Siegler M, Winslade W. *Clinical Ethics: A Practical Approach to Ethical Decisions in Clinical Medicine*. 6th ed. Columbus, OH: McGraw-Hill; 2006.
4. Cassell EJ. *The Nature of Suffering*. 2nd ed. Oxford: Oxford University Press; 2003.
5. Daniels N. Justice, health and health care. *Am J Bioethics*. 2001;1:2–16.
6. Smythe WR, Reznik SI, Putnam JB Jr. Lung. In: Townsend CM Jr, Beauchamp RD, Evers BM, Mattox KL, eds. *Sabiston Textbook of Surgery*. 18th ed. Philadelphia: Elsevier; 2008:ch. 59.
7. Wilper AP, Woolhandler S, Lasser KE, McCormick D, Bor DH, Himmelstein DU. Health insurance and mortality in US adults. *Am J Public Health*. 2009;99:2289–95.

8. Himmelstein DU, Thorne D, Warren E, Woolhandler S. Medical bankruptcy in the United States, 2007: results of a national study. *Am J Med.* 2009;122:741–6.

9. Brett AS. Inappropriate requests for treatments and tests. In: Sugarman J, ed. *Ethics in Primary Care.* New York: McGraw-Hill Health Professions Division; 2000:6.

10. Tung T, Organ CH. Ethics in surgery: historical perspectives. *Arch Surg.* 2000;135:10–13.

11. Kant I. *Foundations of the Metaphysics of Morals.* Lewis White Beck (trans.) New York: Liberal Arts Press; 1959:408.

12. Frankena William K. *Ethics.* 2nd ed. Foundations of Philosophy Series. Englewood Cliffs, NJ: Prentice-Hall; 1973:49.

13. Subjects of biological and behavioral research. The Belmont report. Department of Health, Education, and Welfare Pub. No. (OS) 78-0012, Appendix I, Pub. No. (OS) 78-0013, Appendix II, Pub. No. (OS) 78-0014. Washington, DC: US Government Printing Office; 1978.

14. Beauchamp TL, Childress JF. *Principles of Biomedical Ethics.* New York: Oxford University Press; 1979.

14

Ethical Obligation of Surgeons to Noncompliant Patients

CAN A SURGEON REFUSE TO OPERATE ON AN INTRAVENOUS DRUG–ABUSING PATIENT WITH RECURRENT AORTIC VALVE PROSTHESIS INFECTION?

J. Michael DiMaio, Tomas A. Salerno, Ron Bernstein, Katia Araujo, Marco Ricci, and Robert M. Sade*

Introduction
Robert M. Sade, MD

One of the most frustrating situations confronting a physician is a noncompliant patient. When a patient receives clear instructions, acknowledges those instructions, fails to follow them, and then slips into even worse difficulty than he had before, we sometimes want to throw up our hands and retreat. Surgeons have a special difficulty in this area when, for example, a patient with peripheral vascular disease in need of a bypass operation finds himself unable to stop smoking and therefore unlikely to gain durable benefit from the operation.

Cardiothoracic surgeons are in a parallel situation when a patient who abuses drugs has an operation and then will not or cannot stop using drugs. Personal lifestyles are very difficult to change, whether or not a patient's addiction is involved. Intravenous drug abusers find it particularly difficult to stop using, but resources are available to help those who wish to break an unwanted habit. Particularly nettlesome is the problem of the patient who

*DiMaio JM, Salerno TA, Bernstein R, Araujo K, Ricci M, Sade RM. Ethical obligation of surgeons to non-compliant patients: can a surgeon refuse to operate on an intravenous drug-abusing patient with recurrent aortic valve prosthesis infection? *Ann Thorac Surg.* 2009;88(1):1–8. Copyright Society of Thoracic Surgeons, republished here with permission.

abuses drugs intravenously, develops endocarditis, has a valve replacement, and then, after a drug-free period, reverts to drug use. Two experienced surgeons who have opposing views of what should be done in such a situation consider the following case.

THE CASE OF JAMES SMITH

James Smith is 29 years old and married with 2 children who are 2 and 4 years old. He is frequently absent from home for extended periods and works odd jobs to support himself. He used marijuana when a teenager, and by his early 20s was regularly using cocaine, including intravenously. He is seen in the emergency department with a febrile illness, and is found to have severe aortic insufficiency due to an aortic valve infection.

The chief of cardiothoracic surgery, Dr. William Jones, replaces the aortic valve with a St. Jude Medical prosthesis. Mr. Smith does well postoperatively and is discharged with a warning about the possibility that the infection might come back if he ever uses intravenous drugs again. He understands that he might not be given a second valve if the infection recurs while he is using intravenous drugs. He signs an agreement to this effect.

Mr. Smith is seen intermittently thereafter in the cardiology clinic, where he is found to be doing well, free of intravenous drug abuse. Several months after his last visit, which was 2 years after his valve replacement, he reappears in the emergency department with fever and shaking chills. He has signs of intravenous drug use and admits to using again, starting about 6 months earlier. On the cardiology service, echocardiography and magnetic resonance imaging show severe paravalvular aortic insufficiency, with several small extramural abscesses. The cardiology service's discussions of the case reveal disagreement about whether or not the operation should be done. They send a consultation request to Dr. Jones with the details of Mr. Smith's current condition and laboratory results. Their consult note asks Dr. Jones whether he thinks urgent aortic valve replacement should be done, given the patient's history.

Pro
J. Michael DiMaio, MD

Mr. Smith reinfected his prosthetic aortic valve upon returning to his habit of intravenous drug abuse. He is 29 years old, and he was warned that this might occur. One might think that a surgeon is obligated to operate due to some ethical standard requiring him to do so. But, in fact, there is no such standard. There are plenty of ethical, logical, and moral reasons that allow a surgeon the right to say no.

Some might say that the Hippocratic Oath obligates us to operate. However, careful reading of the oath, which most medical schools have abandoned, at least in its original form, may provide guidance: "I will prescribe regimens for the good of my patients according to my ability and judgment and never do harm to anyone." In this case, a surgeon who offers an operation may be missing the point entirely and may be doing harm to Mr. Smith, himself, his team, and certainly society.

Should all of society's problems be up to the medical profession to repair? Ivan Illich wrote that classifying all the troubles of humanity as medical problems is actually antithetical to true health, in that it limits the ability of people to learn to cope with pain, sickness, and death as integral parts of life.[1] These adversities are natural components of the continuum of life to death. Physicians should not fool themselves into thinking that all problems can and should be fixed. This is not to say that one should never try. Health, he maintains, is not freedom from death, disease, unhappiness, and stress, which are inevitable, but rather the ability to cope with them competently. If this is true, then the more medicine and society direct individual behavior, the less autonomous and, therefore, the less healthy the individual may become.

In 1974, Faith Fitzgerald wrote about social responsibility:

> In the 19th and early 20th centuries, if a person fell ill, had alcoholism or tuberculosis, or abused a spouse or child, it was a pity, but it was a pity for the person and a sadness for his or her family; it was their business. Over the past several decades, however, both the existence of these imperfections and the remedies for them have become society's business, particularly since society began to accept the responsibility to pay for the consequences of the imperfections. Now treatment of drug addiction, prevention of domestic violence, handgun control, and the use of seat belts and helmets are society's responsibility. Concurrently, however, because the imperfections are unhealthy, they are also the responsibility of doctors and nurses. Both health care providers and the commonweal now have a vested interest in certain forms of behavior, previously considered a person's private business, if the behavior impairs a person's "health." Certain failures of self-care have become, in a sense, crimes against society, because society has to pay for their consequences. Society increasingly looks to health care providers for leadership in eliminating behavior that leads to disease.[2]

Individuals need to accept responsibility for their own health and not look to physicians and nurses to relieve them of their duty.

A distinguished professor with whom I discussed this case stated, "You're not fixing the problem, you are fixing the heart!" Ludicrous though it might seem to surgeons who have been trained to fix the heart, Mr. Smith' primary problem is not his heart at all. It is his substance abuse. His destiny was sealed by this problem, which is as lethal as any metastatic cancer. Many longitudinal studies have documented this fact.

DRUG ABUSE MORTALITY

Robert Frater reviewed 57 known drug addicts with endocarditis who were operated on at Montefiore Medical Center from 1977 to 1989.[3] The most common lesion was aortic endocarditis. The 30-day in-hospital mortality rate was 9%, yet during 5 to 10 years of follow-up, the mortality rate was about 90%.

A 33-year follow-up of 471 heroin addicts who had been admitted to a drug addiction program identified three clinical trajectories for these individuals: stable high-level heroine users, late decelerators, and early quitters.[4] A literature review showed mortality rates for the three groups of 50%, 38%, and 25%, respectively. Only 44% of the 471 addicts were early quitters; most continued to use drugs. A separate study of the same cohort showed the addicts lost an average of 18.3 years of life: 22.3% of the years were lost due to heroin overdose, 14% to chronic disease, and 10% to accidents.[5] The average future life expectancy of the addicts was 19 years vs 33 years for comparable men. The estimated monetary value of lost productivity was more than $174 million.

A study of 4200 intravenous drug users in Italy found increased mortality from cardiovascular, respiratory, and gastrointestinal disease as well as violence, overdose, and AIDS. Although most deaths were due to endocarditis, a significant number were due to cirrhosis in men and pneumonia in women.[6] [...]

In a London study of a cohort of 128 addicts, 43 died during a 22-year period. Most deaths were drug related, 18 specifically of drug overdose.[7] Review of the United Kingdom heart valve registry found that the 1-, 5-, and 10-year survival rates after operations for prosthetic valve endocarditis were only 67%, 55%, and 37%, respectively; a dismal prognosis. [...]

PROTECTING THE TEAM

What about the team? Should a surgeon place 10 or more persons at risk, including nurses, perfusionists, and anesthesiologists? Few of them have the right or ability to protest the decision made by a surgeon who feels an obligation to help someone who fails to care for himself.

The risk of infection to health care workers is real. [...]

THE GOOD OF SOCIETY

What about society? Utilitarianism is the idea that the moral worth of an action is determined solely by its contribution to its overall utility: that is, its contribution to happiness or pleasure as summed among all persons, sometimes described by the phrase "the greatest good for the greatest number." According to utilitarian theory, the collective risk of harming many persons shifts the equation to the greatest amount of good to the greatest number of people. Spending time, energy, and resources, which are not unlimited, on one patient who has chosen to do himself harm does not serve the greater good. Although a surgeon might think that he operates simply within a one-on-one relationship with a patient, he denies the good of many others within such a narrow framework.

Allocation of resources in society is also an issue. Time is not unlimited. This is true for the surgeon, but it is equally true for all the members of the operating and care teams. Expending this limited resource on Mr. Smith is wasteful.

What about money? This would certainly be a very costly operation, its reoperative nature potentially including renal failure requiring dialysis and other complications. As surgeons, we can argue that saving money is not our job, but I would strongly argue that it is. We all have a sense of what things cost. We may substitute a less expensive suture or stapler if we believe that it will save money and not cause any difference in patient care. We allocate scarce organs for transplantation because we try to watch out for the greater good of society. Mr. Smith's case is not different. Even if the number of valves is theoretically unlimited, other resources are not. Certainly, if we do not begin to understand how to allocate health care resources more wisely, others will force it upon us.

We do not have an obligation to treat this patient if he is a poor steward of the gifts he has received. Mr. Smith is not unlike someone who has, for example, received a kidney or heart transplant and has stopped taking his graft-preserving medications. We are not obligated to endlessly supply new operations, valves, or organs if the person is a poor steward of the resources charged to his care.

Where does one draw the line? The only principled response is to do the first operation. By that, we mean that there is no principled reason to do more than one operation. One may argue that it is fair to give him one more chance, but that same argument can be made for two, three, or four operations, and there is no end. This is not a slippery slope argument, it merely suggests that a surgeon is obligated to do something once; if it is done right, the obligation falls to the patient to care for his gift.

THE SURGEON AS A PROFESSIONAL

Finally, a surgeon is a professional with professional obligations. He has the right and responsibility to assess the situation, circumstances, probabilities, and likely outcomes and to determine whether he believes an operation is futile. Just because the patient wants a procedure does not require a surgeon to perform it. [...] In this case, Mr. Smith and society would not receive benefit from an operation. Therefore, Dr. Jones has every right to say no!

Con
Tomas A. Salerno, MD, Ron Bernstein, JD, Katia Araujo, PsyD, Marco Ricci, MD

Valve endocarditis represents one of the leading causes of operative mortality in cardiac surgery, ranging from 8% to 37%.[8] Poor outcomes are related to drug resistance, delay in surgical treatment, presence of concomitant risk factors and multiple end-organ dysfunction, acute congestive heart failure, prosthetic valve reinfection, and severity of valve injury.[9] Surgeons are frequently asked to operate on patients who have acquired endocarditis of a native or prosthetic valve resulting from intravenous drug use. Without surgery, the prognosis of this condition is poor, especially when vegetations, annular abscesses, intracardiac fistulas, and severe valve insufficiency develop. [...]

When surgeons face the scenario of a patient with endocarditis related to drug use, what often comes to mind is that all efforts at salvaging the patient's life could be futile should the patient return to drug use. Such is the case of the hypothetical patient, James Smith, discussed in this article. [...] The question [is]: Should the surgeon operate again on this patient? To answer this question, it is important to understand not only the disease process but also the medical issues related to drug addiction and its treatment options. Furthermore, the points of view of a psychologist and a lawyer, in addition to that of a surgeon, may provide further insight into this complex issue.

DEFINITION OF DRUG ADDICTION

In 2001, the American Academy of Pain Medicine, the American Pain Society, and the American Society of Addiction Medicine jointly defined addiction:

> Addiction is a primary, chronic, neurobiologic disease, with genetic, psychosocial, and environmental factors influencing its development and manifestations. It is characterized by behaviors that include one or more of the following: impaired control over drug use, compulsive use, continued use despite harm, and craving.[10]

Drug addiction is a complex but treatable disease, characterized by compulsive drug craving and drug usage that persists despite serious consequences. It may become chronic, with relapses after prolonged periods of abstinence. For this reason, it may require ongoing surveillance and repeated treatments.

PSYCHOLOGIST'S VIEW [KATIA ARAUJO, PSYD]

Mr. Smith did not receive the benefits of an appropriate treatment plan that would target detoxification and relapse prevention and ensure that the patient had an adequate support system for his problem. The physicians involved in the care of this patient should have sought the expertise of a psychiatrist and a clinical psychologist specializing in drug rehabilitation. He should have been treated as a dual-diagnosis patient. Comprehensive alcohol and drug addiction treatment centers provide dual-diagnosis programs specializing in detoxification and relapse prevention. Mental health professionals work with the patient to provide him with emotional tools and psychopharmacology treatments to help him achieve abstinence and prevent relapse.

Many times, due to lack of insight and judgment, addict patients delay medical assistance until their medical conditions reach high levels of severity. [...] In recovery, an addict patient cannot do it alone, so the agreement or demands made of this patient is akin to punishment.

Other issues may also arise: Some professionals may tend to be omnipotent caretakers, and end up deluding themselves into believing that they can do it all, rarely asking for help from other professionals. That might have happened in this case.

LAWYER'S VIEW [RON BERNSTEIN, JD]

One of the greatest risk factors for developing endocarditis is a previous heart operation for endocarditis, along with many other factors, such as poor dental hygiene. Therefore, recurrent endocarditis may result from a problem unrelated to the addiction, even if the patient remains engaged in drug use. Should physicians require lifestyle agreements and contracts or refuse to treat a patient if a condition arises that could be potentially linked to a lifestyle violation or to some other cause? Furthermore, who should decide which lifestyle habits constitute a violation and which do not? In the end, the patient would pay, perhaps with his life, adding to the suffering of his 2 innocent children!

In some medical circumstances, such as that of an alcoholic liver transplant patient, clinicians may have a keen interest in making sure that scarce replacement organs go to those who will care for them the best. Performance contracts are used, and prospective organ recipients must demonstrate lifestyle changes to qualify for a transplant. From a logical and ethical point of view, in organ transplantation the scarcity of organs affects patient selection. In contrast, our case of recurrent endocarditis involves the need for emergency care without withholding essential care from other patients with similar medical problems. The disease mechanism may or may not have been related to a disfavored lifestyle or a breach of "contract," whether enforceable or unenforceable. This should not be viewed as a closed question—to operate or not to operate. Rather, the surgeon should operate or transfer the patient to another surgeon.

Another important issue is the legality of "contracts" between patients and health care professionals. Such contracts should not be incorporated in medical practice, because they could be fraught with both ethical problems and potential legal consequences. Surgeons should provide treatment within the prevailing standard of care to patients, regardless of any contract or previous agreement. Should the patient not abide by care guidelines and recommendations despite the best efforts of health care providers, the consequences are on the patient. But greater consequences would be visited on the health care providers who feel empowered to decide whether a patient is morally worthy of their care. [...]

A contract alone would not insulate the surgeon from a malpractice suit, and the risks of that suit under these circumstances could very well be significant. Such a case would probably not be defensible on the basis of that contract. This would make a strong case for physicians, already exposed to litigation when the care needed is rendered, not to venture into decision-making processes based on anything other than medical need. [...]

The better choice is for the physician to either provide the indicated care or make sure that the patient's care is transferred to another appropriate clinician. [...]

SURGEON'S VIEW [TOMAS A. SALERNO, MD]

We, as physicians, have the ethical responsibility to treat and heal. If we venture into the moral background of patients, then we would spend more time passing judgment on lifestyle choices instead of making the medical decisions we have been trained for.

Additional considerations may also arise: Some health care professionals, at times, tend to feel like omnipotent caretakers, leading them to believe that they can do it all and that they do not need help or advice from other professionals. The clinical scenario described here seems to be one such situation. Treating drug addicts can be overwhelming and frustrating. [...]

Finally, isn't the position of the surgeon refusing to treat the same as that of a physician dealing with a smoker whose lung cancer has been cured, but who would be declared ineligible for further treatment should he continue to smoke and develop a recurrence? Or that of a physician dealing with a morbidly obese patient who would be denied treatment should he develop a complication resulting from recurrent overeating? Does a physician have the authority, the time, and the mission to be a law enforcement agent? After all, should physicians decide not to treat medical conditions that result from exposure to certain risk factors or unsafe behaviors, what would be left for us to treat? A vast number of medical conditions, including heart diseases and infectious disease, may result from exposure to well-known environmental factors. Does the willingness of a patient to be exposed to those factors disqualify him from receiving indicated medical or surgical treatment? In our opinion, that should not be the case.

Concluding Remarks
Robert M. Sade, MD

[...] Dr. Jones's dilemma is clearly complex. Yet, Mr. Smith's story brings to front stage some basic principles of medical ethics. The primary obligation of physicians is to their patients.[11] We have other obligations, of course, to ourselves, to the institutions in which we work, to our colleagues, and to society, but these are all secondary: Consideration of the patient's well-being must come first. In addition, social worth has no place in medical decision making.[12] This became a crucial principle of medical ethics when the bottom of the slippery slope of social worth as an evaluative factor was reached in Europe in the 1930s and 1940s.[13] We often stereotype drug addicts as occupants of the lowest rung of the social ladder, but this social judgment must play no role in deliberations about whether an operation should be done. [...]

As with social worth, several other aspects of Mr. Smith's story are not relevant to making the decision to replace his aortic valve for the second time. He has returned to using intravenous drugs, and this lapse is the most likely cause of his reinfected valve. He has done it to himself, many would say, so does not deserve a second valve. But deciding what is deserved or undeserved is a moral judgment that we, as physicians, are not in a position to make. We see human frailty in action every day. [...]

Mr. Smith's relapse is just such a human failing, whether it is due to unwillingness or to inability to refrain from using drugs. His failure is not different from the biker, the overeater, or the smoker, and we should similarly care for him without hesitation. From a physician's perspective, it does not matter whether a patient with an unambiguous medical need is addicted to traveling on 2 wheels at high-speed in the open air, to eating rich foods, to smoking cigarettes, or to abusing drugs: We are ethically bound to use available resources to provide indicated, proper treatment. In view of the human frailty we as physicians observe daily, a patient's agreement, promise, or contract not to return to abusing drugs cannot justify refusing an indicated operation. [...]

The American Medical Association Code of Medical Ethics discusses resource allocation criteria, and includes this statement: "Nonmedical criteria, such as ... social worth, patient contribution to illness, or past use of resources should not be considered."[14] [...]

An aid to deciding whether to offer an operation to Mr. Smith is to imagine a parallel case, retaining all the features of his case, including availability of resources and predicted survival, but substituting for Mr. Smith a 29-year-old black woman with 2 young children. The woman has systemic lupus erythematosus (SLE) with chronic glomerulonephritis, requiring treatment with immunosuppressive agents. She does not smoke, drink, or use recreational drugs. Yet, her life expectancy is substantially reduced by the combination of SLE, immunosuppression, and cardiac valve infections; it is roughly comparable to that of an intravenous cocaine drug abuser with infective endocarditis.

It seems likely that every surgeon would offer this woman a second operation. Any surgeon who would make such an offer, however, must make the same offer to Mr. Smith. The facts that she leads a praiseworthy life and her acquisition of a cardiac valve infection is "innocent" and that he is a member of a despised group, drug addicts, and his infection is "self-inflicted" are of no relevance to the surgical decision. In making treatment decisions, Dr. Jones must free his mind of biases and moral prejudgment. He must do this to discharge his first responsibility—the care of his patient.

If a surgeon applies the comparison test and finds that he would operate on the innocent patient but still cannot, in good conscience, offer an operation to the drug addict, he can consider alternative courses. He can seek advice from experienced, trusted colleagues or an ethics committee in thinking through the many complexities of the case, or he can refer the patient to another surgeon. He should not, however, simply declare that an operation is not indicated and close the book. He owes more than that to every patient.

References

1. Illich I. Medical nemesis. *Lancet.* 1974;i:918–21.
2. Fitzgerald FT. The tyranny of health. *N Engl J Med.* 1994;331:196–8.
3. Frater RW. Surgical management of endocarditis in drug addicts and long-term results. *J of Card Surg.* 1990;5:63–7.
4. Smyth B, Hoffman V, Fan J, Hser YI. Years of potential life lost among heroin addicts 33 years after treatment. *Prev Med.* 2007;44:369–74.
5. Smyth B, Fan J, Hser YI. Life expectancy and productivity loss among narcotics addicts thirty-three years after index treatment. *J Addict Dis.* 2006;25:37–47.
6. Perucci CA, Forastiere F, Rapiti E, Davoli M, Abeni DD. The impact of intravenous drug use on mortality of young adults in Rome, Italy. *Addict.* 2006;87:1637–41.
7. Oppenheimer E, Tobutt C, Taylor C, Andrew T. Death and survival in a cohort of heroin addicts from London clinics: a 22-year follow-up study. *Addict.* 1994;89:1299–1303.
8. Yamaguchi H, Eishi K. Surgical treatment of active infective mitral valve endocarditis. *Ann Thorac Cardiovasc Surg.* 2007;13:150–5.

9. Delay D, Pellerin, M, Carrier M, et al. Immediate and long-term results of valve replacement for native and prosthetic valve endocarditis. *Ann Thorac Surg.* 2000;70:1219–23.

10. Savage S, Covington EC, Heit HA, Hunt J, Joranson D, Schnoll SH. Definitions related to the use of opioids for the treatment of pain: a consensus document for the American Academy of Pain Medicine, the American Pain Society, and the American Society for Addiction Medicine. Chevy Chase, MD: American Society of Addiction Medicine; February 13, 2001.

11. Sade RM. The primary obligation of physicians should be to their patients, not to society. *J So Carolina Med Assoc.* 2006;102:81–3.

12. Council on Ethical and Judicial Affairs, American Medical Association. Ethical considerations in the allocation of organs and other scarce medical resources among patients. *Arch Int Med.* 1995;155:29–40.

13. Pross C. Nazi doctors, German medicine, and historical truth. In: Annas GJ, Grodin M, eds. *The Nazi Doctors and the Nuremberg Code: Human Rights in Human Experimentation.* New York: Oxford University Press; 1992:32–52.

14. Council on Ethical and Judicial Affairs, American Medical Association. E-2.03: Allocation of limited medical resources. Code of Medical Ethics: current opinions with annotations, 2008–2009 ed. Chicago: American Medical Association; 2008:9–10.

SECTION 4

Innovation and Uses of Technology

Robert M. Sade

Be not the first by whom the New are try'd,
Nor yet the last to lay the Old aside.

—Alexander Pope ("An Essay on Criticism," 1711)

Innovation is constant in surgery, usually arising from incremental changes in a procedure. Most innovation need not be reported to the patient during the informed-consent process; in fact, many improvements cannot be reported to the patient because they occur on-the-fly during an operation. Sometimes, however, planned innovation departs substantially from standard practice and in those cases should be reported to the patient and his or her consent obtained. Innovation is distinguished from research by the absence of systematic collection of data intended to develop or contribute to generalized knowledge. The line between the two often becomes indistinct when a single innovation is repeated several times and data from medical records entered onto a spreadsheet. When a surgeon begins to think about publishing a successful innovation as a series of cases, then the innovation becomes research, and formal application to an institutional review board should be undertaken.

The introduction of a new technology usually results from research rather than innovation. The research may be initiated by a surgeon or by a company—many of the most important technological advances in surgery have been made possible by collaboration between surgeons and industry (see chapter 24).

Technology is the lifeblood of the art and science of surgery—this has been true for millennia. The use of various tools to treat injuries goes back to prehistory, as one of the earliest uses of homo sapiens' ability to use tools was for the treatment of fractures and wounds. Burr holes resulting from trepanning of the skull have been found in human remains from Neolithic times.[1] The earliest record of devices to treat injuries, fractures, and wounds of all kinds is 3,500 years old: the Edwin Smith Papyrus, an Egyptian scroll describing the treatment of forty-eight traumatic injuries.[2] The use of medical devices was described by writers in antiquity and the Middle Ages. From the time of Galen (129–216 CE), the development of clinical technologies was virtually stagnant for more than 1,500 years; for example, the practice of bloodletting from the times of Hippocrates (460–370 BCE) and Galen persisted well into the nineteenth century.[3]

Surgical technologies blossomed in the mid-nineteenth century after the introduction of anesthesia and antisepsis. These were soon followed by the development of artificial ventilation, endotracheal intubation, and a host of innovations that made surgery easier and safer and also led to operations that were not previously possible. Some new technologies were found to work well, were celebrated, and came into wide use. Others appeared to be useful but were later found to be flawed and were abandoned. Operations that later turned out to be passing fads included ligation of the internal thoracic arteries to treat angina pectoris, nephropexy for "floating kidney," colectomy for epilepsy, and laparotomy "to let the air in" for the treatment of abdominal tuberculosis.[4] Recently, a well-known sham-controlled clinical trial demonstrated that arthroscopic surgery for osteoarthritis of the knee had no better results than medical treatment.[5] A procedure that had a brief period of popularity and notoriety before becoming discredited was the neurosurgical procedure of prefrontal lobotomy for treating a range of psychiatric conditions, for which Egas Moniz won the Nobel Prize for Medicine and Physiology in 1949.[6] Gastric freezing to treat ulcer disease had a brief surge of popularity in the 1960s before its harms were found to outweigh its benefits.[7] A wide range of controversial techniques in plastic surgery have been introduced, and many are still in use, seemingly for the central purpose of marketing a surgical practice.[8] Every field of surgery has seen its share of passing fads and failed technologies.

The introduction of new technologies in the mid-twentieth century was largely responsible for the emergence of contemporary biomedical ethics. The introduction of hemodialysis to treat end-stage renal failure in the 1950s and of artificial ventilation to support failing respiratory function in the 1960s resulted in large numbers of patients who would have died in earlier eras but now were on life support from which they could not be removed, especially in cases of neurological injuries. Interestingly, the new field of bioethics was driven less by philosophy and medicine than by the law in cases such as those of Karen Ann Quinlan (a court case in which the New Jersey Supreme Court established the right to refuse life-sustaining medical treatment) and Nancy Beth Cruzan (a case in which the US Supreme Court found that states could require an unusually high level of evidence that the patient would have wanted to die and that nutrition and hydration are medical treatments that can be refused).[9]

The development and implementation of new devices and technologies have produced numerous ethical dilemmas for surgeons. Many such technologies are expensive, raising questions of rationing—should a device be withheld in certain cases where it might be only marginally helpful? Technologies such as ventricular assist devices, da Vinci robots, and transcatheter aortic valve replacement have created a range of ethical dilemmas for surgeons. This section addresses a few such problems.

Chapters

Chapter 15 addresses the regulation and oversight of surgical innovation as distinguished from surgical research, recognizing that the first often shades into the second.[10] The most serious objection to regulating innovation is the potential for it to undermine or obstruct the advances that have been the lifeblood of surgery for many decades. Yet innovation suffers from many of the same conflicts of interest, particularly nonfinancial conflicts, that threaten research. Could innovation be regulated in a way that protects patients but at the same time does not threaten advances in surgery? One of the participants proposes a candidate for such regulation: collegial review of a proposed major innovation by a departmental review committee charged with establishing guidelines for carrying out the innovative procedure safely. The review process would be both prospective before it is initiated and retrospective, examining the results after the new procedure has been carried out. In this way, a stifling bureaucracy can be avoided.

Chapter 16 presents a debate on one of the most controversial technologies to appear in recent years: robotic surgery.[11] A young surgeon's use and promotion of robotic surgery affects the practice of an older colleague in the target vignette. The older surgeon is determined to learn how to do robotic surgery himself, raising several ethically relevant issues: declining mental and physical function related to the age difference between the two surgeons, the propriety of competition serving to motivate learning a complex new technique, and uncertainties about the effectiveness of robotic surgery. Is the older surgeon wrong to seek training in a new technology as a response to competition?

Several of the sessions sponsored by the Ethics Forum are related to a recent, fast-spreading surgical technology, transcatheter aortic valve replacement (TAVR). This technique involves the transcatheter insertion of a device that replaces the function of the aortic valve by way of percutaneous vascular access or the left ventricular apex. TAVR initially was reserved for patients with comorbidities or severity of disease that contraindicated standard aortic-valve replacement. The ethical questions raised by TAVR are relevant to all fields of surgery, as they all encounter problems related to sophisticated new technologies. **Chapter 17** explores contemporary implications of a decades-old observation: the positive association between high volumes of certain diseases and procedures by hospitals and surgeons and positive outcomes in terms of mortality and morbidity.[12] But should access to TAVR be limited to high-volume surgical centers because of this positive association? Evidence is produced to support and oppose limitation of access to TAVR. Also addressed is the question of whether access to surgical procedures should be limited by consideration of excellence of performance or of surgical competence. Nearly all of the many reports exploring volume–outcome associations are cross-sectional analyses; should such snapshots be used as a rationale for limiting access, given that surgical volumes and outcomes are not static but rather are moving targets?

Questions regarding rationing of expensive technologies have been prominent in ethics-related publications for decades, beginning in the 1950s with hemodialysis machines to treat renal failure. In **chapter 18**, the discussion of rationing focuses on an elderly man who was rejected for transcatheter aortic valve implantation (TAVI, an early acronym of TAVR) because of his lack of a social support system and the expense of the procedure.[13] One of the essayists asserts that explicit rationing would not be ethical at this time, although it might become a reality in the future; the other believes that use of the technology should be controlled and monitored by the medical profession, which he believes will result in patients and physicians making wise decisions that will effectively limit its use. One of the essayists asserts that the first concern of physicians must be the patient's best interests, and withholding a particular technology from one's patient despite a positive benefit–harm balance is inconsistent with this responsibility.

References

1. Brothwell DR. *Digging up Bones: The Excavation, Treatment and Study of Human Skeletal Remains*. London: British Museum of Natural History; 1963:126.
2. Nunn JF. *Ancient Egyptian Medicine*. Norman: University of Oklahoma Press; 1996: 26–28.
3. Wooton D. *Bad Medicine*. New York: Oxford University Press; 2007.
4. Johnson AG. Surgery as a placebo. *Lancet* 1994;344:1140–1142.

5. Moseley JB, O'Malley K, Petersen NJ, et al. A controlled trial of arthroscopic surgery for osteoarthritis of the knee. *New Engl J Med.* 2002;337:81–88.

6. Jansson B. Controversial Psychosurgery resulted in a Nobel Prize. http://www.nobelprize.org/nobel_prizes/medicine/laureates/1949/moniz-Chapter.html. Accessed March 19, 2014.

7. Edmonson JM. Gastric freezing: the view a quarter century later. *J Lab Clin Med.* 1989;114(5):613–614.

8. Bosshardt R. Whatever happened to . . .? Passing fads in plastic surgery. House Calls, March 11, 2014. http://www.hypeorlando.com/house-calls/2014/03/11/whatever-to-happened-to-passing-fads-in-plastic-surgery/. Accessed March 20, 2014.

9. Annas GJ. *Standard of Care: the Law of American Bioethics.* New York: Oxford University Press; 1993:3–12.

10. Morreim EH, Mack M, Sade RM. Is surgical innovation too dangerous to remain unregulated? *Ann Thorac Surg.* 2006;82:1957–1965.

11. Smyth JK, Deveney KE, Sade RM. Who should adopt robotic surgery, and when? *Ann Thorac Surg.* 2013;96(4):1132–1137.

12. Sade RM. Should access to transcatheter aortic valve replacement be limited to high-volume surgical centers? *J Thorac Cardiovasc Surg.* 2013;145(1):1439–1440; Bavaria JE. Access to transcatheter aortic valve replacement should be limited to high volume centers. *J Thorac Cardiovasc Surg.* 2013;145:1441–1443; Green P, Rosner GF. Leon MB, Schwartz A. Access to TAVR should not be limited to high volume surgical centers. *J Thorac Cardiovasc Surg.* 2013;145:1444–1445.

13. Sade RM. Should use of transcatheter aortic valve implantation be rationed? *J Thorac Cardiovasc Surg.* 2012;143(4):769–770; Mayer JE Jr. Transcatheter aortic valve implantation should be controlled and monitored by the medical profession. *J Thorac Cardiovasc Surg.* 2012;143(4):771–773; Wheatley GH III. Use of transcatheter valve should not be rationed. *J Thorac Cardiovasc Surg.* 2012;143(4):774–775.

15

Surgical Innovation

TOO RISKY TO REMAIN UNREGULATED?

Haavi Morreim, Michael J. Mack,
and Robert M. Sade*

Introduction

Robert M. Sade, MD

A recent investigation of cardiothoracic surgical studies involving human
subjects [...] showed that only 10% of such studies are randomized clinical
trials, the gold standard for human research. This should not be surprising,
because surgical studies are qualitatively different from medical investigations, for example, drug trials, in a number of ways. Surgical trial protocols
that use placebo controls or controls with no treatment are often not ethical
or not desirable, or both. Target populations for many surgical procedures
are often quite small, so series large enough for accurate statistical evaluation may be difficult to develop. Double-blind studies are usually not possible
because the surgeon-investigator must always know what he is doing. Most
importantly, surgical procedures are characterized by a learning curve that
leads to progressively improving skill in performing the procedure, and small
incremental changes in the procedure itself lead to progressive improvement
in results.

Most progress in surgery comes from innovation that does not fit
into the category of surgical research. A commonly accepted definition of
research is that contained in federal regulations regarding human subject
research: "Research means a systematic investigation, including research
development, testing, and evaluation, designed to develop or contribute to

*Morreim EH, Mack M, Sade RM. Is surgical innovation too dangerous to remain unregu-
lated? *Ann Thorac Surg.* 2006;82:1957–65. Copyright Society of Thoracic Surgeons, republished
here with permission.

generalized knowledge." Innovative surgery is often not systematic but is designed to benefit individual patients; there is often no intent to publish the surgical series at a later time, or such intent is secondary. Thus, most surgical innovation is outside the scope of "research" and not subject to oversight by institutional review boards (IRB).

A surgeon's decision-making is generally motivated by pursuit of the patient's best interests, yet other motivators lurk in the shadows; for example, pursuit of the surgeon's interests, such as increasing personal income. Most surgeons recognize the importance of placing the patient's interests above their own and reject even the intimation of any temptation to recommend unjustified operations for personal gain.

Surgeons who wish to be innovative, however, may have additional interests of their own to pursue ahead of those of their patients: the intangible reward of emotional excitement from breaking new ground and making new discoveries, the possibility of enhanced reputation and of academic advancement through discovery of new information and its publication; the possibility of obtaining grants, awards, or contracts to create a formal clinical trial if an innovation is successful, and perhaps the satisfaction of very strong personal dedication to advancing the science of medicine.

The following case illustrates surgical innovation that is clearly not research, is outside the domain of the IRB, but perhaps requires some kind of oversight.

CASE

At general surgery grand rounds, Dr. Outinfrunt, a cardiothoracic surgeon at Far South University Health Sciences Center, learns of FlexTexPatch, a new tightly woven polymeric fabric that is used as a covering for abdominal wall defects and as a vascular patch. It has been available for several years in Europe and recently became available in the United States. A few reports in European journals regarding its use as a vascular patch indicate that the material does not calcify as other patch materials do and seems particularly resistant to thrombosis. Dr. Outinfrunt looks up the material's technical specifications and finds that it is resistant to tearing, supple, easy to suture, dimensionally stable, and highly durable, as well as resistant to calcification and thrombosis.

[…] He obtains samples of several different thicknesses of the material and brings them to the autopsy room where he uses them to augment human mitral and aortic valve tissue. He is very pleased with the handling of the material and its strength in holding sutures. This experience, combined with what he learned about FlexTexPatch's technical specifications and its performance as a vascular patch, leads him to believe that this will be an excellent material to use for valve reconstruction.

The following week, Dr. Outinfrunt has a patient with severe aortic insufficiency who has been scheduled for valvuloplasty. Preoperatively, he conducts his usual discussion with the patient about the benefits and risks of the operation. He also explains in some detail that he intends to use a new material, FlexTexPatch, rather than the pericardium that he has used in the past, because he believes it may be superior in the long run. The patient understands and agrees to the plan, and signs an operative consent form.

Dr. Outinfrunt completes the operation and is satisfied with the result. He decides to use this material for such operations in the future. If it works out as satisfactorily as he believes it will, he may even be able to publish his results.

A month later, the patient is readmitted to the hospital with progressive fatigue and dyspnea and echocardiographic findings of severe aortic incompetence. The patch is intact, but the adjacent thin aortic leaflet has torn, due in part to its fixation to a stiffer artificial material and the stresses of frequent opening and closing of the valve. Dr. Outinfrunt reoperates, performing an aortic valve replacement. [. . .]

Dr. Outinfrunt's approach to surgical innovation in this case is repeated daily in different forms by cardiothoracic surgeons throughout the United States. Should there be some form of oversight for surgical innovation?

Pro
Haavi Morreim, PhD

Surgery isn't medicine. On this we can agree, and much more. As Dr. Sade points out in his introduction, advances in surgery often do not lend themselves to evaluation by way of the gold standard of clinical trials: double-blind, randomized, (placebo-)controlled. As he also points out, the real work of surgical advancement often comes through incremental innovations, not the decisive sweeps of change that may more obviously require—and permit—a clinical trial. [. . .]

Just as importantly, we can agree that this surgeon is highly conscientious and serious about undertaking this innovation in an ethically sound way. He has identified a clear problem with the current standard of care, namely, the significant inadequacies of using pericardium for valve reconstruction. He has done his homework, from evaluating the new FlexTexPatch's technical specifications and its performance in Europe, to hands-on work in the cadaver lab. And he has ensured that his patient knows that part of the proposed surgery is innovative, and the patient agrees to try it. [. . .]

THE DOWNSIDE OF SURGICAL INNOVATION

We also know that surgical innovations can fail, even those that initially appear very promising. As noted by Henry Beecher in 1961, "[v]arious surgical procedures have been recommended and carried out for the relief of angina pectoris," including ligation of the internal mammary arteries—a procedure that became widely used until finally shown to be no better than placebo.[1] Indeed, "[t]he history of surgery abounds with examples of operations that were fashionable at the time and then abandoned after being found to have no specific effect. Examples include nephropexy for so-called 'floating-kidney,' colectomy for epilepsy, and laparotomy for abdominal tuberculosis 'to let the air in'."[2] Even well-accepted contemporary surgical procedures have been shown, on closer and more rigorous examination, to be no better than placebo.[3] As suggested by some commentators, surgery may itself be the placebo. As the case before us in this debate would indicate, even theoretically attractive, thoughtfully conducted innovations can bring nasty surprises.[4]

Nothing—not the greatest care nor the most extensive regulation—can avoid all the risks and adverse outcomes that can accompany surgical innovation. And yet, the fact that we cannot avoid all risk does not mean we cannot reduce it. Where a surgeon contemplates a significant change from prevailing practice, he may needlessly exacerbate the risks when he declines to seek an honest evaluation from colleagues. Moreover, the one who is most enthused about the idea may be least likely to see its potential drawbacks, and the one who has been the most immersed in the idea can, at a certain point, be least likely to see its alternatives and potentially helpful improvements.

Martin McKneally has discussed the need for "a systematic approach to the introduction and evaluation of new surgical procedures."[5] He does not recommend formal regulation such as government might impose, but rather a collegial sort of oversight in which such procedures would be reviewed and quite possibly improved before introduction on patients. [...]

Amplifying on McKneally's lead, I shall propose a mechanism considerably less formal than an IRB process, yet potentially as or more effective in protecting those patients who may be early recipients of surgical innovation. I will describe, first, what kinds of innovations should be subjected to formal collegial review before human implementation; second, what should be included in such a review; and third, how such a review process should be enforced within the profession.

This proposal does not suggest that surgical innovations should routinely be subjected to the rigors of formal clinical research (which would then require IRB review). [...] Rather, I will recommend a fairly informal collegial review of major innovations, a kind of in-house "curbside consult" designed to improve good ideas and weed out those that fellow surgeons consider too risky or still too unrefined to try on patients. [...]

A MECHANISM FOR REDUCING RISKS BY REQUIRING REVIEW

What to Review

Clearly, it would be unwieldy, unnecessary, and in most cases, impossible to review every prospective innovation in surgery. A good surgeon must adapt procedures to any patient's anatomic anomalies and idiosyncrasies, a process of "custom innovation" that often cannot even be anticipated, let alone prospectively reviewed. And many other modifications are incremental refinements more than significant changes. Evolving practical experience often shows the need for such refinements and renders their desirability obvious. And because they are small, they rarely bring significant unanticipated risks.

Rather, the collegial review I propose would be applied to the major innovations—those that are substantial enough that a conscientious surgeon must think them through in advance, conceive of them from start to finish (including potential problems and their solutions), and likely test them in the laboratory. These are the innovations that, if successful, would be good candidates for publication in a professional journal, to share with colleagues, and hopefully, improve practices to help patients elsewhere. [...]

Hence, we might suggest a rule of thumb: if a contemplated innovation would be important enough to share after the fact if successful, then it is significant enough to be evaluated before the fact to increase its chances of success and reduce its odds of adverse outcomes.

How to Review

The surgery departments within any institution in which significant surgical innovations are likely to be contemplated should establish a mechanism for assembling a group with the appropriate expertise to evaluate prospectively the kinds of innovations just described. Mainly, these institutions will be academic hospitals. [...]

The review should include, though not be limited to:

- ensuring that current management truly is inadequate or problematic;
- ensuring that the theoretical merits of the proposed innovation withstand scrutiny;
- identifying any need for further theoretical examination, and specifying improvements that might reduce risk and enhance likelihood of success;
- assuring that preparatory studies with animals or cadavers, or both, are adequate and identifying any need for further testing;
- making appropriate refinements on the original idea;
- crafting suitable criteria for patient selection and for surgeon selection (the surgeon who conceives the idea may not always be the best one to undertake it);

◻ determining the kind and amount of training that should be undertaken by the surgical team before human testing;

◻ determining the adequacy of local resources such as equipment and nursing personnel;

◻ stipulating what sort of information should be provided in the consent process (the review committee may wish to approve a written consent form); and

◻ specifying a reasonable interval(s) at which to require follow-up information about each patient's outcome.

As suggested by the last element, the review process should not just be prospective. It should be retrospective. When the innovative procedure is completed and a patient's outcome is reasonably clear, the same group should reassemble to discuss:

◻ how well the realities matched the hopes;

◻ any unanticipated problems;

◻ whether this innovation warrants repetition; and

◻ if so, what sort of patient would be suitable, and how best to address whatever problems arose during the prior patient's operative procedure and postoperative care.

Enforcement Options

Enforcement mechanisms would not inquire into the details of whether the review group has performed adequately, but rather would inquire whether the review has taken place in good faith. [...]

Various mechanisms could ensure reviews are conducted. Theoretically, government could issue regulations, or large agencies such as the Joint Commission on Accreditation of Healthcare Organizations (JCAHO) might step in. I would not recommend either, however. If the collegial review process described above were mandated from outside the surgical realm, it could easily spawn inflexible bureaucracy and the gamesmanship that often follow. Quickly, form could dominate substance.

I would prefer essentially market-based structures that could foster genuinely effective review, based on mutual respect and collegiality. For instance, professional organizations such as the American College of Surgeons, the American Association for Thoracic Surgery, and the Society of Thoracic Surgeons could state clearly that they expect institutions whose surgeons engage in significant innovation to establish such review mechanisms. [...]

In addition, because many innovative procedures will take place at academic institutions, residency accrediting bodies could require such a mechanism in any program undergoing the (re)accreditation process. Detecting failure to comply could be relatively straightforward. [...] Sanctions for noncompliance can mirror those applied to any other significant failure within a residency program, from remedial actions to probation to, if warranted for repeated and un-remediated violations, loss of accreditation.

One other source of informal enforcement can come from the broader community. Business firms increasingly encourage their employees to seek health care at the best institutions in the belief that higher quality health care is not only medically better but, in the long run, also more economic. The LeapFrog Group, for instance, [...] disseminates information about hospital quality ratings to member organizations, [...] and gives employees incentives to seek higher quality care.[6] Once IRCs are established as a best practice, it is reasonable to expect that corporations such as those belonging to LeapFrog or any similar organization may include IRCs as a criterion for identifying its preferred providers.

CONCLUSION

Surgery cannot progress without the creative efforts of its best surgeons constantly considering how to improve patients' care. Even as these efforts should be encouraged, major innovations can carry significant hazards. Surgeons need to monitor and guide that progress. Truly, two minds are better than one, and collective wisdom should be sought before a surgeon exposes a patient to the risks that inevitably accompany the potential benefits of a new procedure or a new use of an existing device. The innovation review process described here does not represent a stifling bureaucracy imposed from outside. Rather, it calls upon surgeons to collect their best wisdom as they push forward the boundaries of professional practice.

Con
Michael J. Mack, MD

Surgical innovation has resulted in remarkable advances in the treatment of human disease and suffering. This is particularly true in the past 50 years of cardiac surgery, from the invention of the heart-lung machine, development of heart and lung transplantation, and ventricular assist device therapy to coronary artery bypass and valve surgery. These advances have occurred through a complex system that strikes an effective and productive balance of fostering innovation and introducing new therapy into clinical medicine in an efficacious manner while ensuring patient safety. Professor Morreim is now proposing to upset that delicate balance between innovation and regulation by introducing another bureaucratic layer of committees, which I am afraid, will stifle the innovative process.

[...] [I]t strikes me that although it is hard to argue with the concept of an IRC in theory, the barriers that would be constructed to successful adoption and implementation of innovation by these regulatory bodies, however informal, are such that what will be created is a quagmire of ineffectiveness. Idealism is directly proportional to the distance from an issue. Although the proposal is well intentioned and sensible in theory, my view is that it is an unnecessary intrusion into an intricate, balanced system that is already working and serving patients well.

INNOVATION VERSUS RESEARCH

[...] Innovation is defined as a change in therapy to benefit an individual, whereas research is a "protocolized" study, the goal of which is to gain knowledge but not necessarily benefit the individual being treated. [...] Innovative therapies are characterized by being both novel and nonvalidated, which have attributes of both research and clinical practice. [...]

I would rather submit that this is an artificial distinction, and both processes—whether innovation or research, no matter how informal or formalized—are in fact embodiments of the scientific method. [...] The scientific method is the bedrock of every innovation that occurs in surgery, either informal in the surgeon's mind or formalized in a research protocol. To create a "gray zone" between what constitutes clinical practice and research endeavors that requires regulation is at least nonproductive and at most counterproductive. As Chalmers has stated: "The practice of medicine is in effect the conduct of clinical research ... Every practicing physician conducts clinical trials daily as he is seeing patients. The research discipline known as the 'clinical trial' is the formalization of this daily process."[7]

EVALUATION OF NEW TECHNOLOGY AND TECHNIQUES IN SURGERY

To dissect this issue further, it may be helpful to examine how new technology and techniques are introduced into surgery. Innovation in surgery is a complex process that is different from the introduction of new therapies in other areas of medicine. In the world of drug therapy, a standardized treatment—a pill—can be introduced into a study population and its effect, beneficial or otherwise, be determined by appropriate trial design; however, the evaluation of effectiveness is much more complex and difficult in surgery. Variables that need to be accounted for in surgery include not only the innovative technique or device and subsequent iterations of both but also surgeon expertise, the procedural learning curve, the disease being treated, and the ability to distinguish the effects of the therapy from the disease being treated. Operations are not standardized, and one cannot separate the operative procedure from the surgeon performing it. Surgery is a not a pill and, therefore, cannot be evaluated as a pill; it is an iterative process, as is the sustaining technology to facilitate it.

The standards applied to nonsurgical medical research are not generally applicable to the design of surgical research. These difficulties impact the ethics of surgical innovation. Whereas the randomized clinical trial is the highest order of evidence-based medicine, here are many factors that make implementation of that research tool difficult in surgery:[8]

◻ First, it is generally impossible to achieve full blinding in surgical research.

◻ Second, surgery has a powerful placebo effect that may exist independently of the general efficacy of an operation.

◻ Third, as Francis D. Moore has observed, "the most remarkable and effective extensions of surgery have often not required elaborate statistical analysis for their establishment."

◻ Fourth, there are situations in which randomized clinical trials may be both impractical and ethically dubious. The advisability of a trial is open to serious questions when thousands of patients must be treated to establish statistically significant but otherwise small differences.

◻ Fifth, randomized clinical trials may be impossible when the newer treatment for a given condition is in a state of rapid evolution. The introduction of off-pump coronary bypass surgery is a case in point here.

◻ Sixth, it is often difficult to launch controlled studies of surgical innovation after the new device or technique has become popular. This has been commonly termed "lost opportunity."

◻ Seventh, it is often difficult to justify the use of a "placebo," that is a sham procedure in surgery despite its scientific desirability. [...]

REGULATION OF SURGICAL INNOVATION

Innovation involves iterations of both device and techniques and significant oversight is already in place to regulate both. The US Food and Drug Administration (FDA) at the federal level, medical boards at the state level, and credentialing committees at the local hospital level provide appropriate oversight of medical practice and innovation. Furthermore, professional societies provide practice guidelines for the adoption and implementation of new technologies and techniques. [...] IRBs provide oversight of research at universities and community hospitals alike. [...] Lastly, research studies include data safety monitoring boards to adequately protect patient safety.

The FDA, according to its mission statement, is responsible for "protecting public health assuring the safety, efficacy, and security of ... medical devices...." The FDA is also responsible for "advancing public health by helping to speed innovation...."[9]

In recognition of the different levels of significance, there are different regulatory paths providing different levels of scrutiny by which new devices are approved by the FDA. The most stringent of these is the Pre-Market Approval, which is the process by which the FDA evaluates and regulates the safety and effectiveness of medical devices that support and sustain human life and are of substantial importance in preventing impairment of human health. Clinical studies on human subjects are less stringently regulated by the Individual Device Exemption (IDE) pathway. A more lenient regulatory process (510K) is available for devices that are substantially equivalent to already legally marketed devices. [...]

INNOVATION REVIEW COMMITTEES

Into this elaborate and effective regulatory structure, we now must consider adding another layer of review, the IRC. Morreim makes a number of assumptions of the practicality of implementing IRCs that are simply not true.

First, she claims that innovations are most likely to be contemplated in academic institutions, and therefore, appropriate personnel would be available to form committees. Although that may have been true in a bygone era, nonacademic institutions are frequently at the forefront of innovation and research, from laparoscopic cholecystectomy to coronary stent trials to off-pump coronary artery bypass surgery, because academicians and patients have moved to private practice settings.

Second is the assumption that the review would be collegial and altruistic. Many motivations form opinion—not all of which are consensus, expressed, and beneficial. The assumption that there would be unbiased, beneficent peers willing to "curbside consult" in the current practice environment is not realistic. [...]

Next is the opinion that the noninnovator would add balance to the assessment. The spectrum of practitioners range from the innovators to the early adopters to the late majority and the laggards. An IRC composed of laggards would be counterproductive to the process and not only not balance innovation, but would halt progress.

OPINION REGARDING THE HYPOTHETICAL CASE

My opinion regarding the hypothetical case presentation posed to us of Dr. Outinfrunt is that he acted in a moral and ethical manner despite the fact that his innovation did not work. He used an approved device in an off label use, which is legal and ethical. He was experienced and knew the shortcomings of the current therapy. He performed appropriate due diligence to test the device in the new application in a cadaver lab before the procedure, and he obtained informed consent from the patient about the use of this innovative device. He had a reasonable expectation of success that was based on the experience in the use of the device by others in other indications. The failure indeed may not have been related to the device itself, but rather to the suturing technique, to the disease process, or other patient factors. There is no evidence that he did this for self-gain, and he acted by all accounts in his own patient's best interest. [...]

Innovation is hard work. The easy path is to perform the standard proven operation despite its known inadequacies. The extra effort Dr. Outinfrunt expended in his attempt to improve his patient's outcome was laudable and the ultimate expression of individualization of care. It arose from the drive to make a difference and make a contribution to the human condition.

CONCLUSION

The expansion of oversight systems to surgical innovation that does not fall into the category of research will serve only to stifle the advancement of surgical science. [...] To promote innovation, one needs a regulatory environment that allows an easy start and adjustment to changing circumstances and opportunities and the ability to innovate. Lack of economic development in many African and Middle Eastern countries can be traced to excessive regulation. The same dynamics hold true for surgical innovation as they do for economic development. Adequate regulation of surgical research and innovation that does not fall in to the category of research already exists. Let's not fix something that isn't broken.

Concluding Remarks
Robert M. Sade, MD

Dr. Morreim has proposed an intriguing idea aimed at improving outcomes for patients who undergo innovative surgical procedures: prior review of the innovative idea by a suitably expert group, which she calls an Innovation Review Committee (IRC). [...]

Dr. Mack [...] suggests that IRCs with noninnovator members would be counterproductive and bring progress to a halt. Ultimately, he sees the IRC as regulatory excess attempting to fix a well-functioning system that is not broken.

Dr. Morreim, however, does not claim that the system is broken; rather, she recites evidence of unanticipated adverse consequences of several well-known innovative procedures and suggests that the IRC could be part of an overall effort to improve the quality of surgical care. Clearly, her intention is benevolent; however, one might ask: Which alternative weighs more heavily in the balance of benefits and harms: the potential benefit (improved outcomes) of innovative procedures or the potential harms (a stifling new layer of review)? A glimpse backward into the mid-20th century might be instructive.

An urgent need for oversight of clinical research was recognized in the wake of World War II. The Nuremberg trials of 1947–48 shed light on atrocious human experimentation during the Nazi regime. The revelations of those trials resulted in drafting of the Nuremberg Code, the first international guide to the ethics of human research.[10] Building on that foundation, the Declaration of Helsinki in 1964 promulgated more detailed guidelines.[11] In 1966, Beecher reported a study of 22 human experiments published in several of our foremost journals, conducted in leading medical schools, and funded by federal agencies and major foundations.[12] All were done without the consent of the subjects, mostly children and institutionalized mentally deficient adults, few of whom could have understood the nature of the experiment. [...]

Both the Nuremberg trials and the Beecher paper revealed horrific, unethical human experimentation and provided great impetus for the regulation of human subjects research and the development of IRBs. This brief retrospective prompts the question: What is the impetus for the development of IRCs? Is there evidence of widespread misdeeds associated with surgical innovation? Certainly, all innovations do not result in positive advances; many have failed in their intended outcomes, and some have resulted in fatalities. But such uncertainty of outcomes is to be expected whenever new territory is explored. If we must have some sort of prior review or regulation of innovative surgery, Dr. Morreim's suggestion makes sense—but must we have prior review?

The horns of the dilemma presented by this debate are two unpleasant choices, both arising from inadequate information: we are impaled on one horn by the discomfort of abandoning a well-known, comfortable process of innovation that we believe has served our patients well and on the other horn by the possibility that our process has serious flaws that might be easily repaired with a relatively innocuous fix. Unlike research, our current process of innovation operates almost entirely under the radar screen. It provides no information about the nature of major innovations actually attempted, how many there are, and their outcomes. The only innovations we hear about (outside of weekly service conferences) are the successes, and then only those that are important enough to warrant publishing. As a result, Dr. Morreim has no horrendous Nuremberg or Beecher experiences to support her case, and Dr. Mack has no recounting of the (hopefully) negligible number and severity of harms of innovations-gone-bad to bolster his. Dr. Mack cannot confidently assure us [...] that the system is not broken, nor can Dr. Morreim persuade us that it is.

The resolution of this dilemma, like that of all clinical conflicts, lies in choosing the alternative that will ultimately be best for our patients. But which is the right alternative? There seems only one objective way to make the choice. Some brave soul or institution that is committed to attempting to improve the lot of patients and is persuaded by the case Dr. Morreim has made must undertake a major innovation, an administrative trial, so to speak: designing and executing a study of an innovation review process such as she has suggested. I have neither the skill nor the temerity to suggest what the design ought to be, how or which outcomes ought to be measured, or what, if any, controls would be appropriate. Until the results of such an administrative trial are available, however, I am afraid we are stuck with (or on) the horns of this dilemma.

References

1. Beecher HK. Surgery as placebo. *JAMA*. 1961;176:88–93.
2. Johnson AG. Surgery as a placebo. *Lancet*. 1994;344:1140–2.
3. Moseley JB, O'Malley K, Petersen NJ, et al. A controlled trial of arthroscopic surgery for osteoarthritis of the knee. *New Engl J Med*. 2002;337:81–8.
4. Strasberg SM, Ludbrook PA. Who oversees innovative practice? *J Am Coll Surg*. 2003;196:938–48.
5. McKneally MF. Ethical problems in surgery: innovation leading to unforeseen complications. *World J Surg*. 1999;23:786–8.
6. LeapFrog group. http://www.leapfroggroup.org/. Accessed July 7–10, 2006.
7. Miller F, Rosenstein DL. The therapeutic orientation to clinical trials. *N Engl J Med*. 2003;348:1383–6.
8. Roy DJ, Black P, McPeek B, McKneally MF. Ethical principles in research. In: Troidl H, McKneally MF, Mulder DS, et al, eds. *Textbook on Surgical Research*. New York: Springer; 1997:581–604.
9. US Food and Drug Administration. Mission statement. Washington, DC: US Food and Drug Administration. http://www.fda.gov/opacom/morechoices/mission.html. Accessed December 19, 2005.
10. Annas GJ, Grodin MA. *The Nazi Doctors and the Nuremberg Code: Human Rights in Human Experimentation*. New York: Oxford University Press; 1992.
11. World Medical Association Declaration of Helsinki. Ethical principles for medical research involving human subjects. *JAMA*. 2000;284:3043–5.
12. Beecher HK. Ethics and clinical research. *N Engl J Med*. 1966;274:1354–60.

16

Who Should Adopt Robotic Surgery and When?

Jessica K. Smyth, Karen E. Deveney,
and Robert M. Sade*

Introduction
Robert M. Sade, MD

New technologies abound in the surgical specialties, cardiothoracic surgery
in particular. One of the more highly visible and controversial new technologies is robotic surgery—some claim that it is a useful adjunct to surgery, others that it is mostly a marketing tool. Assuming that it has a high utility value,
however, when should it be adopted in practice, and by whom? The following
case serves to focus discussion of opposing points of view.

CASE

Dr Pierre Jaloux, a 55-year-old highly respected cardiothoracic surgeon,
hires Dr Woody Randolph, a young well-trained surgeon who has recently
finished fellowship training in robotic surgery. The older surgeon plans to
cut back on his practice in about 10 years to work part time. Six months
later, Dr Randolph has developed a busy practice in robotic surgery and has
a growing reputation for very good outcomes. Dr Jaloux finds his patient
load declining because referring physicians and patients are impressed by
the robotic procedures. He has feelings of competitiveness and even jealousy
toward his new colleague, although they remain friendly and Dr Randolph
is, by any measure, clearly doing a great job. The older surgeon decides to

---

*Smyth JK, Deveney KE, Sade RM. Who should adopt robotic surgery, and when? *Ann
Thorac Surg.* 2013;96(4):1132–7. Copyright Society of Thoracic Surgeons, republished here with
permission.

take a 2-week course in robotic surgery and use the technology in his own practice to better compete with his young colleague. Should Dr Jaloux carry out his plan?

Pro
Jessica K. Smyth, MD

Presented with the case of Dr Jaloux, you may ask yourself, "How can any surgeon justify performing an operation when there is another surgeon available who is more experienced or skilled?" The mistake in this line of thinking is twofold. The first error is equating technical skill or experience with competence. Based solely on technical skill, one may falsely conclude that the best technician is the best surgeon. However, competence includes more than technical proficiency. Competence is the exercise of the required knowledge, judgment, and skill to perform a particular task reliably to produce an appropriate outcome.

The second flaw in this line of thinking is equating competence with perfection. At each institution in this country, it is likely there are a great number of competent surgeons. Sound quality assurance in surgery should provide patients with surgical care that is above the morally required threshold of competence, similar to the safety standards for aircraft pilots and bridge builders. Fine-grained distinctions of proficiency and expertise may be helpful in identifying appropriate surgeons for unusually complex cases, but it is unnecessary, and may be counterproductive, to make expertise rather than competence the reference standard for all surgical care.

As a highly respected academic surgeon, Dr Jaloux has likely demonstrated a high degree of competence, not only in his own performance, but also in his ability to oversee and train others. We can assume that over the course of his career, he has integrated new evidence and technology into his practice. Surgeons of all specialties are integrating evidence-based medicine and new technologies they mastered after residency training into their current practices. For example, neurosurgeons and otolaryngologists are now using an endoscopic transnasal transsphenoidal approach for the resection of many pituitary adenomas.[1] In orthopedic surgery, treatment of femoral shaft fractures has evolved from traction and casting to locked intramedullary nailing.[2] Cardiothoracic surgeons are rapidly adopting the recently approved technology of transcatheter aortic valve replacement for use when open replacement is deemed high risk.[3] Leading practitioners must incorporate new techniques after their formal training is complete to employ current best practices.

And isn't this one of the greatest draws of medicine—to be challenged, to continually learn and refine our expertise?

The daily responsibility for successfully performing invasive procedures on another human being distinguishes surgery from other branches of medicine. This is a sobering reminder. What allows an individual surgeon to do this? Our ability to operate comes not only from knowledge and technical expertise, but also through connecting with patients in such a way that they have confidence in our capabilities.

Over the course of his career, Dr Jaloux has assuredly developed significant relationships with his patients and their families. This supportive environment adds to the overall care he provides to them. Given that the number of patients has decreased, it is clear that his current scope of practice is not meeting their expectations. How many times has one of your patients said to you, "Well, I read on the Internet that this technique was better than that technique or that this course of treatment was better for my illness." Gaining this skill set will enable the senior physician to not only offer robotic surgery, but also enable him to discuss its advantages and disadvantages and to counsel his patients on the best treatment choice for their particular situation.

Ultimately the decision to pursue further training to effectively incorporate advanced technology into his practice should not stem from personal interests, but from what is in the best interest of the patients he serves. The scenario suggests that he is motivated by feelings of jealousy and competitiveness; however, the question to ask yourself is this: how many can boast of only altruistic motivation for every choice made along their career path? Oftentimes, decisions or actions are based on personal motives. However, further training and education most commonly result in better performance and better outcomes for the patient. The patient and the public may be harmed if physicians make clinical decisions based on factors other that what is best for the patient. That being said, having the capability to offer his patients multiple treatment options may be in the best interest of the patient.

So the crux of the scenario remains: how can a surgeon safely incorporate evolving technology into his practice?

Across the globe, health care delivery is undergoing a major evolution. The introduction of new technologies, the use of telemedicine to deliver health care remotely, and the evolving restrictions in work hours of trainee physicians are changing the face of medicine. Training physicians and surgeons in more specialized techniques, in shorter periods of time, while maintaining the highest levels of patient safety and in a cost-effective manner is a challenging order. This introduction of new technology and evolution of education and health care delivery should lead to improvement without harming patients in the process.

Robotic surgery was developed in response to the limitations and drawbacks of laparoscopic surgery. Since 1997 when the first robotic procedure was performed, various papers have been published highlighting the advantages of this technique. The robotic system offers several features, including intuitive movements, tremor filtration, stereoscopic vision, and motion scaling, which are thought to contribute to making robotic-assisted surgery more intuitive to conceptualize and master.

In a study performed by Kaul and colleagues,[4] operative times and learning curves were drawn for three surgeons: an experienced laparoscopic surgeon who had performed more than 1,000 procedures; an experienced open surgeon who was performing his or her first robotic radical prostatectomy; and a fellow who started performing robotic radical prostatectomies after having assisted and observed during more than 100 robotic procedures.

The robot decreased the learning curve for the experienced open surgeon so that by the seventh case, the operative times using the robot were faster than those of the experienced laparoscopic surgeon, who had performed more than 1,000 laparoscopic procedures. The fellow, who was mentored in robotics, performed his first robotic case faster than surgeons A and B, both of whom were more experienced surgeons.

Although our scenario implies that Dr Jaloux intends to go to a 2-week course and then introduce the technology into his own practice, there are professional standards and likely institutional requirements before he would be able to incorporate this technology in the operating room. He could begin with the course and then be mentored at his home institution by other surgeons already trained in robotics before he would be allowed to practice independently. Additionally, some institutions are now purchasing robotic simulators to aid staff in acquiring robotic skills.

Finally, this discussion wouldn't be complete without touching on the subject of age. What weight should be placed on the fact that the senior surgeon is 55? It is not uncommon for professionals to work well into their 60s and 70s. As a gauge, the average age of an incoming president is 55. Age is not, in and of itself, impairing. Studies on learning and age demonstrate that motivation and positive self-perception are directly linked to our capability to learn.

But let us be guided by words of the English physician, Dr Thomas Percival: "Let both the Physician and Surgeon never forget that their professions are public trusts, properly rendered lucrative whilst they fulfill them, but which they are bound by honor and probity to relinquish as soon as they find themselves unequal to their adequate and faithful execution."[5]

As I conclude, let me summarize: surgical care involves lifelong learning that should be directed to improving patient outcomes and may continue as long as there is due diligence to our professional obligations.

Con
Karen E. Deveney, MD

No, it would be wrong for Dr Jaloux to take a 2-week course in robotic surgery to compete with his younger, fellowship-trained colleague.

I base my opinion on three diverse arguments: (1) the effects of age on cognitive function, dexterity, and ability to learn new technologies; (2) the inappropriate, unethical reasons that are motivating him to learn robotics; and (3) the increased cost and lack of demonstrated superiority of robotic procedures.

Studies on cognitive function have demonstrated unequivocally that measured IQ declines in adults as they age. The average IQ of 100 in the 25- to 34-year-old person decreases to 90 by age 55 to 64, to 82 by age 65 to 74, and to 73 for persons over age 75 years.[6] Although these data apply to a general population and not MD's, studies that compare the abilities of non-MDs and MDs of varying ages performing tests measuring physical and mental traits such as reactivity, attention, numeric recall, verbal memory, visiospatial facility, reasoning, and mental calculation show that MDs decline with age more slowly, but still show a decrease of 5% in their total scores by age 60, and 10% by age 70.[7]

A study that looked specifically at cognitive and physical function of surgeons as they age was conducted using surgeon volunteers aged 45 years and older who were attending the Clinical Congress of the American College of Surgeons (ACS) between 2001 and 2006. Surgeons took a battery of tests measuring attention, reaction times, visual learning, and memory. The studies showed a gradual decline in all areas with aging.[8]

Studies of general surgeons recertifying on the American Board of Surgery examination show that the failure rate on the examination dramatically increases with age, from a mean of 3.6% on the first recertification taken 10 years after initial Board certification to 10.3% at 20 years and to 16.9% at 30 years.[9]

Although the above studies show that age is associated with a decline in cognition and knowledge and skill on surrogate tests of physical functioning, some would argue that the increased surgical experience with age can compensate for the decreased mental agility and manual dexterity that accompany aging. In fact, the effects of age and experience were studied as factors in outcomes of inguinal hernia repair in the much-quoted randomized, controlled, multi-institutional Veterans Affairs cooperative study of laparoscopic versus open inguinal hernia repair. In that study surgeons older than age 45 who had performed fewer than 250 laparoscopic repairs had a mean hernia recurrence rate of 18%, compared with 3.4% for surgeons younger than age 45.[10] This finding is consistent with results of a systematic review by Choudhry and associates[11] in which all but one of 59 studies found some decline in performance with increasing age or time in practice. Are these poorer outcomes fair to patients?

Opportunities for fully trained, older surgeons to learn new procedures are often limited to short courses with their inherent limitations on opportunities to practice a procedure longitudinally as is seen over the course of a several-year residency or even a 2-year fellowship. To perform robotic procedures requires not only a course, but also practice time on a trainer and proctoring in active practice. The steep learning curve of robotic cardiothoracic surgery has been explored in a few small studies in the literature. In one study of robotic coronary artery bypass graft surgery, four of five adverse graft outcomes occurred in the first quintile of cases. These investigators reviewed the reported experience at other centers and concluded that "even in the most experienced hands limited-access, telerobotic CABG involves a significant learning curve."[12] The steep learning curve has been looked at for complex robotic operations in other surgical specialties such as urology. After initial robotic training performing prostatectomy, it was found that 110 to 200 cases were necessary for a surgeon experienced in open procedures to achieve the level of competence that would demonstrate mastery of the robotic procedure.[13] The long learning curve for complex robotic procedures certainly takes it beyond a 2-week course, especially for an older surgeon with diminishing cognitive and physical skills.

Privileging to perform robotic procedures requires not only a formal course, but also a period of proctoring in practice. Who would be willing to provide such proctoring? The older surgeon's younger partner would be the natural person to proctor him, but for him to do so would detract from his own practice and also set up an awkward dynamic in which the younger surgeon may feel obligated to approve of the older surgeon's technical skills prematurely because they are partners. Finding a surgeon from elsewhere to proctor him for an adequate time would be difficult.

Finally, it may be anecdotal, but a prominent and famous academic endocrine surgeon, Atul Gawande, recently confessed that his outcomes had plateaued and he was no longer "beating the averages."[14] He wondered that "maybe this is what happens when you turn forty-five." He went on to say, "Surgery is, at least, a relatively late-peaking career"—not like mathematics, baseball, or pop music (which peak at age 30), but more like Standard & Poor's 500 CEOs (average age of hire, 52) or age of maximum productivity for geologists, 54. "Surgeons apparently fall somewhere between the extremes, requiring both physical stamina and the judgment that comes with experience. Apparently, I'd arrived at that middle point."

The second argument against the older surgeon's learning robotic surgery to compete with his younger partner is that his motivation is self-serving. Self-interest should never be an ethical justification for any action in the practice of medicine. One need look no further than the motto of the American College of Surgeons (ACS): "Omnibus per artem fidemque prodesse" (To serve all with skill and fidelity). Furthermore, the ACS mission statement maintains that "The American College of Surgeons is dedicated to improving the care of the surgical patient and to safeguarding standards of care in an optimal and ethical practice environment."[15] The basic principles of medical ethics require that one place the interests of the patient above those of one's own interest such as personal gain, promotion, or fame.

The third and last issue in this case is to query whether robotic surgery has even been shown to improve the care of the surgical patient. To date there is no evidence to support the superiority of robotic surgery over open surgery for any procedure. Although potential advantages of robotic procedures include better "3-D" vision, better magnification, decreased hand tremor, and facilitated suturing in a small space, robotic procedures also take longer, cost more, and are at best equivalent to open procedures in outcomes.[16] The role of robots in cardiac surgery has not been fully defined and, although it has "immense long-term potential to minimize morbidity and improve the outcomes of CABG procedures," only "highly specialized centers" can afford the cost and garner adequate experience to justify its use. In one study,[17] the researcher surveyed all US institutions that owned a da Vinci robot concerning the yearly volume of robotic heart operations and found that only an average of 7.3 cardiac operations were performed annually per robot, representing only 0.5% of all cardiac operations. Only 12% of programs performed more than 50 robotic procedures yearly. Although some centers did report good outcomes with robotic cardiac procedures, the outcomes did not exceed those of comparable minimally invasive methods.

For all of the above reasons, then, it would be wrong for the older surgeon to attend a 2-week robotic surgery course with the goal of competing with his younger, fellowship-trained colleague.

Concluding Remarks
Robert M. Sade, MD

Smyth and Deveney address three broad ethically relevant areas: mental and physical functioning, motivation, and effectiveness of robotic surgery. I would add a fourth to those three: marketing.

MENTAL AND PHYSICAL FUNCTION RELATED TO AGE

The debaters agree that 2 weeks of robotic training is inadequate to develop clinical competence; additional training on a simulator and a period of proctoring will be necessary. Deveney points to declining cognitive and physical functioning with age, although less so for physicians than others. Smyth does not challenge those findings but emphasizes the importance of noncognitive traits, such as experience, judgment, and adaptability, in determining competence. Both essayists analyze the question in general terms, but neither mentions the importance of individual variation. What should Dr. Jaloux, specifically, do? Much depends on his individual characteristics; for example, a highly intelligent and dexterous surgeon can lose 5% or 10% of his IQ and dexterity and still be highly intelligent and dexterous. On this point, I believe Smyth makes the stronger case.

MOTIVATION

Deveney finds Dr. Jaloux's motivation to be self-serving and asserts, "Self-interest should never be an ethical justification for any action in the practice of medicine." "Never" is a strong word, and it seems likely that we can never entirely rid ourselves of self-interest. One wonders whether attempting to maintain one's practice volume and the income it generates crosses an ethical line into unacceptable territory. Arguing to the contrary, Smyth suggests that jealousy and competitiveness may not be such a bad thing because, for surgeons, "Oftentimes, decisions or actions are based on personal motives." She softens this statement by pointing out that adopting new technologies commonly improves patient outcomes, but we can wonder whether it is right to base decisions on personal motives. Underlying motives are notoriously difficult to analyze and are seldom uncomplicated. Dr. Jaloux's motivation probably is not simple and includes concern for the safety and benefit of his patients. Most decisions surrounding patient care have complex motivations; ethically, the greatest weight must be given to the interests of the patient.[18] I believe Deveney has made the better case on this point.

EFFECTIVENESS OF ROBOTIC SURGERY

Ethical decision making in clinical medicine often requires weighing of benefits and harms first to the patient, then balancing benefits and harms to others, such as the physician, his partners, the hospital, and society in general. Dr. Jaloux faced this balancing act in deciding whether to learn robotic surgery. A critical factor is the potential for harm to his patients. For reasons Smyth enumerates, it seems likely that Dr. Jaloux can become competent at robotic lobectomy, and if he does not, the training and proctoring processes should inform him and others that he should not use this technique clinically.

Are the outcomes after robotic lobectomy better than, similar to, or worse than those after more standard approaches? Early reports suggest that initial survival and other outcome measures may be similar to standard approaches, but follow-up reports have been sparse, and comparisons of lobectomy techniques could be the topic of another debate that is beyond the scope of the present one. For our purposes, there seems to be no decisive clinical advantage or disadvantage to robotic lobectomy compared with open and video-assisted thoracic surgery approaches.

MARKETING

Much of the growth in robotic surgery may be driven by marketing efforts of hospitals and surgery programs.[19] Is there something intrinsically wrong with using new technologies to preserve or increase the patient base of a hospital or practice?

At one time, marketing was considered to be unethical, typified by this statement in the Principles of the American Medical Association (AMA) Code of Medical Ethics of 1957, Section 5: "A physician should not solicit patients."[20] This was taken to mean that all forms of advertising other than a simple public statement of name, address, telephone number, and nature of practice were unethical. A lawsuit alleging restraint of trade against the AMA by the Federal Trade Commission in 1975 resulted in an agreement in 1988 that included the AMA's removal of the prohibition against solicitation of patients from the Code of Medical Ethics.[21] For the last 25 years, advertising and other forms of marketing that are not false, deceptive, or misleading are deemed to be legal and are increasingly felt to be ethically acceptable. For many, however, some forms of legal marketing, such as using new technologies to build surgical volume, fail the sniff test. Yet, as long as new technologies are used competently, full and accurate information about advantages and disadvantages is provided, and patients are not harmed, there seems to be nothing intrinsically wrong with marketing.

Surgeons using robotic technology could be flirting with ethical boundaries, however, if they become involved with certain kinds of promotional activities; such issues are beyond the scope of the present case.

CONCLUSION

Dr. Jaloux has already made his decision to seek training in robotic surgery. The essayists both gave persuasive reasons why he should or should not decide to seek robotic training. They were not asked to advise him on what decision he should make, however; rather, they were asked to determine whether he should carry out the plan he has already made. We should assume that this highly respected surgeon's decision was based on adequate self-assessment of his own strengths and limitations and that he knows the only partially understood advantages and disadvantages of robotic lobectomy. Without good reason to believe his patients will be harmed, we seem not to have sufficient evidence to tell Dr. Jaloux that the decision he has made was wrong.

References

1. Loyo-Varela M, Herrada-Pineda T, Revilla-Pacheco F, et al. Pituitary tumor surgery: a review of 3004 patients. *World Neurosurg.* 2013;79(2):33–6.

2. Blasier RB. The problem of the aging surgeon: when surgeon age becomes a surgical risk factor. *Clin Orthop Relat Res.* 2009;467:402–11.

3. Stone ML, Kern JA, Sade RM. Transcatheter aortic valve replacement: clinical aspects and ethical considerations. *Ann Thorac Surg.* 2012;94(6):1791–5.

4. Kaul S, Shah NL, Menon M. Learning curve using robotic surgery. *Curr Urol Rep.* 2006;7:125–9.

5. Percival T. *Medical Ethics, or, a Code of Institutes and Precepts, Adapted to the Professional Conduct of Physicians and Surgeons.* London: Johnson & Bickerstaff; 1803.

6. Kaufman AS. *Assessing Adolescent and Adult Intelligence.* Boston: Allyn & Bacon; 1990.

7. Powell D. *Profiles in Cognitive Aging.* Cambridge, MA: Harvard University Press; 1994.

8. Bieliauskas LA, Langenacker S, Graver C, et al. Cognitive changes and retirement among senior surgeons: results from the CCRASS study. *J Am Coll Surg.* 2008;207:69–79.

9. Rhodes RS, Biester TW. Certification and maintenance of certification in surgery. *Surg Clin North Am.* 2007;87:825–36.

10. Neumayer LA, Gawande AA, Wang J, et al. Proficiency of surgeons in inguinal hernia repair: effect of experience and age. *Ann Surg.* 2005;242:344–52.

11. Choudhry NK, Fletcher RH, Soumerai SB. Systematic review: the relationship between clinical experience and quality of health care. *Ann Intern Med.* 2005;142:260–73.

12. Novick RJ, Fox SA, Klail BB, et al. Analysis of the learning curve in telerobotic, beating heart coronary artery bypass grafting: a 90 patient experience. *Ann Thorac Surg.* 2003;76:749–53.

13. Doumerc N, Yuen C, Saudie R, et al. Should experienced open prostatic surgeons convert to robotic surgery? The real learning curve for one surgeon over three years. *Br J Urol Int* 2010;106:378–84.

14. Gawande AA. Personal best. *The New Yorker*, October 3, 2011.

15. American College of Surgeons Bulletin. www.facs.org. Accessed November 2012.

16. Rawlings AL, Woodland JH, Vegunta K, et al. Robotic versus laparoscopic colectomy. *Surg Endosc.* 2007;21:1701–8.

17. Robicsek F. Robotic cardiac surgery: time told! *J Thorac Cardiovasc Surg.* 2008;135:243–6.

18. Council on Ethical and Judicial Affairs. Principle VIII. In: Code of Medical Ethics of the American Medical Association, 2012–2013 ed. Chicago: American Medical Association; 2012:lxxi–xxv.

19. Schiavone MB, Kuo EC, Naumann RW, et al. The commercialization of robotic surgery: unsubstantiated marketing of gynecologic surgery by hospitals. *Am Obstet Gynecol.* 2012;207:174.

20. Judicial Council, American Medical Association. Principles of medical ethics. Chicago: American Medical Association; 1957. http://www.ama-assn.org/resources/doc/ethics/1957_principles.pdf. Accessed February 13, 2013.

21. Hirsh BD. Antitrust and medical ethics. *JAMA.* 1983;250: 2759–60.

17

Should Access to Transcatheter Aortic Valve Replacement Be Limited to High-Volume Surgical Centers?

Joseph E. Bavaria, Philip Green, Gregg F. Rosner,
Martin B. Leon, Allan Schwartz, and Robert M. Sade*

Introduction
Robert M. Sade, MD

[...] This discussion is a new incarnation of the long-standing volume–outcome relationship debate, placed this time in the context of a new technology that is shared by cardiac surgeons and interventional cardiologists. Bavaria presents a great deal of data based on published literature over the last 3 decades; these data generally show that larger volume programs and individual surgeons are associated with better outcomes in terms of mortality and morbidity, with a few exceptions. Green and colleagues present arguments based on recent studies that show no volume–outcome associations and a number of other arguments suggesting that limiting access to transcatheter aortic valve replacement is not a good idea.

Pro
Joseph E. Bavaria, MD

A document describing characteristics of the heart team to perform transcatheter aortic valve replacement (TAVR) was recently developed for the

*Sade RM. Should access to transcatheter aortic valve replacement be limited to high-volume surgical centers? *J Thorac Cardiovasc Surg* 2013;145(1):1439–40; Bavaria JE. Access to transcatheter aortic valve replacement should be limited to high-volume centers. *J Thorac Cardiovasc Surg.* 2013;145:1441–3. Green P, Rosner GF. Leon MB, Schwartz A. Access to TAVR should not be limited to high-volume surgical centers. *J Thorac Cardiovasc Surg.* 2013;145:1444–5. Copyright American Association for Thoracic Surgery, republished here with permission.

Centers for Medicare and Medicaid Services and the Food and Drug Administration.[1] Among those characteristics were three that are relevant to this discussion: cardiac surgeon criteria, interventional cardiologist criteria, and institutional requirements for programmatic volumes. These three characteristics are germane to the question of whether there is a relationship between the volume of procedures performed by a program/surgeon and patient outcomes.

The association of volume with outcomes was first noted in 1979 when hospital surgical volume was associated with better outcomes.[2] The same relationship was found [...] in urological oncology. The most complex cystectomy operations had two to three times lower mortality rates in high than in low-volume centers. This outcome was not found in simple urological procedures, leading to the idea that big procedures should be performed at big hospitals and small procedures should be performed at small hospitals.[3] One study of the volume outcomes metric showed that approximately 39% of the effect is related to the surgeon and 61% is the institutional effect.[4] Other factors drive the association between volume and outcomes as well: hospital size, urban location, teaching mission, staffing ratios, and patient demographic factors, such as age, length of stay, and accompanying procedures.

An early article that used Medicare data to evaluate 12 major cancer and major cardiovascular surgical procedures showed a significant inverse relationship between hospital volume and mortality rates. When the same group looked at surgeon volume in an analysis of more than 500,000 patients, the results were dramatic and even more conclusive, showing that surgeon volume is inversely related to operative mortality for all procedures examined.[4] The authors concluded: "In the absence of other information about the quality of surgery at the hospitals near them, Medicare patients undergoing selected cardiovascular or cancer procedures can significantly reduce their risk of operative death by selecting a high-volume hospital." The excess of deaths associated with lower-volume hospitals, according to one analysis, is 10,000 lives that could be saved by selective referral to high-volume hospitals.[5] [...]

Specific cardiovascular procedure volume–outcome relationships have been investigated. A study of carotid endarterectomy showed dramatic decreases in the incidence of death, stroke, and length of stay as a function of surgeon volume.[6] Procedural volume as a marker for coronary artery bypass graft (CABG) surgery has similar results: approximately a 3% reduction in mortality rate for CABG surgery in high-volume hospitals and approximately a 15% reduction in morbidity and mortality from highest to lowest quartile volume.[7] High surgeon volume was also associated with approximately a 30% reduction in 30-day mortality rate. This article similarly studied the outcomes in many patients in the Society of Thoracic Surgeons database and found significantly better outcomes for patients older than 65 years undergoing CABG, but no difference in lower risk and younger patients. The article concluded that hospital volume had limited value as a quality metric for CABG.

Data from the New York State database show that hospitals with a higher CABG surgery volume also have lower risk-adjusted mortality rates; high-volume hospitals and surgeons both had a 30% to 40% reduction in risk-adjusted mortality rates.[8] The combination of a high-volume surgeon and a high-volume hospital had far better results than the combination of a low-volume surgeon and a low-volume hospital. As a result, New York developed a policy intended to enhance outcomes, setting specific CABG requirements of 200 a year for hospitals and 50 a year for surgeons. Pennsylvania also mandated reporting of outcomes, and analysis showed nearly identical volume–outcome relations.[9]

The surgeon volume-mortality relationship showed lower mortality rates with greater surgical volume, and this relationship was stronger than hospital volumes.

Another indication that the surgeon's experience in CABG procedures is a critical factor in determining outcomes is provided by the observation that when the same surgical team uses the same systems in high- and low-volume hospitals, the survival outcomes are not statistically different.[10]

In aortic valve replacement (AVR) surgery, higher surgeon volumes are associated with better outcomes, and the effect is substantially augmented in the case of complex operations, such as reoperative AVR.[11] Similar results were found when hospital volume was related to outcomes of CABG, AVR, and mitral valve replacement: the surgeon-volume relationship was robust.[12]

Elective thoracic aortic aneurysm surgery shows the same volume–outcome relationship—mortality for all aortic operations is much better in high-volume centers. It is interesting that thoracoabdominal operations were not performed by the low-volume centers at all; they referred all those procedures to high-volume centers.[13] Heart transplantation shows the same thing: heart transplant outcomes are worse at low-volume centers.[14] Type A aortic dissection outcomes show further proof of this concept; as volume increases, outcomes improve for this operation.[15]

Clearly, the volume–outcome relationship advantage in high-volume centers disproportionately benefits high-risk patients, but one study reached the counterintuitive conclusion that operations in high-volume programs benefited low-risk patients more than high-risk patients. In this study, even very-low-risk patients had substantially better outcomes in high-volumes centers.[16] It seems logical that poor results in one type of operation could correlate with poor results in others as well. This logic has been confirmed: hospitals that performed badly with CABG surgery also performed badly with AVR and mitral valve replacement, both by institution and by surgeon.[17] This suggests that suboptimal results in percutaneous coronary interventions (PCIs) and AVR might predict suboptimal results in TAVR.

Regarding the interventional volume–outcome relationship, the international PCI community does well in fairly simple interventions, but in the more complicated interventions, the volume–outcome relationship is robust. High-volume PCI centers had dramatically better outcomes and mortality rates versus low-volume centers. The same is true of patients going to emergency CABG surgery.[18] The authors concluded that there is no doubt in the PCI literature that the volume–outcome relationship remains strong. [...]

Data from the early experience with TAVR clearly show that as experience increases, results also improve.[19] This holds true for patients undergoing TAVR by the transapical approach, which shows far better outcomes in the second 150 cases in a series than in the initial 150 cases.[20] There is no question that as one gains experience, one gets better at TAVR.

This information has substantial implications for health policy. The National Agenda to Improve Patient Safety of the Agency for Healthcare Research and Quality says this: "Localizing specific surgeries and procedures to high-volume centers"' is a high priority area for patient safety research.[21] The data overwhelmingly support the volume–outcome relationship. Therefore, the complex cardiovascular procedure of TAVR should be limited to high-volume centers.

Con
Philip Green, MD, Gregg F. Rosner, MD, Martin B. Leon, MD, Allan Schwartz, MD

Transcatheter aortic valve replacement (TAVR) has transformed the treatment of aortic stenosis in high-risk older adults in Europe and has begun to do so in the United States. Recent Food and Drug Administration approval of the Edwards Lifesciences SAPIEN Transcatheter Heart Valve (Irvine, Calif) in inoperable and high-risk patients led to enthusiasm for widespread implementation of this technology. Experts have highlighted the central role of the multidisciplinary heart team in implementing a successful TAVR program.[22] Other experts, such as Joseph Bavaria, have suggested that access to TAVR should be restricted to high-volume surgical aortic valve replacement centers. In our opinion, access to TAVR should not be limited to high-volume surgical centers for the following reasons. First, high surgical volume does not ensure good outcomes in complex interventional procedures. Second, centers with low or no surgical volume can have excellent interventional results. Third, new multidisciplinary heart teams have achieved excellent results in part because of the transmission of accumulated knowledge from experienced centers. Finally, in the absence of evidence suggesting that high-volume surgical centers produce superior TAVR results, therapeutic options for patients should not be limited.

HIGH SURGICAL VOLUME DOES NOT ENSURE GOOD
INTERVENTIONAL OUTCOMES

The Synergy between Percutaneous Coronary Angio-plasty with Taxus and Cardiac Surgery (SYNTAX) trial[23] randomized 1800 patients with multivessel disease across sites in 17 countries. Participants were randomized to coronary artery bypass surgery or a Taxus stent (Boston Scientific Corporation, Natick, Mass) implantation. Analysis of rates of major adverse cardiac events by site showed that there was no relationship between volume and outcomes for both the Taxus stent and coronary bypass arm of the trial. This indicates that high volume, surgical or percutaneous, does not guarantee excellent outcomes and therefore volume alone should not be treated as a sufficient marker of high-quality care.

CENTERS WITH LOW OR NO SURGICAL VOLUME CAN HAVE EXCELLENT
INTERVENTIONAL RESULTS

Recent data from the Cardiovascular Patient Outcomes Research Team–Elective Angioplasty Study (CPORT-E) trial confirmed that surgical backup is not necessary for excellent interventional outcomes.[24] In the CPORT-E study, approximately 1900 patients were randomized to percutaneous coronary intervention with surgery on site versus no surgery onsite. The overall 6-week and 9-month adverse cardiac event rates were low and there were no significant differences between the sites with and without surgical backup. These findings underscore the belief that high surgical volume is not essential for excellent interventional cardiology results.

GROUP LEARNING CAN ATTENUATE THE LEARNING CURVE

Data from the Columbia HeartSource experience have shown that high-volume centers of excellence can transmit expertise to outlying centers. This can be achieved through targeted physician recruitment, a focus on continuous quality improvement through regular oversight and peer review, and formal and informal didactics. Most importantly, expert consultation is available to all participating sites at all times, including nights and weekends. The use of this approach to transmit knowledge across sites has enabled low-volume sites to achieve cardiac surgical risk-adjusted outcomes that are comparable with high-volumes affiliates.[25]

This group-learning phenomena has been replicated on a larger scale in the transcatheter arena in Europe and in the United States. In the European Edwards SAPIEN Aortic Bioprosthesis European Outcome (SOURCE) Registry, the early [...] and later [...] transapical TAVR results were compared. Despite comparable baseline risk characteristics, outcomes in the early group were as good as outcomes in the later group. Specifically, there were no differences in 30-day rates of death, stroke, bleeding, or vascular complications.[26]

The absence of a demonstrable learning curve is a result of shared knowledge across sites, enabling each site to rapidly integrate the collective experience to achieve results comparable with more experienced sites. The early US TAVR experience also showed that group learning can attenuate the learning curve. Dewey and colleagues (STS presentation; January, 2012) analyzed the randomized and nonrandomized continued-access transfemoral TAVR Placement of Aortic Transcatheter Valve (PARTNER) trial experience and showed the following: (1) 30-day and 1-year mortality rates among the TAVR subjects were not different when high-enrolling sites were compared with low-enrolling sites, and (2) the 30-day and 1-year mortality rates were similar for the first set of 20, the second set of 20, and the third set of 20 valve implantations at each site (PARTNER Executive Committee presentation; April, 2012). This suggests that early lessons learned were integrated rapidly into the group experience and through formal and informal educational initiatives and hands-on proctoring, excellent results were achieved in low-volume sites and among the first cases at new sites.

Finally, although we applaud the careful assimilation of TAVR technology to clinical care to ensure optimal outcomes for the highest-risk patients, restricting this kind of therapy to centers with high surgical aortic valve replacement volume is unprecedented in the surgical community. Bolling and colleagues[27] highlighted that most mitral valve surgery occurs at low-volume sites, despite the increased likelihood of successful mitral valve repair at high-volume centers. Furthermore, Dewey and colleagues[28] showed that the discordance between observed and expected outcomes after aortic valve replacement decreases as surgical volume increases. However, according to data from the Society of Thoracic Surgery database, the median number of sole aortic valve replacements per center is 20 per year, and per cardiac surgeon is 8 per year (Society of Thoracic Surgery database; 2010). Despite evidence of better outcomes at high-volume surgical centers, heart valve surgery is not restricted to high-volume centers. In TAVR, in which the available evidence suggests that an excellent heart team with the support of national experts and regional centers can achieve excellent results despite low volume, there is no rationale to restrict the availability of this transformative technology to patients cared for at high-volume surgical centers.

Concluding Remarks
Robert M. Sade, MD

Several important issues related to the volume–outcomes ongoing debate are not addressed by either side of this discussion [...]. These are related to excellence, well-controlled studies, and moving targets.

EXCELLENCE

All physicians aspire to be the best that they can be and to provide every patient with the highest quality care. These are aspirations, however, not requirements. The requirement for surgeons is not perfection and is not even excellence—it is competence.[29] Certification and maintenance of certification in a medical specialty are measures of competence; the programmatic requirements of the various specialty boards are the 6 core *competencies* that are well known to us[30]—they have never been designated the 6 core *excellences*. Requiring that every patient be sent to centers associated with the best outcomes is ethically questionable, and making such a requirement a matter of policy seems overreaching. If a surgeon is competent, his or her results may not measure up to those of a master surgeon, but that should not in itself justify depriving potential patients of his or her services.

WELL-CONTROLLED STUDIES

Existing studies of the volume–outcome association suffer from the biases that plague all retrospective studies. For example, wide variation in study methodology makes meta-analysis of the volume–outcome relation impossible and is probably responsible for much of the great variation in conclusions reached by those studies.[31] Moreover, the data in most studies come from administrative databases, which are notoriously unreliable regarding their clinical accuracy and are not risk adjusted.[32] These important flaws make the conclusions of such studies unreliable grounds for making policy decisions that might make referral lines unreasonably rigid. The need is for studies that are designed for prospective collection of clinically accurate risk-adjusted data. Such studies seem unlikely to take place in the near future.

MOVING TARGETS

The studies of volume–outcome associations that have been done to date are snapshots; that is, they measure relations between surgeon or center volume compared with outcomes over a specified time period. But it might be the case that those relations vary substantially over time. Some small centers have become bigger centers over several years by demonstrating improved results. Many examples of this could be cited, but in my own institution, the volume of aortic aneurysm/dissection surgery has tripled since Dr John Ikonomidis joined our faculty immediately after finishing his training 12 years ago. The volume increase has been a result of his interest in such surgery and his excellent results. This growth would not have occurred if aortic surgery had been regionalized to high-volume centers in the late 1990s. Surgical volumes and outcomes are moving targets. It would be helpful to know how many large-volume programs have become smaller and low-volume programs larger over 1 or 2 decades and how these changes correlated with outcomes. Such a study has not yet been done.

CONCLUSIONS

The volume–outcome controversy is likely to continue in the future, partly in an effort to find ways to optimize outcomes for patients and perhaps partly as a means for large programs to increase market share. There are good arguments to be made on both sides of this question, and Bavaria and Green and colleagues have presented some of them. This editorial attempts to fill in some of the gaps in their presentations.

References

1. Centers for Medicare and Medicaid Services. Characteristics of the heart team to perform TAVI for best patient outcomes. Baltimore, MD: Centers for Medicare and Medicaid Services. http://www.cms.gov. Accessed May 20, 2014.

2. Luft HS, Bunker J, Enthoven AC. Should operations be regionalized? An empirical study of the relation between surgical volume and mortality. *N Engl J Med.* 1979;301:1364–9.

3. Konety BR, Allareddy V, Modak S, Smith B. Mortality after major surgery for urologic cancers in specialized urology hospitals: are they any better? *J Clin Oncol.* 2006;24:2006–12.

4. Birkmeyer JD, Stukel TA, Siewers AE, et al. Surgeon volume and operative mortality in the United States. *N Engl J Med.* 2003;349:2117–27.

5. Dudley RA, Johansen KL, Brand R, et al. Selective referral to high-volume hospitals: estimating potentially avoidable deaths. *JAMA.* 2000; 283:1159–66.

6. Cowan JA, Dimick JB, Thompson BG, et al. Surgeon volume as an indicator of outcomes after carotid endarterectomy: an effect independent of specialty practice and hospital volume. *J Am Coll Surg.* 2002;195:814–21.

7. Peterson ED, Coombs LP, DeLong ER, et al. Procedural volume as a marker of quality for CABG surgery. *JAMA.* 2004;291:195–201.

8. Hannan EL, Wu C, Ryan TJ, et al. Do hospitals and surgeons with higher coronary artery bypass graft surgery volumes still have lower risk-adjusted mortality rates? *Circulation.* 2003;108:795–801.

9. Gorton CP, Jones JL, Hollenbeak CS, et al. Variation in volume–outcome relationships for hospitals and surgeons performing CABG surgery: Pennsylvania Health Care Council Containment Council. http://www.academyhealth.org/. les/2005/ppt/gorton.ppt. Washington, DC: Academy Health. Accessed October 16, 2012.

10. Zacharias A, Schwann TA, Riordan CJ, et al. Is hospital procedure volume a reliable marker of quality for coronary artery bypass surgery? *Ann Thorac Surg.* 2005;79:1961–9.

11. Dewey TM, Herbert MA, Ryan WH, et al. Influence of surgeon volume on outcomes with aortic valve replacement. *Ann Thorac Surg.* 2012;93:1107–12.

12. Goodney PP, Lucas FL, Birkmeyer JD. Should volume standards for cardiovascular surgery focus only on high-risk patients? *Circulation.* 2003;107:384–7.

13. Gazoni LM, Speir AM, Kron IL, et al. Elective thoracic aortic aneurysm surgery: better outcomes from high-volume centers. *J Am Coll Surg.* 2010;210:855–9; discussion 859–60.

14. Russo MJ, Iribarne A, Easterwood R, et al. Post-heart transplant survival is inferior at low-volume centers across all risk strata. *Circulation.* 2010;122(Suppl.):S85–91.

15. Knipp BS, Deeb GM, Prager RL, et al. A contemporary analysis of outcomes for operative repair of type A aortic dissection in the United States. [published correction appears in *Surgery.* 2008;143:301]. *Surgery.* 2007;142:524–8.

16. Glance LG, Dick AW, Mukamel DB, Osler TM. Is the hospital volume–mortality relationship in coronary artery bypass surgery the same for low-risk versus high-risk patients? *Ann Thorac Surg.* 2003;76:1155–62.

17. Goodney PP, O'Connor GT, Wennberg DE, Birkmeyer JD. Do hospitals with low mortality rates in coronary artery bypass also perform well in valve replacement? *Ann Thorac Surg.* 2003;76:1131–6.

18. McGrath PD, Wennberg DE, Dickens JD Jr, et al. Relation between operator and hospital volume and outcomes following percutaneous coronary interventions in the era of the coronary stent. *JAMA.* 2000;284:3139–44.

19. Gurvitch R, Tay EL, Wijesinghe N, et al. Transcatheter aortic valve implantation: lessons from the learning curve of the first 270 high-risk patients. *Catheter Cardiovasc Interv.* 2011;78:977–84.

20. Kempfert J, Rastan A, Holzhey D, et al. Transapical aortic valve implantation: analysis of risk factors and learning experience in 299 patients. *Circulation.* 2011;124(Suppl.):S124–9.

21. Agency for Healthcare Research and Quality. Evidence Report/Technology Assessment No. 43. Making health care safer: a critical analysis of patient safety practices. Rockville, MD: Agency for Healthcare Research and Quality. http://www.ahrq.gov/clinic/ptsafety/pdf/ptsafety.pdf. Accessed October 16, 2012.

22. Holmes DR Jr, Mack MJ, Kaul S, et al. 2012 ACCF/AATS/SCAI/STS expert consensus document on transcatheter aortic valve replacement. *J Am Coll Cardiol.* 2012;59:1200–54.

23. Serruys PW, Morice M-C, Kappetein AP, et al. Percutaneous coronary intervention versus coronary-artery bypass grafting for severe coronary artery disease. *N Engl J Med.* 2009;360:961–72.

24. Aversano T, Lemmon CC, Liu L. Outcomes of PCI at hospitals with or without on-site cardiac surgery. *N Engl J Med.* 2012;366:1792–802.

25. Kurlansky PA, Argenziano M, Dunton R, et al. Quality, not volume, determines outcome of coronary artery bypass surgery in a university-based community hospital network. *J Thorac Cardiovasc Surg.* 2012;143:287–93.

26. Wendler O, Walther T, Schroefel H, et al. The SOURCE Registry: what is the learning curve in transapical aortic valve implantation? *Eur J Cardiothoracic Surg.* 2011;39:853–60.

27. Bolling SF, Li S, O'Brien SM, et al. Predictors of mitral valve repair: clinical and surgeon factors. *Ann Thorac Surg.* 2010;90: 1904–12.

28. Dewey TM, Herbert MA, Ryan WH, et al. Influence of surgeon volume on outcomes with aortic valve replacement. *Ann Thorac Surg.* 2012;93:1107–13.

29. Council on Ethical and Judicial Affairs. Principles of Medical Ethics, Principle I. Code of Medical Ethics of the American Medical Association, current opinions with annotations. 2012–2013 ed. Chicago: American Medical Association; 2012:xx–xxvi.

30. American Board of Medical Specialties. MOC competencies and criteria. Chicago: American Board of Medical Specialties. http://www.abms.org/maintenance_of_certification/MOC_competencies.aspx. Accessed February 5, 2013.

31. Halm EA,Lee C, Chassin MR.Is volume related to outcome in healthcare? A systematic review and methodologic critique of the literature. *Ann Intern Med.* 2002;137:511–20.

32. Cerfolio RJ, Jacobs JP. Sade RM. The ethics of transparency: publication of cardiothoracic surgical outcomes in the lay press. *Ann Thorac Surg.* 2009;87:679–86.

18

Should the Use of Transcatheter Aortic Valve Implantation Be Rationed?

John E. Mayer, Jr., Grayson H. Wheatley III, and Robert M. Sade*

Introduction

Robert M. Sade, MD

Transcatheter aortic valve implantation (TAVI) has great promise of helping patients with severe aortic valve disease who are not candidates for open surgery. It is an expensive technology, however, and some believe it should not be offered to every patient who is medically suitable to receive it—in other words, its use should be rationed.

The Ethics Forum [. . .] sponsored a debate on rationing TAVI at the 2011 Annual Meeting of the American Association for Thoracic Surgery. John E. Mayer, Jr, MD, argued the proponent position, Grayson H. Wheatley, MD, the contrariant regarding a hypothetical case, constructed to focus on the question of whether the offer of TAVI should be withheld from an elderly patient.

THE CASE OF THE OLD MAN AND HIS VALVE

The patient is 75 years old, and 10 years ago he received a 4-vessel coronary artery bypass graft, including the left internal thoracic artery to the

---

*Sade RM. Should use of transcatheter aortic valve implantation be rationed? *J Thorac Cardiovasc Surg.* 2012;143(4):769–70; Mayer JE Jr. Transcatheter aortic valve implantation should be controlled and monitored by the medical profession. *J Thorac Cardiovasc Surg.* 2012;143(4):771–3; Wheatley GH III. Use of transcatheter valve should not be rationed. *J Thorac Cardiovasc Surg.* 2012;143(4):774–5. Copyright American Association for Thoracic Surgery, republished here with permission.

left anterior descending coronary artery. He did well thereafter but has lived alone since his wife died 2 years ago; he has no children and no close relatives. Significant heart failure symptoms recently developed in the patient. Echocardiographic assessment now shows evidence of severe aortic stenosis with a calculated valve area of 0.8 cm^2 and a mean gradient across the valve of 60 mm Hg. There is left ventricular hypertrophy, and the left ventricular ejection fraction is 40%. Coronary catheterization shows severe native coronary disease with all grafts patent and no new native coronary obstructions. Computed tomography scan reveals evidence of moderate to severe calcification of the ascending aorta, and the left internal thoracic artery passes directly under the sternum, and thus is at high risk of being damaged during reoperative sternotomy. In addition, the patient has moderate to severe chronic obstructive pulmonary disease (forced expiratory volume in1 second 45% of normal) and a baseline creatinine of 1.8 mg/d.

The patient is referred to Dr. Sloan, an established cardiothoracic surgeon who participated in the initial Sapien (Edwards Lifesciences, Irvine, Calif) TAVI trial and has significant expertise with the procedure. Although Dr. Sloan has determined that the patient is a medically acceptable candidate for TAVI, but not for aortic valve replacement, he wonders whether some advanced technologies such as this one are expanding the scope of health care beyond sustainable limits. He knows that the only reason to deny TAVI to this particular patient is consideration of nonmedical issues, that is, the patient's advanced age and lack of a social support system, and the expense of the procedure, and is undecided whether he should offer the procedure or, for the greater good, deny him its benefits.

Pro
John E. Mayer, Jr, MD

On the basis of the accompanying case presentation of a 75-year-old widowed male nursing home resident with hemodynamically significant aortic stenosis, heart failure, angina, and a high surgical risk for a conventional aortic valve replacement, I support the proposition that the newly emerging transcatheter aortic valve implantation (TAVI) should be "rationed," or at least monitored and controlled. The placement of aortic transcatheter valve (PARTNER) trial assessed both the clinical outcomes and resource use results from this multicenter prospective, randomized trial of transcatheter aortic valve insertion in both patients at "high risk" for open heart aortic valve replacement and in surgically "inoperable" patients. The results of the trial indicated that in surgically inoperable patients receiving a transcatheter aortic valve compared with "medically treated" patients (most with balloon valvotomy alone), the 1-year mortality for patients undergoing

TAVI was 30.7% versus 50.4% for "medically treated" patients. The stroke rate was 5% in the patients undergoing TAVI versus 1.1% in the medical group, and the major vascular complication rates were 16.2% versus 1.1% for TAVI and medically treated patients, respectively.[1] The average total cost for the TAVI procedure itself was $46,238, and the average total hospitalization cost for the admission at which TAVI was performed was $78,540. The 1-year average resource use after the TAVI admission was $29,352 versus $52,724 for those treated medically. The study showed that this therapy added on average 1.59 incremental life years at a cost of $50,212 per added life year. The increment in quality-adjusted life years was 1.29 years at a cost of $61,889 per added quality-adjusted life year.[2] For this patient, my recommendation regarding the use of TAVI would rest on an assessment of his "frailty" and the presence of other comorbidities that would exert the dominant impact on his survival and quality of life. Being a widower and living in a nursing home alone do not represent sufficient comorbid conditions to preclude treatment.

However, I also conclude, on the basis of these data, that the diffusion of this technology should be carefully monitored and controlled by the medical profession. Some may argue that "monitoring and control" is a distinction without a difference from "rationing," but uncontrolled diffusion of new medical technology has been a major source of the current crisis in funding for medical care in the United States, with approximately 18% of the gross domestic product now devoted to health care.[3] Given the growing elderly population in this country and the incidence of aortic valve sclerosis in this aging population, there is a significant likelihood that use of TAVI for all elderly patients with aortic valve disease could add significantly to the Medicare expenditures for cardiovascular disease.

I[4] and others[5] have argued that it is a responsibility of the medical profession to wisely allocate societal health care resources, but if TAVI results in improved 1-year survival, how could an ethical physician or surgeon, or an entire society, "deny" a given individual patient access to this technology. Consideration of this dilemma reveals some fundamental conflicts both within the value structures of the medical profession and within the value structures of American society, which I will attempt to briefly describe. I will then offer my own thoughts on how to address some of these dilemmas.

As a starting point, it is important to distinguish between efficacy and effectiveness. Assessment of the efficacy and safety of medical devices is the province of the US Food and Drug Administration, which is tasked with determining whether a new device safely accomplishes the stated purpose of the device. This efficacy assessment is typically based on randomized clinical trials, such as the PARTNER trial, in carefully defined clinical populations. Effectiveness has been described as the outcome when this same device is deployed in the general population by the medical profession. The Food and Drug Administration does not have (or want) the legal mandate to regulate the practice of medicine, and thus the assessment of the effectiveness of a device has traditionally been the responsibility of the medical profession, although health services researchers increasingly have inserted themselves into this domain. The assessments of effectiveness involve the medical profession's obligations to society to self-regulate and to wisely allocate what is now becoming a scarce societal resource. I have argued that if the medical profession does not actively engage in this effectiveness assessment, then major resource allocation decisions will be made by those who do not take care of patients, and then the medical profession will have forfeited an important role and responsibility in American society.[6] Krause, in Death of the Guilds,[7] has pointed out that professions are granted privileges and prerogatives by a society only so long as society believes that the profession is acting in the society's interest and not in its own interest. In the context of other erosions of medicine's prerogatives and privileges that have occurred in recent years, including managed care constraints on diagnostic testing, medication use, and procedures, I believe that failure to address the effectiveness question by the profession, even if it means that professional income will suffer, will be a major mistake that will affect the ability of medicine to continue to function as a profession.

The overriding issue for this debate, however, is reconciliation of the 2 roles that physicians have: "healer of the sick" and "member of a profession." These 2 roles have different historical roots and can potentially come into conflict, as in the case that served as the topic for this debate. Should a "healer of the sick" choose not to offer a potentially beneficial therapy to any patient? Should a member of a profession disregard the profession's responsibilities to the society that it serves by failing to self-regulate or to wisely allocate societal resources? If physicians and surgeons indiscriminately apply a new and expensive technology to any patient who might benefit, even if it will minimally prolong life or marginally reduce suffering, can the medical profession argue that there has been a wise use of society's health care dollar? Is there a means by which both of these responsibilities of the physician can be fulfilled? I submit that there is, and I believe that the solution to this dilemma must rest on a rigorous, controlled collection and analysis of data on both the clinical and the resource use outcomes for this transcatheter valve therapy. I submit that outcomes data have the greatest impact on physician practice, and these outcomes must include both clinical outcomes and resource use outcomes for the procedure itself and for at least several years after the procedure. I believe that this approach will, of necessity, require a controlled dissemination of this technology and linkage of clinical databases with administrative claims databases so that resource use over time can be assessed after device insertion. [...]

The ASCERT (American College of Cardiology Foundation–The Society of Thoracic Surgeons Collaboration on the Comparative Effectiveness of Revascularization Strategies) study[8] [...] attempts to compare coronary bypass surgery with percutaneous coronary interventions and has used the Society of Thoracic Surgeons' Adult Cardiac Database and the American College of Cardiology interventional catheterization database with linkage of both databases to the Medicare claims database. This study has demonstrated that such database linkages can be accomplished and that long-term outcomes, including resource use, can be assessed through linkage of these datasets. We cannot ignore the simple notion that value equals quality divided by cost, and society must ultimately believe that the deployment of its resources is providing real value to its members and not just to the profession that provides the services.

It is my expectation that the information from an ongoing study of TAVI will provide direction to cardiologists and surgeons involved in this therapy to identify subgroups of patients for whom this therapy will provide little benefit and could result in significant harm, particularly neurologic injury. In addition, it will be critical that the patients be provided this information so that each may make his or her own decision. It is this type of rigorously collected and analyzed information that will provide a pathway through the dilemma posed by the coexisting roles of healer of the sick and member of a profession that must wisely allocate societal resources. I anticipate that the patient characteristics that will indicate little benefit from TAVI will be in the realm of noncardiac comorbidities and "frailty." There will always be differences of professional opinion in a given case, but the information on the outcomes and effectiveness of any therapy will enable physicians, surgeons, and patients to make the wisest choices both for the patient and for society to ensure that both patient and society recognize the value of the therapy.

It is for these reasons that I believe the diffusion of the transcatheter aortic valve replacement technology should be controlled and monitored by the profession. I believe that such a process is distinctly different from "rationing," particularly because rationing implies that the process would be carried out by an entity that is not directly involved in the interaction between patient and physician. If physicians, surgeons, and patients can rationally assess rigorously collected and analyzed information, then I am confident that the profession can be true to its responsibilities to both patients and society, and we in the profession can make the right recommendations to our patients regarding the application of this new technology. In so doing, we and our patients will be able to limit the application of this new technology to those who will best benefit by it and spare society, through its governmental representatives, from making ill-advised, blanket judgments about the wisdom of applying TAVI to individual patients or to an entire population.

Con

Grayson H. Wheatley III, MD

The emergence of new technologies for the treatment of aortic valve disorders has brought with it a host of medical and ethical challenges regarding patient selection and choice of treatment. Because of the uncertainty around the safety of new transcatheter aortic valve implantation (TAVI) technologies, early device trials have focused on enrolling and treating patients at high surgical risk who are "nonoperative" candidates. Although outcomes for open surgical repair of critical aortic stenosis are improving, early results with TAVI are encouraging and have led to expanded patient selection criteria.[9] Although some clinicians believe that the use of TAVI should be rationed in these non-operative patients, there is a strong argument to make that these patients ethically deserve the same treatment options (when medically appropriate) as younger, less high-risk patients.

ETHICAL AND TREATMENT DECISIONS

Our hypothetical 75-year-old patient with critical aortic stenosis, multiple comorbidities, and a prior coronary artery revascularization with patent bypass grafts has been determined by the surgical team to be a non-operative candidate, and this patient's situation is becoming increasingly common. Recent data have shown that there are a growing number of similar patients who are denied surgical therapy because of comorbidities. Iung and colleagues[10] retrospectively showed that 33% of patients referred for aortic valve replacement were denied surgical repair because of their high surgical risk. The benefits of aortic valve treatment with relief of physiologic gradient across the stenotic aortic valve drastically alters the survival curve of patients compared with medical management.[11] However, in patients with end-stage disease, TAVI has shown promise of extending life an average of 6 months.[12] The fundamental question becomes, should we? Or in other terms, should we ration health care to patients?

There are 3 different ethical frameworks for which to consider this case: need principles, maximizing principles, and egalitarian principles.[13] The need principle is based on "rules of rescue," in which the immediate and long-term medical needs of the patient are the highest priority and supersede all other considerations. This is standard operating practice for most physician–patient interactions in today's healthcare environment. This is the perspective that all of our patients expect from us when making difficult and complex decisions. This traditional approach is intended to offer the best possible outcome and intervention for any patient in need. In this case, it would look simply at the patient and the feasibility of implanting a percutaneous aortic valve. If the patient were deemed a suitable candidate, he or she would be offered this intervention. Because the patient is a candidate for TAVI, it should be offered to the patient to improve his or her quality of life and to relieve suffering. A majority of clinicians would follow this principle of justice. The facts that the patient did not have a well-developed support structure to assist him or her after the procedure and that the patient's life expectancy is short are not important drivers of this ethical and moral framework. Essentially, rationing of care is not a consideration with the need principle, and the patient should be offered a TAVI procedure.

The second principle of justice in rationing health care is the maximizing principle. This principle seeks to achieve the best possible consequences, both for the patient and for society as a whole. This slightly broader perspective takes into consideration that this patient has limited support at home and after TAVI would most likely not return to being a productive member of society. The total economic burden of the TAVI procedure, hospitalization, and subsequent care facility is a sizable amount and would certainly have an overall impact on total health care costs. It is difficult for patients to actively engage in this broader perspective because it is difficult for them to fully comprehend the consequences of the therapy in relation to their own debilitated state. The intent here is to maximize well-being for the patient. A TAVI procedure in this patient would certainly improve his or her well-being, and therefore TAVI would meet the threshold for rationing in this patient's case using the maximizing principle and should be offered to the patient.

Finally, the egalitarian principle of justice in health care considers in equalities in health care, and every effort should be made to reduce these inequalities. The total cost of the procedure and rehabilitation is sizeable primarily because of the costs of the percutaneous valve technology compared with a standard aortic valve replacement. From this perspective, the total costs used in the last several months of this patient's life might be better served going to a pediatric patient who has a long prosperous life ahead. As a result, the egalitarian principle would most likely support rationing care to this patient, and using this moral framework, the physician should make this informed decision without much input from the patient. This is also the hardest decision to make for the physician because the health care system as a whole is being considered and the patient is left out of this decision-making process. The physician standing at the patient's bedside must look at society's costs in light of the total costs for the patient relative to the expected outcome. Although this type of decision process may be best for the health care system in the long run to help decrease health care expenditures, it is a framework with which we as clinicians are not yet comfortable. With the passage of the US health care reform, tough choices are mandatory to help counteract the increasing health care costs, and rationing of health care will most likely be a new part of providing care.[14] New technologies, such as TAVI, will certainly receive a great deal of pushback to ration.

In terms of the possibility of rationing TAVI procedures, the costs of this procedure need to be compared with other existing technologies and treatments. Wu and colleagues[15] have looked at the cost-effective ratio (CER) of standard aortic valve replacement and shown that for a 75-year-old patient the average CER is $16,500. This is compared with a CER of $50,000 for TAVI procedures.[16] These costs take into consideration the quality of life, hospital costs, and need for extended care. Although this difference is substantial, a CER between $20,000 and $100,000 is acceptable to the US health care system.[12] As a result, TAVI procedures are justifiable from a cost analysis.

TAVI has already proven to be a successful and useful technology for high-risk surgical patients with critical aortic stenosis. The increased procedural and device costs of TAVI compared with a surgical aortic valve prosthesis and replacement surgery put TAVI procedures at risk for future health care rationing as part of health care reform to minimize growing health care costs in the United States. The CER of TAVI procedures is in line with other existing technologies and therefore should not be singled out as an "expensive" new technology. The principles of justice in health care rationing also support continued use of TAVI procedures in high-risk patients. Future new technologies must face continued evaluation and scrutiny, and physicians must be prepared to be involved in some degree of health care rationing in the future.

Concluding Remarks
Robert M. Sade, MD

[...] Bedside rationing is a relatively new role for physicians, yet the foundation of the healing relationship is the patient's trust that physicians will be primarily concerned for the patient's interests rather than their own or society's interests. Nearly every current code of ethics [...] places the interests of the patient as physicians' paramount responsibility. Bedside rationing—withholding the offer of a particular therapy from one's own patient despite a positive benefit–harm balance—is prima facie inconsistent with this responsibility. Both discussants recognize the primary obligation of physicians to patients. Wheatley believes [...] expensive new technologies will likely have to be rationed in the future.

Mayer, however, believes rationing can be avoided if rigorous data provided by the profession's monitoring of TAVI are used by physicians and patients for rational consideration, enabling the physician and patient together to limit TAVI to those who will benefit most. In the case presented, TAVI was medically indicated, but Dr. Sloan wondered about how to weigh age, social situation, and cost in deciding whether to offer the procedure to the patient. Both discussants agree that age and social status are not determinants of suitability for TAVI, so cost remains as the central nonmedical issue. Mayer couples "control" of TAVI with monitoring, but it is unclear what it means to control a technology when "it will be critical that the patients be provided this information so that each may make their own decisions." In the presence of a positive benefit–harm balance, it is difficult to imagine patients refusing an offer of a life-prolonging, quality of life–improving procedure on the basis of avoiding an expense that will not be borne by either them or their survivors.

Critical to this discussion is current law and future policy development. The legislative battles over revisions of the Patient Protection and Affordable Care Act that are currently underway in Washington will eventually produce a health care system that will ultimately determine the shape and nature of the patient–physician relationship. Some reforms will empower physicians and patients to make clinical decisions, and others will relegate much decision-making to external agencies. Resolution of the rationing debate awaits the precise configuration of our developing health care system.

References

1. Leon MB, Smith CR, Mack M, et al. Transcatheter aortic valve implantation for aortic stenosis in patients who cannot undergo surgery. *N Engl J Med*. 2010;363:1597–607.
2. Reynolds MR, Magnuson EA, Wang K, et al. Lifetime cost effectiveness of trans-catheter aortic valve replacement compared with standard care among inoperable patients with severe aortic stenosis: results from the PARTNER Trial (Cohort B). *Circulation*. 2012;125:1102–9.
3. Martin A, Lassman D, Whittle L, Catlin A. National Health Expenditure Accounts Team. Recession contributes to slowest annual rate of increase in health spending in five decades. *Health Aff* (Milwood). 2011;30:11–22.
4. Mayer JE. Is there a role for the medical profession in solving the problems of the American health care system? *Ann Thorac Surg*. 2009;87:1655–61.
5. ABIM Foundation, American Board of Internal Medicine, American College of Physicians–American Society of Internal Medicine, European Federation of Internal Medicine. Medical professionalism in the new millennium: a physician charter. *Ann Intern Med*. 2002;136:243–6.
6. Mayer JE. The American health care system and the role of the medical profession in solving its problems. *Ann Thorac Surg*. 2007;84:1432–4.
7. Krause EA. The United States: capitalism dominant, professions pressured. In: *Death of the Guilds*. New Haven, CT: Yale University Press; 1995:29–49.
8. Holmes DR, Mack MJ. Transcatheter valve therapy: a professional society overview from the American College of Cardiology Foundation and the Society of Thoracic Surgeons. *Ann Thorac Surg*. 2011;91:714–5.
9. Finks JF, Osborne NH, Birkmeyer JD. Trends in hospital volume and operative mortality for high-risk surgery. *N Engl J Med*. 2011;364:2128–37.

10. Iung B, Cachier A, Baron G, et al. Decision-making in elderly patients with severe aortic stenosis: why are so many denied surgery? *Eur Heart J.* 2005;26:2714–20.

11. Brown ML, Schaff HV, Sarano ME, et al. Is the European System for Cardiac Operative Risk Evaluation model valid for estimating the operative risk of patients considered for percutaneous aortic valve replacement? *J Thorac Cardiovasc Surg.* 2008;136:566–71.

12. Lefevre T, Kappetein AP, Wolner E, et al. One-year follow-up of the multi-centre European PARTNER transcatheter heart valve study. *Eur Heart J.* 2011;32:148–57.

13. Cookson R, Dolan P. Principles of justice in health care rationing. *J Med Ethics.* 2000;26:323–9.

14. Groeneveld PW, Polsky D, Yang F, et al. The impact of new cardiovascular device technology on health care costs. *Arch Intern Med.* 2011;171:1289–91.

15. Wu Y, Jin R, Gao G, Grunkemeier GL, Starr A. Cost-effectiveness of aortic valve replacement in the elderly: an introductory study. *J Thorac Cardiovasc Surg.* 2007;133:608–13.

16. Reynolds MR. Lifetime cost effectiveness of implantation compared with standard care in inoperable patients: results from the PARTNER Trial (Cohort B). Paper presented at the American College Cardiology ACC.11/i2 summit; April 2-5, 2011; New Orleans, LA.

Organ Donation and Transplantation

Robert M. Sade

> *What you leave behind is not what is engraved in stone monuments, but what is woven into the lives of others.*
>
> —*Pericles (495–429 BCE), according to Thucydides (460–395 BCE)*

Ethical issues related to organ donation and transplantation abound. Most are related to the scarcity of organs available for transplantation—there are simply not enough organs to supply the needs of patients on the national transplant waiting lists. These problems originate in the inadequacy of our national organ-donation policy and create the most vexing difficulty of organ transplantation: allocation of this scarce resource.

After the first successful kidney transplantation in 1954, the growth of transplantation was severely hindered by the lack of effective immunosuppression regimens to prevent rejection of donor tissues. The field of transplantation began to grow rapidly after the introduction of the first highly effective immunosuppressive drug, cyclosporine, in the early 1980s. The US Congress recognized the need for national policy on organ donation and transplantation and in 1984 addressed the issue by enacting the National Organ Transplantation Act. This law created the framework for organ-procurement organizations and established a national clearinghouse for organ allocation, the Organ Procurement and Transplantation Network. The network was initially contracted to the United Network for Organ Sharing. In response to the early development of an organ-brokerage firm, the National Organ Transplantation Act prohibited the exchange of any "valuable consideration" for organs intended for transplantation.[1]

As the field of transplantation expanded rapidly, a growing gap was recognized between the number of organs needed for transplantation and the number available from donors. Since the earliest days of organ transplantation, at least twenty-six laws and regulations at the state and federal levels have been passed, with the intent of facilitating organ donation, including, for example, the Uniform Anatomical Gift Act (1968, 1987, 2006), the Uniform Determination of Death Act (1980), the National Organ Transplantation Act (1984), the Federal Omnibus Budget Reconciliation Act (1986), the Health Omnibus Programs Extension (1988), the Organ Donor Leave Act (1999), and the federal Hospital Conditions of Participation Regulations (1998, 2006). None of them has been effective in narrowing the gap.

In 2003 the Department of Health and Human Services funded a program intended to develop best practices for organ procurement organizations to improve rates of organ donation, the Organ Donation Breakthrough Collaborative. As shown in Figure S5.1, the collaborative was initially effective—rate of organ donation increased from 2003 to 2006 but then leveled off, so that by 2013 the rate was the same as it would have been if the temporary uptick in donation rates had not occurred. Meanwhile, the size of the waiting list continued to grow at a constant rate that was nearly three times faster than the rate of increase in donors, paralleled by an increasing rate of deaths related to the organ shortage (calculated as deaths on the waiting list plus candidates who became too sick to transplant removed from the waiting list). This figure extends the donation and transplantation data presented in chapter 20 (1988–2008 extended to 1993–2013).

Over the past twenty years, an increasing chorus of voices in the medical,[2] economics,[3] and ethics[4] literatures have spoken out against the absolute prohibition of valuable considerations for organ donors, arguing that a reward of some kind for organ donors has the potential to wipe out waiting lists and the deaths associated with the shortage of organs. Economists at Auburn University, arguing in 1991 for the use of financial incentives for organ donation, prophetically wrote: "We have never encountered a single policy more at odds with public welfare than the current [altruism-only] organ procurement policy in the United States. . . . If the current policy is maintained the shortage will continue to grow worse, as will the needless suffering."[5]

The shortage of organs is the central problem that generates the vast majority of ethical issues in transplantation, as well as organ donation—the shortage has fed the ongoing debate that focuses on the question of fairness in the distribution of available organs. The responsibility for developing policies regarding organ allocation lies with the Organ Procurement and Transplantation Network/United Network for Organ Sharing, which considers such factors as severity of the patient's medical

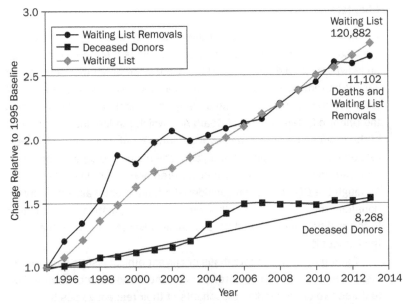

FIGURE S5.1 Relative Change in Transplant Data. This graph depicts the change in deceased donors, all-organ waiting list, and deaths plus waiting-list removals (virtually all are patients who became too sick to transplant and died off the list) relative to 1995 baseline. The sharp rise in deceased donors in 2003–2006 reflects the results of intensive efforts to increase donation by the Organ Donation Breakthrough Collaborative. (Source of data: Health Resources and Services Administration. Donation and Transplantation Community of Practice, http://organdonor.gov/dtcp/dtcp.html. Accessed May 8, 2014). The trend line shows that after the collaborative ended, donation plateaued, placing the 2013 donation rate where it would have been if the collaborative had not occurred. (Source of data: Health Resources and Services Administration. Data reports: National data, http://optn.transplant.hrsa.gov/latestData/step2.asp. Accessed May 8, 2014.)

condition and age, likelihood of benefit from receiving an organ, maximizing expected years of survival, maximizing relief from suffering, time on the waiting list, and likelihood of organ longevity based on immunological laboratory examinations, among others.[6] Commentators representing different perspectives of ethical analysis arrive at different conclusions regarding how organs should be allocated; consequentialist, deontological, teleological, and many other perspectives have a voice in this debate. Policy is developed by the United Network for Organ Sharing in an open process that includes public commentary, as well as expert opinion, but in the end almost everyone dislikes something about the policies guiding the distribution of organs. Nearly all of those disagreements and ethical disputes would disappear if the supply of organs were sufficient to eliminate the waiting list.

Chapters

The dead-donor rule(DDR) lies at the core of organ-donation policy and is the focus of **chapter 19.**[7] The basis of this rule is the widespread belief that an individual should not be killed to save the life of another, so vital organs cannot be removed before a person is already dead, since this act would kill that person. The DDR is the underlying rationale for the development of the Uniform Determination of Death Act, which renders loss of all functions of the brain and brain stem a legal determinant of death. It is also the reason for a required period of organ ischemia before organs can be removed from the patient who has suffered permanent loss of circulation. Although the DDR has been considered a fundamental aspect of organ donation, the first chapter in this section raises questions of its relation to the realities of death and its potentially adverse effects on the way we think about death.

Perhaps the most contentious of current ethical issues in regard to organ donation and transplantation is incentives to donate. **Chapter 20** features two of the leading proponents of their respective positions regarding the question of whether financial incentives should be used to increase organ donation.[8] In support of financial incentives, the argument is made that individuals in a liberal democracy, which characterizes most industrialized countries, should not be prohibited from choosing among three options: to donate altruistically (no additional benefit), to donate for a financial reward in a regulated market for organs, or not to donate at all. The opposing argument focuses on distributive justice as the basis for public policy, thus prohibiting financial incentives on the grounds of exploitation of the poor; instead, to increase organ donation, public health and preventive health measures aimed at reducing the development of kidney failure should be intensified.

A highly publicized case of a prisoner on death row who wanted to be an organ donor serves as the basis for **chapter 21**, a debate on using legally executed prisoners as a source of organs.[9] The main argument in support of allowing death-row prisoners to donate organs is made on practical and ethical grounds: Physicians' primary concern is helping patients, and any medically suitable source of organs should be pursued. The argument against permitting such donations is the potential damage to organs related to the logistics of causing death by legal execution, making them less suitable for transplantation, as well as the position of the potential donor as a prisoner, which entails unavoidable coercion. Using organs from executed prisoners who volunteer as donors would not be a high-yield policy, but it raises questions central to physician responsibilities and medical ethics.

References

1. Joralemon D. Shifting ethics: debating the incentive question in organ transplantation. *J Med Ethics*. 2001;27:30–5.
2. Working Group on Incentives for Living Donation, Matas AJ, Satel S, et al. Incentives for organ donation: proposed standards for an internationally acceptable system. *Am J Transplant*. 2012;12(2):306–12.
3. Becker GJ, Elias JJ. Cash for kidneys: The case for a market for organs. *Wall Street Journal*, January 18, 2014.
4. Hippen BE. Introduction: symposium on a regulated market in transplantable organs. *J Med Philos*. 2009;34(6):545–51.
5. Blair RD, Kaserman DL; The economics and ethics of alternative cadaveric organ procurement policies. *Yale J. Regul*. 1991;8:403–52.
6. Health Research Support Agency. Policy 3.5. Allocation of kidneys. Washington, DC: US Department of Health & Human Services, 2013. http://optn.transplant.hrsa.gov/PoliciesandBylaws2/policies/pdfs/policy_7.pdf. Accessed March 31, 2014.
7. Sade RM, Miller F. Patients declared dead for organ donation are not really dead—the dead donor rule should be abandoned. *Ann Thorac Surg*. 2014;97(4):1131–4.
8. Hippen B, Ross LF, Sade RM. Saving lives is more important than abstract moral concerns: financial incentives should be use to increase organ donation. *Ann Thorac Surg*. 2009;88:1053–61.
9. Lin SS, Rich L, Pal JD, Sade RM. Prisoners on death row should be accepted as organ donors. *Ann Thorac Surg*. 2012;93:1773–9.

19

Heart Donation Without the Dead-Donor Rule

Franklin G. Miller and Robert M. Sade*

Introduction
Robert M. Sade, MD

A discussion of the Dead Donor Rule (DDR) was presented at the 49th Annual Meeting of the Society of Thoracic Surgeons in 2013. Prior to Dr. Franklin Miller's paper, the following case was presented.

THE CASE OF THE REJECTED HEART DONOR

Terry Sklavin is 49 years old and was a successful investment banker before he sustained a severe head injury in an automobile accident. A week after the accident, the patient is ventilator-dependent in the intensive care unit. Dr. P.V. Staat, the consulting neurologist, determines that only minimal brainstem function is present, and estimates that Mr. Sklavin's chance of recovery is negligible. The patient's wife has produced her husband's living will and durable power of attorney for health care; she is his health care agent. Both documents specify that if he were ever in an incapacitated condition from which he is unlikely to recover substantially, he does not want to be kept alive but wants to donate any organs that are medically suitable for transplantation. His hand-written instruction emphasizes that his heart especially should be used if at all possible.

The patient and his wife have had several conversations about end-of-life preferences, and she says that he felt very strongly about his clearly documented wishes. Dr. Staat informs her that organ donation might be feasible

*Sade RM, Miller F. Patients declared dead for organ donation are not really dead—the dead-donor rule should be abandoned. 2014;97(4):1131–2. Copyright Society of Thoracic Surgeons, republished here with permission.

under the hospital's donation after cardiac death protocol, but even if DCD were successful, it's highly unlikely that the heart could be used. Mrs. Sklavin says that her husband is as good as dead, will die soon, and can't understand why all of his medically suitable organs won't be used, particularly why his heart will most likely be buried with him. She wants his heart and other organs to be recovered while they're still in good condition for transplantation.

Dr. Staat explains that the dead donor rule does not permit recovery of organs until the patient has been declared dead after withdrawal of life support. He's aware of recent challenges to the current concepts of death and organ donation, and wonders whether it's time to replace the dead donor rule with one that permits donation by persons who are not dead but are facing inevitable imminent death.

COMMENTARY

A person who has irreversibly lost function of the entire brain, including the brain stem, is dead. The concept of brain death seems simple enough, but there is a great deal of confusion about it. For example, two out of three people think that someone who is brain dead is not legally dead, and more than half think that a patient in coma is brain dead.[1] Both beliefs are wrong. Because of such misunderstandings, controversy has been ongoing for many years about the relation between declaration of death and organ donation.

As the field of organ transplantation grew, demand mounted for increasing numbers of organs, especially from the recently deceased, producing a paradox: "the need for both a living body and a dead donor."[2] To resolve this paradox, the Uniform Determination of Death Act (UDDA) was promulgated in 1981 and was subsequently adopted by all the states:

> An individual who has sustained either (1) irreversible cessation of circulatory and respiratory functions, or (2) irreversible cessation of all functions of the entire brain, including the brain stem, is dead. A determination of death must be made in accordance with accepted medical standards.

Although death is unitary, the law allows its determination in two different ways. Legally, an individual who is brain dead and is warm and pink with intact circulation and ventilation is just as dead as a cadaver that has turned cold and stiff after permanent circulatory arrest.

The "Dead Donor Rule" (DDR) lies at the heart of current organ procurement policy.[3] It is not a legal statute; rather, it reflects the widely held belief that it is wrong to kill one person to save the life of another. On those grounds, an organ donor must already be dead before vital organs are removed. The DDR is therefore an ethical norm: vital organs may be removed only after the organ donor is dead. The UDDA assures patients, families, physicians, and other health professionals that a patient who is brain dead is in fact dead, so the combination with the DDR makes removal of organs for life-saving transplantation legally and ethically acceptable.

Brain death under the UDDA undoubtedly increased the supply of organs for transplantation, but the demand has grown much faster than the supply. Because of the growing waiting list and annual deaths, there has been increasing emphasis on donation after cardiac death (DCD) over the last 20 years. A protocol for DCD allows organ donation by patients who are near death and are ventilator-dependent but will not progress to brain death.[4] After a valid decision is made to discontinue life support, the option of organ donation may be offered. If the patient expressed a wish to be a donor or if the family agrees to donation, DCD may be carried out. The patient is brought to the operating room, the ventilator is removed so ventilation stops, circulation stops within 60 minutes, and when there has been no circulation for 2–5 minutes, the patient is pronounced dead and organs are rapidly removed. Kidneys and liver can often be used for transplantation, but because of the ischemic time, the heart is seldom transplanted. If circulation does not stop within 60 minutes, the organs are deemed to be too damaged for transplant and the patient dies without donating organs.

A problem that arises from the DDR is that it may frustrate the express wishes of an individual to be an organ donor. An example is Terry Sklavin, the patient in our scenario. He wants to donate his heart as well as other organs, but he cannot because of the DDR. He is near death and will certainly be dead very soon. The DCD protocol requires up to 60 minutes of diminishing circulation, several minutes of no circulation, and the additional time it takes to open the body cavities, administer tissue preservation fluids, and remove the organs. This extended period of ischemia means that his heart will almost certainly not be used for transplant, although his kidneys and liver probably will be used, as they are less sensitive to ischemic damage than the heart. In cases in which the time requirements are not met, all organs are lost.

Although the DDR is well-established in transplantation policy and practice, it has been challenged in recent years as an unnecessary fiction that results in lost lives.[5,6] According to this position, without the DDR, Mr. Sklavin's heart, as well as other organs could have been donated without violating basic ethical and legal principles, as Dr. Miller explains in the accompanying paper.

Heart Donation Without the Dead Donor Rule
Franklin G. Miller, PhD

Donation of vital organs is currently governed by the "dead donor rule" (DDR). Donors must be determined to be dead according to established legal criteria and medical standards prior to procurement of vital organs for transplantation. Most donors are determined to be dead on neurological criteria: the irreversible cessation of all functions of the entire brain. In response to a shortage of "brain dead" donors, vital organs increasingly have been procured from donors declared dead according to circulatory criteria following withdrawal of life-sustaining treatment (LST). Protocols for donation after circulatory death (DCD) typically involve patients on mechanical ventilation with severe neurological damage short of "brain death," as in the case of Mr. Sklavin. After withdrawal of life support and cessation of circulation, a waiting period of usually 2-5 minutes is required before organs are retrieved. Hearts rarely have been procured under DCD protocols, although hearts of infants have been transplanted successfully in some controversial cases.[7]

Rethinking the ethics of vital organ donation is imperative because there are compelling reasons for calling into question compliance of current practices of transplantation with the DDR. The first criterion for determining death under the Uniform Determination of Death Act—the operative law in most states in the U.S.—is "irreversible cessation of circulatory and respiratory functions." Can we be confident that these functions are *irreversible* a very short interval after cessation of heart beat? The fact that circulation has ceased 2–5 minutes (or even less in some cases) does not mean that the cessation of circulation is irreversible. To satisfy the criterion of "irreversibility" in its ordinary meaning, it must be impossible to restore circulation with available means of medical intervention. Although decisions have been made not to undertake cardiopulmonary resuscitation (CPR) following withdrawal of LST in DCD cases, the use of CPR might be successful in restoring circulation if it were initiated. Hence, donors under DCD protocols are not known to be dead at the time of organ procurement. Some commentators have contended that the permanent cessation of circulation is sufficient to satisfy the DDR. However, "permanent" does not mean the same as "irreversible." If cessation of circulation is irreversible, then it also is permanent; but the converse is not necessarily true.[8]

There are even more compelling reasons to argue that the DDR is routinely being violated in the case of "brain dead" donors. With mechanical ventilation, "brain dead" individuals maintain a wide array of biological functions, including circulation, respiration, wound healing, infection fighting, temperature regulation, secretion of neurohormones, and even gestation of a fetus for up to three months. They are not dead according to the established biological conception of death. While detailed examination of the status of "brain dead" donors lies outside the scope of this essay, it is mentioned here to indicate that compliance with the DDR is systemically problematic—the problem is not limited to the practice of transplantation under DCD protocols.

What is the upshot if vital organ donors under DCD protocols (and "brain dead donors) are not really dead, or not known to be dead, at the time of organ procurement? Strict compliance with the DDR would dictate that we stop transplanting vital organs from these donors. However, this would lead to many desperately ill patients failing to receive life-saving, or life-enhancing, organ transplantations—a drastic outcome that few people would endorse. To be sure, it is possible to sustain the status quo by muddling through, relying on the fiction, which is not officially acknowledged, that vital organ donors are dead at the time of organ procurement. Instead of relying on a legal and moral fiction, however, we can seek an ethically sound justification for vital organ transplantation from donors who are not known to be dead. Space limitations permit only a sketch of the argument, which has been developed in detail elsewhere.[9]

The key to justifying vital organ donation without the DDR is to acknowledge the causal force of withdrawing LST, particularly mechanical ventilation. The conventional view is that withdrawing mechanical ventilation, or other means of life support, merely allows the patient to die, but does not cause the patient's death. Rather, the patient's underlying medical condition causes death. This view, however, is not credible and fails to withstand critical scrutiny.

Consider the following case. Debbie, aged 50 years, was thrown from her horse in a horse-show event. She sustained a high level spinal cord injury. The accident left her quadriplegic and ventilator-dependent. Two years later, following rehabilitation and return home, she decided that her life was no longer worth living. She arranged to be admitted to the intensive care unit of an academic medical center for the purpose of withdrawing her ventilator. Thirty minutes after being sedated and extubated, Debbie died.[10] What caused Debbie's death? Was it the spinal cord injury? Despite her spinal cord injury, Debbie likely could have lived for many years with continued mechanical ventilation and personal care. Withdrawing the ventilator set in motion the causal chain leading to her death, given her inability to breathe spontaneously due to the spinal cord injury. In other words, the treatment withdrawal was the proximate cause of Debbie's death. Based on our common-sense understanding of causation, withdrawing mechanical ventilation causes death in patients unable to breathe spontaneously.

The same causal account pertains to patients on mechanical ventilation with a much more grim prognosis than that of Debbie, as in the case of Mr. Sklavin. According to his advance directive and conversations with his wife, it is clear that Mr. Sklavin would not want to live with no hope of recovery from profound neurological injury and would want to donate his heart, along with his other vital organs. Successful heart donation is considered highly unlikely for him under a DCD protocol. Would there be anything wrong from an ethical perspective in procuring Mr. Sklavin's heart and other vital organs prior to stopping mechanical ventilation? Through Mrs. Sklavin's surrogate decision-making, in light of Mr. Sklavin's prior expressed preferences, valid decisions have been made to stop life support and donate organs. Moreover, Mr. Sklavin would be dead following withdrawal of LST regardless of whether his organs are procured. Accordingly, no harm or wrong would be done to Mr. Sklavin by procuring his heart and other organs under anesthesia *prior* to withdrawing the ventilator. In this set of circumstances, absence of harm to the donor and valid consent to donation justify organ procurement prior to stopping life support. This not only would make possible a life-saving heart transplantation that otherwise would not occur; it also would provide greater assurance of viability for his other organs, which would be continuously perfused until they were retrieved.

Once we see that withdrawing LST, in service of patient self-determination and relief of suffering, causes the death of patients, there is no sound ethical reason for concern about procuring vital organs prior to treatment withdrawal. The patient is on a planned trajectory, with death as the imminent outcome. Procuring vital organs with valid consent before treatment withdrawal does not change this trajectory; nor does it wrong the patient, who soon will be dead whether or not the organs are procured.

It might be objected that withdrawing mechanical ventilation does not necessarily cause death. While this is true, the possibility of surviving withdrawal of life support does not reflect the medical conditions of current candidates for DCD. In two recent prospective multi-centered studies of potential DCD donors in the Netherlands and the U.K., including 402 cases, all the patients died after treatment withdrawal.[11,12] The median times to death were 20-36 minutes, and the longest times to death were less than four days. Viable organs could not be retrieved in 17% of the potential donors in one of the studies, and 38% in the other. However, under the approach recommended here, vital organs could have been donated from all of these potential donors with procurement prior to withdrawing LST, and heart donation likely would have been possible in many of the cases.

The scope and limits of vital organ donation from still-living patients should be carefully defined. Limiting this practice to patients with valid decisions to stop LST and to donate organs would assure that the interests of patients are not being sacrificed in order to save the lives of others.

Unbiased examination of the practice of withdrawing LST, which causes the death of patients, underwrites a rethinking of the ethics of vital organ donation. From an ethical perspective, we do not need to uphold the DDR. Abandoning the DDR and procuring organs prior to withdrawing LST will potentially lead to many more lives saved from transplantation and greater respect for the donation preferences of individuals like Mr. Sklavin. Realizing this potential, however, will require policy changes predicated on honestly facing up to the realities of withdrawing LST and vital organ donation.

References

1. Siminoff LA, Burant C, Youngner SJ. Death and organ procurement: public beliefs and attitudes. *Kennedy Inst Ethics J.* 2004;14(3):217–34.
2. Greenberg G. As good as dead. *The New Yorker*, August 13, 2001:36.
3. Iltis AS, Cherry MJ. Death revisited: rethinking death and the dead donor rule. *J Med Philos.* 2010;35:223–41.
4. Bernat JL, D'Alessandro AM, Port FK, et al. Report of a national conference on donation after cardiac death. *Am J Transplant.* 2006;6:281–91.
5. Truog RD, Robinson WM. Role of brain death and the dead donor rule in the ethics of organ donation. *Critical Care Med.* 2003;31:2391–6.
6. Miller FG, Truog RD, Rethinking the ethics of vital organ donations. *Hastings Center Rep.* 2008;38(6):38–46.
7. Sade RM. Consequences of the dead donor rule. *Ann Thorac Surg.* 2014;97(4):1131–2.
8. Marquis D. Are DCD donors dead? *Hastings Center Rep.* 2010;40(3):24–31.
9. Miller FG, Truog RD. *Death, Dying, and Organ Transplantation: Reconstructing Medical Ethics at the End of Life.* New York: Oxford University Press; 2012.
10. Miller FG. Heart donation without the dead donor rule. *Ann Thorac Surg.* 2014;97:1133–4.
11. Wind J, Snoeijs MGJ, Brugman CA, et al. Prediction of time of death after withdrawal of life-sustaining treatment in potential donors after cardiac death. *Crit Care Med.* 2012;40:766–9.
12. Suntharalingam C, Sharples L, Dudley C, et al. Time to cardiac death after withdrawal of life-sustaining treatment in potential organ donors. *Am J Transplant* 2009;9:2157–65.

20

Saving Lives Is More Important Than Abstract Moral Concerns

FINANCIAL INCENTIVES SHOULD BE USED TO INCREASE ORGAN DONATION

Benjamin Hippen, Lainie Friedman Ross, and Robert M. Sade*

Ever since organ donation became clinically feasible, there have not been enough organs to go around. Figure 20.1 shows the rate of change from a base value in 1995 through 2008, of three variables: (1) the number of deceased donors, (2) the number of patients with end-stage organ failure who are waiting for an organ, and (3) the number of waiting list patients who either die before an organ becomes available (i.e., death on the waiting list or after removal from the waiting list as "too sick to transplant").[1] The number of potential recipients on transplant waiting lists has more than doubled, and now stands at over 100,000, whereas the number of deceased donors has increased by only half. Meanwhile, the numbers of deaths related to the organ shortage, which is now greater than 9,000 a year, has grown in parallel with the waiting list. Thus, the gap between supply and demand has grown every year for the past 15 years. [...]

How can we increase the number of donors? When a difficult or dangerous job has to be done, such as working on high-rise construction projects, we give workers an added incentive to take these jobs by offering them more benefits, such as salary supplements. Perhaps offering a financial incentive for organ donation would increase the number of willing donors. But if offering

*Hippen B, Ross LF, Sade RM. Saving lives is more important than abstract moral concerns: financial incentives should be used to increase organ donation. *Ann Thorac Surg.* 2009;88:1053–61. Copyright Society of Thoracic Surgeons, republished here with permission.

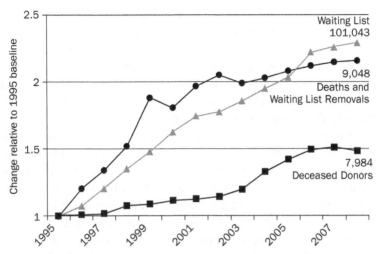

FIGURE 20.1 Relative change (from 1988 baseline data) in the number of patients on organ waiting lists, deaths on the waiting list, and number of donors each year, 1988–2008. Graph derived from Organ Procurement and Transplantation Network data (Removal reasons by year; Removed from the Waiting List: January, 1995–March 31, 2009. OPTN: Organ Procurement and Transplantation Network. http://optn.transplant.hrsa.gov/latestData/rptData.asp. Accessed June 16, 2009)

people financial incentives could increase the supply of organs, should we do it? Would it be morally appropriate? [. . .]

The debate is rendered more concrete by focusing on the case of a United States senator who has a decision to make.

THE CASE OF THE CONSCIENTIOUS SENATOR

Senator Alexis Murray is a member of the Senate's Committee on Health, Education, Labor, and Pensions, which is holding a hearing on a bill that will permit payment of up to $10,000 plus in reimbursement for expenses to living kidney, liver, or lung donors. Senator Murray listened to testimony by a few individuals and by representatives of organizations that either support or oppose the bill. He is particularly struck by the story told by George Cranford, a computer repair technician.

Mr Cranford's 25-year-old daughter, Karen, has diabetic nephropathy and has suffered from end-stage renal disease for 5 years. On renal dialysis, she has had frequent bloodstream infections, several of which have been nearly fatal. She is currently hospitalized, recover-ing from her latest methicillin-resistant Staphylococcus aureus infection. The recurrence rate of such infections is high, and the mortality rate is between 50% and 75%. Karen is an only child; her parents and other relatives are unsuitable to donate a kidney. She is waiting for an organ from a deceased donor, but her place on the waiting list makes it likely that she will be among the 9,000 patients who die each year because of the shortage of organs for transplantation.

Mr Cranford has several friends and acquaintances who have said they have considered donating a kidney for Karen, but have decided not to do so because of concerns for lost income from time away from work, the possibility of losing their jobs, possible health consequences from having only one kidney, and the stress, pain, and physical risks of the donor operation. He expresses the belief that these concerns could be outweighed by the offer of an award of some kind, such as payment for health insurance, an income tax credit, or cash payment of a few thousand dollars. If some of his friends and perhaps many others around the country could be persuaded by such incentives to donate a vital organ, thousands of lives could be saved each year.

Senator Murray is impressed by the story, but is concerned about potential negative consequences of permitting a market in human organs. After the hearing, he seeks the advice of two thoughtful physician-ethicists, Benjamin Hippen, MD, and Lainie Friedman Ross, MD, PhD.

Pro
Benjamin Hippen, MD

The number of people with kidney failure in the United States is increasing. By 2010 it is expected to be 591,000, with more than 80,000 patients waiting for a kidney transplant.[2] Incremental improvements in immunosuppression have rendered kidney transplantation a superior therapeutic modality for more and more patients with kidney failure. Unfortunately, despite our best efforts, the supply of transplantable kidneys has not and will not keep up with the growing demand.

The current state of affairs is responsible for several unintended, but foreseeable, consequences. Longer waiting times for transplant candidates result in patients who are sicker at the time of transplantation. This factor, combined with an increased reliance on extended criteria donors (i.e., marginal donors), results in inferior graft survival. Longer waiting times also serve to increase emotional pressure on any available living donor. Longer waiting times and few available options have contributed to an upsurge in international organ trafficking. [...]

Various solutions to this problem have either proven to be inadequate or are unlikely to succeed. [...] Despite the aggressive efforts of the Organ Donor Collaborative to increase the number of available organs, the total number of procured organs during the last 10 years has been flat relative to the growing demand and a sizeable fraction of "new" organs, which are from extended criteria donors. These organs afford shorter graft survival, increasing the likelihood that recipients of these kidneys will return to dialysis. A policy of involuntary organ conscription is morally problematic, and countries that have such policies ensconced in law have not been able to successfully procure more organs than countries that rely on consent for donation.[3]

The costs of this public policy failure is high, measurable in the unnecessary loss of human life, the vast expenditure of public treasure on a suboptimal therapy (dialysis), and the spread of desperation among waiting recipients and their families. This state of affairs supports arguments in favor of pilot trials of incentives to increase organ procurement from living donors.

The central argument in favor of incentives is patient autonomy. Free societies typically do not interfere with competent adults making choices that affect their lives and do not significantly harm themselves or others. Free societies rely on this principle for ethically defensible uncompensated living donation and (rightly) look askance at those who would abridge this liberty. Opponents of a regulated market in organs encourage us to view this proposal through the lens of the manifest harms to vendors and recipients who participate in underground organ trafficking, without lingering on the fact that organ trafficking in developing countries would not be economically sustainable, except for the shortage of available organs in developed countries. Because organ trafficking continues unfettered by existing laws prohibiting the practice, those who are authentically committed to reducing organ trafficking can find the most straightforward solution in reducing the incentive for recipients in wealthy, developed countries to economically support trafficking. Our public policy failure merely ensures the continued health of international organ trafficking abroad.

Regulated organ markets also may be safer than the current system of living donation. It is true, but trivially so, that organ donors become, in some sense, a patient. The obligations that physicians have to their patients would not change because some donors are compensated and others are not. The existing literature on donor outcomes, however incomplete, nonetheless, supports the premise that donating a kidney is safe for the long term.[4] By vastly expanding the number of potential living donors, one can cherry-pick to identify people who everyone agrees would be at the lowest risk for long-term harm from donation. Incentives would also helpfully eliminate the psychological pressures brought to bear on living donors, borne of their recipient's desperate plight. Far from suppressing altruism, the authentic altruism of those who still choose to donate (uncompensated) would thereby be clarified and preserved.

In itself, low socioeconomic status is an independent risk factor for the development of kidney disease over time, a fact which constitutes sufficient reason to exclude the poorest among us from participation in organ vending (or for that matter, in living organ donation). Exclusion of the very poor is justified not because poor donors and vendors are somehow incapable of autonomous judgment. [...] Rather, exclusion is justified because the purpose of a regulated market in organs is to increase the number of available organs without increasing harm to others. The "right to sell" does not impose an "obligation to buy," and the interests of all involved entail an exchange that benefits recipients without harming sellers.

Any system of incentives requires regulation and oversight, and it is a caricature to suppose that there is a contradiction between free exchange and the strictures of law. Law outlines the conceptual space for articulating obligations to donors and vendors, and the law explains the means whereby the legitimacy and enforcement of these obligations are possible. Among the necessary protections to be included would be the assurances of safety for both donors and recipients; transparency in regard to the risk of a living kidney donation for both the compensated and uncompensated donors; institutional integrity to protect donors, recipients, healthcare providers, and institutions who choose to participate or abstain from compensation arrangements; and the rule of law, to define how the arrangements for exchange could take place for mutual benefit.[5]

These protections morally distinguish a regulated system of incentives for organ procurement from the significant harms generated by organ trafficking, and they would provide a useful guide to the construction of pilot trials for incentives in this country, as well as a means of assessing the conditions in other countries. Along these lines, the United States has something to learn from Iran, which is the only country in the world with a legal pseudo-market in organs from living donors, and the 22-year legacy of that institution provides useful lessons and cautionary tales.[6] No evidence is perfect, but the peer-reviewed evidence we have from several sources supports the following facts: (1) for the last decade, Iran has not had a waiting list for transplantable kidneys; (2) the long-term outcomes of recipients of purchased organs is not significantly different from the outcomes of recipients of donated kidneys (a useful surrogate marker for the health of organ vendors); (3) the existence of a flourishing market has not resulted in attrition of the number of kidneys donated by biological relatives; and (4) uncompensated organ donation from the deceased has increased 10-fold since 2000, when laws recognizing brain-death as death were approved by the Iranian Parliament. On the other hand, the following is also true: (1) organ vendors are disproportionately impoverished and poorly educated; (2) the data on long-term outcomes for organ vendors is conflicting and mixed, but at any rate it is substantially incomplete. It does not follow that a system of incentives inexorably leads to bad outcomes for vendors. What does follow is that a defensible system of incentives must offer plausible assurances that the long-term consequences for organ vendors are at least as safe as for organ donors.

A broader view of what might constitute "compensation" will be instrumentally useful in beginning to provide some of these assurances.

Compensations need not be limited only to cash payment. Providing a non-fungible, lifelong, comprehensive healthcare benefit for donors would intersect with the desire of the transplant community for a long-term, prospective study of outcomes after donation. Compensation might take the form of a deposit in a donor's health savings account, retirement account, favorite charity, or any number of possible permutations. The specific nature of the incentive is less important than the following: (1) a successfully functioning incentive by making more organs available, and (2) an incentive that would not give rise to further harms.[7]

The point is that our current system brings harm to recipients who are dying by the thousands every year on a waiting list, harm to donors who (correctly) understand the dire consequences of their choice not to donate for their recipient, and harm to legions of victims of organ trafficking who silently shoulder the true costs of our ongoing public policy failure. Incentives can be structured in a way to decisively answer moral objections. Whether the transplant community and our political leaders see fit to understand this point in practice, or whether the needless suffering and economic boondoggle of the status quo will simply continue, remains an open question.

Con
Lainie Friedman Ross, MD, PhD

We are posed with the hypothetical case of a senator who is considering a bill that will permit payment for living donors. [...] Karen's story is sad, but so is the story of every individual in end-stage renal disease on dialysis. [...] Although the National Organ Transplant Act made it illegal to buy or sell organs in the United States in 1984, and the World Health Organization recommended a similar ban in 1991, support for a kidney market has blossomed in the past decade.[8] In this article, I argue that the market is not an ethical solution to the organ shortage. I argue this position using the bioethical framework developed by Beauchamp and Childress.[9] [...]

THE FOUR PRINCIPLES

[...] Beauchamp and Childress explicate four fundamental principles of bioethics: (1) autonomy, (2) beneficence, (3) nonmaleficence, and (4) justice. The principle of autonomy (or more accurately, the principle of respect for autonomy) refers to the right of self-determination. In medical ethics, we say that the competent patient (an individual who has decision-making capacity) has the right to accept or refuse medical care, even lifesaving medical care. The principle of beneficence addresses the obligation of physicians to act in their patient's best interest, whereas the principle of nonmaleficence states that physicians should avoid, when possible, harming a patient. Neither of these principles is absolute in that we often cause some harm with our treatments, with chemotherapy for cancer being a case in point. Rather, these principles are understood to mean that the benefits should outweigh the risks of harm.

The fourth principle, the principle of justice, is the most complicated one, because it refers to obligations beyond the doctor–patient relationship. Jonsen and colleagues[10] discuss the importance of justice in policy decisions, but that it should not be used to make distribution decisions at the bedside. There are two main competing conceptions of justice in medical ethics: (1) utilitarian justice and (2) deontological or principle-based justice. Utilitarian justice focuses on utility or efficiency. A distribution scheme of organs is just if it maximizes the number of lives or the number of life-years gained. That is, the focus is on maximizing the well-being of the greatest number. In contrast, egalitarian justice focuses on equity and a fair distribution of resources, even at the expense of efficiency. In general, in the realm of organ transplantation, the practice has been to use policies and practices that balance equity and efficiency.[11] For example, the current deceased donor allocation system focuses on ABO blood type matching (efficiency) and on waiting time (equity). [...]

First, let us look at the principle of autonomy. The principle of autonomy is not absolute, as with all guiding bioethics principles. There are moral constraints on autonomy. As Oliver Wendell Holmes remarked, "The right to swing my fist ends where the other man's nose begins."[12] That is, one moral constraint on autonomy is harm to others. But the harm to the organ vendor is to himself, not to others, except insofar as one believes that we as a society are worse off if we allow vulnerable individuals to sell their body parts on the grounds of commodification.[13] The argument from commodification holds that market valuation has a degrading effect on certain goods and practices if they are bought and sold, even if fair bargaining positions exist (a most unlikely position).

[...] Respect for autonomy [...] permits one to challenge an individual's decision when it is contrary to the individual's best interest. There are many reasons why an individual may make a decision that is contrary to their interests: misinformation, miscalculation, coercion, or even undue influence (an offer that seems too good to be true). Thus, to the extent that one believes that individuals who are willing to sell their kidneys are not acting voluntarily, it would be morally imperative to prohibit them from doing so. [...]

What is interesting about the autonomy debate, however, is that all of the market supporters do not discuss a free market. [...] [T]he proponents of an organ market reject a free market (on grounds of its potential to be exploitative) and focus instead on a regulated market [...].[14] It is not clear if those who promote this believe they are protecting recipients or vendors. The answer is probably both. They are protecting recipients because of the greater risks of infectious diseases in potential vendors abroad.[15] They claim to be protecting the vendors because a market price of $10,000 in the United States would bring hundreds of thousands, if not millions, of individuals from third-world countries for whom the dollar amount would be undue inducement. If vendors were not restricted to citizens of the United States, then the market value could fall to less than $1,000.[16] This may not be a large enough incentive for Mr Cranford's friends, but $1,000 could go a long way in China and India. In addition, if this is the only way for the individual to escape poverty, it is not clear how our protection helps them. The same arguments regarding the opportunity to escape poverty should hold true for citizens in the United States who are poor and for poor citizens of China and India. [...]

It is also the case that autonomy must be understood within a social context. In a society in which great disparities exist in wealth and opportunities, the claim that poor people should have the right to sell their kidney as one more option to escape poverty denies any social responsibility we may have to prevent such a tragic option. [...]

The argument that beneficence requires physicians to help treat the thousands of patients in organ failure at any price also fails. First, we must remember that in transplantation with living sources, the vendor or donor becomes a patient as well.[17] It is not the case that taking an organ in a setting of exploitation is acting in the vendor's best interest. This argument also ignores the fact that the whole focus of organ failure is about how to procure more organs without consideration of our failure in the public health and preventive health mission to reduce organ failure in the first place. [...]

The concerns of harm (nonmaleficence) cannot be pushed aside on the grounds that we take kidneys from family members and view the harms as acceptable. As previously explained, the principles of beneficence and nonmaleficence must be understood in tandem and evaluated as benefit-to-harm ratio. Then, here is why there may be a difference between exposing a paid kidney vendor to the risks of surgery and long-term psychological and clinical risks of unilateral nephrectomy compared with the altruistic donor. That is, we believe that the altruistic donor gains significant psychological benefits by aiding an emotionally related family member or friend.[18] In contrast, data (from Iran and India) show that the paid vendors do not reap the benefits they expected (improved financial circumstances);in fact, data show they experience many emotional and social harms in the stigma that they face for having sold a part of their body.[19] [...]

Even if we assume the current state of affairs, many justice theorists reject utilitarianism because of a theory limited to maximizing good consequences that could allow for significant harm to specific subpopulations. That is, it could be allowed for one adult to sacrifice himself to serve as an organ donor for 10 individuals on the waiting list for financial gain to his next of kin. Worse yet, it might justify lotteries in which individuals were sacrificed to maximize the well-being of 10 individuals per sacrifice! Rather, most justice theorists would argue that in organ transplantation, as in many areas of medicine, we need to consider the distribution of goods and not just the maximization of goods. One widely accepted theory of egalitarian justice was developed by John Rawls.[20] It would permit policies that increase organ transplantation using living vendors if this policy would be accepted behind a veil of ignorance where one was not aware of one's personal traits but did have knowledge of the social and political state of affairs. Behind the veil of ignorance, an individual would know that demand for organs greatly outstripped supply. Behind the veil, the rational Rawlsian individual would adopt policies to increase organ transplants provided that the new policies were not harmful to those who are already "worse off." A market in organs would be most attractive to those who are poor without other alternatives. Then, Rawlsian justice would judge those who are willing to vend as some of the "worst off" members of society. Such a market would be exploitative and not permissible. The market proponents who seek to restrict the kidney market to citizens of the United States are conceding this point. They are failing to acknowledge that if this practice were to be legalized in the United States, then other countries could quickly follow suit, and it would be hard to restrict trade across borders. Even if we could restrict border trades, we could be doing great harm to the "worst off" in poor countries who may now feel that this is an opportunity that they cannot resist, even if it leaves them no better off in the long-run. [...]

CONCLUSION

Although proponents try to use the "Four Principles of Bioethics" to support a market in organs, I have shown that the four principles, when properly operationalized, do not support a market. Rather, I have shown that the pro-market interpretation fails to understand that the principles need to be understood within a particular conception of justice. In a liberal society that values human rights and the dignity of man, an egalitarian conception of justice is the most appropriate conception of justice for public policy. An egalitarian theory of justice must prohibit the sale of organs on grounds of exploitation! The concern of exploitation makes the vendor's autonomy suspect, and it clearly does not minimize the harms to which we expose any living source of organs nor does it ensure that they truly benefit from the procurement.

Bad cases make bad laws. I am sympathetic to Karen, but I am also sympathetic to all individuals with chronic renal failure, even if their illness is somewhat self-induced. A policy to pay Karen's father's friends may resolve the stress, pain and risks of donation, but they do not address the risk of death, which is a real but rare event. If Mr Cranford's friends really thought about the risk of mortality, they would realize that $10,000 is too little, given the real but remote risk of death. They should also realize that money should not fully resolve their reluctance. In fact, the risk of mortality should give us reason to pause and realize that the solution to our organ shortage should not be based on increasing the number of living donors. Rather, we need to focus on prevention, to maximize voluntary deceased donation, to develop alternative organ sources (such as therapeutic organ cloning), and even to promote research in xenotransplantation.

Concluding Remarks
Robert M. Sade, MD

[...] The conclusions readers should draw from these opposing positions, which start with mostly identical facts but reach radically different conclusions, depend largely on how they weigh the two central facts of the issue at hand in the context of their own personal value systems. The central facts are: (1) in this country more than 9,000 patients in need of a transplant die each year because the number of available organs is inadequate; and (2) financial incentives in a regulated market would increase the supply of organs (a fact asserted by Hippen and not denied by Ross).

A reader will support Hippen's position if persuaded that people in a mature liberal democracy, such as the United States, should be allowed the freedom to choose among three options (in the context of a carefully regulated market that excludes poor people as donors and ensures safety for all participants): that is, to donate altruistically, to donate for financial benefit, or not to donate at all.

A reader will support Ross's position if persuaded that egalitarian (distributive) justice is the best guide for public policy, that financial incentives for organ donations must therefore be prohibited on grounds of exploitation of the poor, and that we should not attempt to increase the number of living donors but should pursue alternative strategies, including a greater emphasis on public health and preventive health measures that may reduce or retard the development of kidney failure.

The heat generated by the public debate on financial incentives for organ donors has been rising as more voices join each side. Congress has shown interest in this issue, including Representative James Greenwood in 2003,[21] and most recently Senator Arlen Specter by way of his proposed bill, the Organ Donor Clarification Act.[22] How public policy makers respond to the opposing views presented in this debate will have long-term effects on the quality and duration of the lives of many patients and on the moral foundations of our society.

References

1. Removal reasons by year; removed from the waiting list: January, 1995–March 31, 2009. OPTN: Organ Procurement and Transplantation Network. Washington, DC: US Department of Health & Human Services. http://optn.transplant.hrsa.gov/latestData/rptData.asp. Accessed June 16, 2009.
2. Gilbertson DT, Liu J, Xue JL. Projecting the number of patients with end-stage renal disease in the United States to the year 2015. *J Am Soc Nephrol.* 2005;16:3736–41.
3. Healy K. Do presumed consent laws raise organ procure-ment rates? *De Paul Law Rev.* 2006;55:1017–43.
4. Ibrahim HN, Foley R, Tan L. Long-term consequences of kidney donation. *New Eng J of Med.* 2009;360:459–69.
5. Hippen BE. In defense of a regulated market in kidneys from living vendors. *J Med Philos.* 2005;30:593–626.
6. Hippen B. Organ sales and moral travails: lessons from the living kidney vendor program in Iran. Cato Policy Analysis No. 614. 2008. Washington, DC: Cato Institute. http://www.cato.org/pub_display.php?pub_id=9273. Accessed July 31, 2009.
7. Hippen BE. The case for kidney markets. *The New Atlantis* 2006;14:47–1461. http://www.thenewatlantis.com/archive/14/hippen.htm. Accessed July 31, 2009.
8. Taylor JS. *Stakes and Kidneys: Why Markets in Human Body Parts Are Morally Imperative.* Hampshire. UK: Ashgate; 2005.
9. Beauchamp TL, Childress JF. *Principles of Biomedical Ethics,* 5th ed. New York: Oxford University Press; 2001.
10. Jonsen A, Siegler M, Winslade W. *Clinical Ethics: A Practical Approach to Ethical Decisions in Clinical Medicine,* 6th ed. New York: McGraw-Hill; 2006.
11. Veatch RM. *Transplantation Ethics.* Washington, DC: Georgetown University Press; 2000.
12. Holmes OW Jr. http://thinkexist.com/quotation/the_right_to_swing_my_.st_ends_where_the_other/217369.html. Accessed August 1, 2009.
13. Sandel MJ. What money can't buy: the moral limits of markets. The Tanner Lectures on Human Values. Paper presented at, Brasenose College, Oxford, May 11–12, 1998. http://www.tannerlectures.utah.edu/lectures/documents/sandel00.pdf.   Accessed August 1, 2009.
14. Erin CA, Harris J. An ethical market in human organs. *J Med Ethics.* 2003;29:137–8.
15. Rizvi SNS, Zafar M, Ahmed E, et al. Health status and renal function evaluation of kidney venders: a report from Pakistan. *Am J Transplant.* 2008;13:453–76.
16. Adams AF, Barnett AH, Kaserman DL. Markets of organs: the question of supply. *Contemp Econ Policy.* 1999;17:147–55.
17. Danovitch GM. The doctor–patient relationship in living donor kidney transplantation. *Curr Opin Nephrol Hypertens.* 2007;16:503–5.
18. Frade IC, Fonseca I, Dias L, et al. Impact assessment in living kidney donation: psychosocial aspects in the donor. *Transplant Proc* 2008;40:677–81.
19. Goyal M, Mehta RL, Schneiderman LJ, Sehgal AR. Economic and health consequences of selling a kidney in India. *JAMA.* 2002;288:1589–93.
20. Rawls J. *A Theory of Justice.* Cambridge, MA: Belknap Press of Harvard University Press; 1971.

21. Assessing initiatives to increase organ donations: hearing before the Subcommittee on Oversight and Investigations of the Committee on Energy and Commerce, House of Representatives. June 3, 2003. http://archives.energycommerce.house.gov/repar-chives/108/Hearings/06032003hearing946/print.htm. Accessed June 16, 2009.
22. Pitney JJ. Incentives for organ donation. Politicalmavens.com. December 2, 2008. http://politicalmavens.com/index.php/2008/12/02/incentives-for-organ-donation/. Accessed June 16, 2009.

21

Prisoners on Death Row Should Be Accepted as Organ Donors

Shu S. Lin, Lauren Rich, Jay D. Pal, and Robert M. Sade*

Introduction

Robert M. Sade, MD

Ten years ago, Christian Longo had been deeply enmeshed in a career of minor crimes and crushing financial burdens that had led to bankruptcy. He saw only one way out: relieving his family, his wife Mary Jane and their three children, of their dependency on him. He strangled Mary Jane and 2-year old daughter Madison, put them into suitcases and threw them into Yaquina Bay in Newport, Oregon. He stuffed his 3-year old daughter Sadie and 4-year old son Zachery into pillowcases, weighted them down with rocks, and threw them, still alive, into a nearby pond where they drowned.

His crime was discovered when Zachery's body floated to the surface of the pond. He was placed on the FBI's 10 most wanted list, was found 2 years later living with his girlfriend in Cancun, Mexico, and was arrested, brought back to Oregon, put on trial, found guilty on four counts of murder, and sentenced to death.

In March 2011, Longo wrote an editorial that was published in the New York Times: "Giving Life After Death Row."[1] The editorial began with these words: "Eight years ago I was sentenced to death for the murders of my wife and three children. I am guilty. I once thought that I could fool others into believing this was not true. Failing that, I tried to convince myself that

---

*Lin SS, Rich L, Pal JD, Sade RM. Prisoners on death row should be accepted as organ donors. *Ann Thorac Surg.* 2012;93:1773–9. Copyright Society of Thoracic Surgeons, republished here with permission.

it didn't matter. But gradually, the enormity of what I did seeped in; that was followed by remorse and then a wish to make amends."

He continued: "There is no way to atone for my crimes, but I believe that a profound benefit to society can come from my circumstances. I have asked to end my remaining appeals, and then donate my organs after my execution to those who need them." He went on to say, "And yet, the prison authority's response to my latest appeal to donate was this: 'The interests of the public and condemned inmates are best served by denying the petition.'"

Longo claimed that half of the other inmates on death row wanted to do the same and that there was no valid reason to prohibit them from donating. The question: [...] who was right, the condemned prisoner or the prison parole board [...]?

Pro
Shu S. Lin, MD, PhD, Lauren Rich, RN, BSN

The shortage of donor organs often seems insurmountable. As a transplant surgeon, I understand the importance of seizing every appropriate opportunity to help patients with end-stage organ failure. When I learned that prisoners on death row have been denied their desire to donate their organs after execution, I asked myself, "Why not allow it?"

WHY NOT ALLOW DEATH ROW INMATES TO DONATE?

Each organ donor means at least one or more lives saved. Pursuing every opportunity for organ donation is not merely an attempt to "close the ever-widening gap between demand and supply of organs" in transplantation, as some have charged.[2] It is, quite simply, to help individuals suffering from end-stage organ disease. The center of attention, in my mind, should be the patient, and how we, as health care providers, can help them. There is no question that, when there is a therapy with known benefits to the patients we serve, it is reasonable that we should attempt to implement that therapy pending evaluation of the risks or the drawbacks of that therapy.

Organ donation is legally governed in the United States by two documents—the National Organ Transplantation Act (NOTA) of 1984, a federal law, and the Uniform Anatomical Gift Act (UAGA), a state law—neither explicitly prohibits organ donation by death row inmates. NOTA stipulates that organ donation cannot be made for "valuable considerations," including any monetary or material benefit or, for prisoners, a shorter sentence—obviously not an issue for death row inmates. Under the UAGA, any adult can commit to being an organ donor simply by saying so in a document, such as a donor card or a symbol on a driver's license. Therefore, the critical question here is what are the reasons not to permit donation by condemned prisoners?

WHY PROHIBIT PRISONER DONATION?

Objections to allowing death row inmates to be organ donors can be categorized into those caused by *practical barriers* and those involving *ethical or moral concerns*

Wide cultural differences require that this discussion be considered in the context of US law and culture, not necessarily those of other countries.[3]

Practical Barriers

Small number of potential organ donors. *Even if death row inmates are allowed to donate their organs, this practice "cannot yield anything more than a tiny number of organs for those in need."*[2] Whether or not this statement is true, the point of using consenting death row inmates as organ donors is not to solve the problem of organ shortage but to help patients who are in dire need of transplantable organs. The number of patients directly helped is not relevant, given the hugely significant impact on the recipients and their families.

Quality of donor. *On the basis of the medical and social history of these individuals, many of these prisoners "would not be eligible to serve as donors due to age, ill health, obesity, or communicable disease."*[2] Yet, so-called marginal donors have yielded perfectly usable organs for transplantation, and donor variables rarely have significant adverse effects on the outcome of transplant recipients. Although all might not be suitable donors, exclusion of all prisoners as donors would result in missed opportunities to transplant acceptable organs.

In addition, the idea that transmission of infectious diseases is a great risk if prisoners donate, while seemly legitimate, is refuted by the fact that there would be more time for screening death row inmates than typical brain-dead donors in hospitals. Thus, the rate of disease transmission might actually be lower when death row inmates donate because of the possibility of more thorough screening processes.

Difficulties from method of execution. *Organ donation by condemned prisoners will be less successful than donation in a hospital setting because of the "legal and practical requirements of the execution."*[2] The most common method of execution in the United States is injection of a three-drug combination (sodium thiopental to induce unconsciousness, pancuronium bromide to cause muscle paralysis and respiratory arrest, and potassium chloride to achieve cardiac arrest), so donation by death row inmates will be more like donation after cardiac death (DCD) than typical brain-death donation. The speculation that a prisoner's DCD organs would be qualitatively inferior is flawed, however, because DCD in hospitals is associated with more or less lengthy periods of hypoxemia before death is declared, up to 60 minutes after extubation, and the procurement process begins after an additional waiting period of up to 5 minutes. Thus, the potential for ischemic damage to various organs may actually be greater in hospital DCD than in the setting of execution, which has an ischemic time of only 10 to 15 minutes before organ recovery can begin. [...]

Respecting the dead donor rule. The question, "Could organ removal be used as the mode of execution?"[2]*, is a cynical polemic, not an argument.* The dead donor rule requires that procuring organs not cause death; that rule has governed the transplant field for decades and is likely to continue to do so. Moreover, death and donation are consistently observed as two distinct processes, and in accordance with current guidelines, physicians must not be involved in the execution of the prisoner-donor.[4]

Ethical or Moral Concerns

Coercion is inevitable in donation by death row inmates. Coercion can be "subtle" and "even without an explicit reward like early parole in exchange for a promise of organ donation, prisoners will understand themselves to be making an implicit exchange for their generosity, and policymakers will take advantage of that unspoken expectation." Moreover, "free and voluntary consent is compromised *by the prison environment."*[5]

Although this argument may be relevant to ordinary inmates, it does not apply to condemned prisoners, such as Christian Longo, who willingly and voluntarily ask to donate after execution. Precedent for allowing donation by non–death row inmates already exists (although the arguments for and against this practice are just as heated),[6] so why not permit it in condemned prisoners, in whom coercion is less of an issue?

Although Christian Longo is not the first condemned prisoner to request organ donation after his execution, his case is the most publicized in recent memory. As far as we know, no one approached Longo to ask him to consider donating his organs after the execution; he voluntarily thought of this plan and wrote his editorial in *The New York Times* after its rejection. In at least 14 earlier cases, death row inmates or their lawyers sought opportunities to donate their organs but were denied. Clearly, death row inmates are requesting to donate their organs for transplantation, indicating their willingness to consent to this process. It is hypocritical to argue that organ donation by death row inmates is morally wrong because the prisoners' autonomy is undermined by a subtle form of coercion, because denying the prisoners' requests to donate is an even greater compromise of their autonomy.

Organ donation by death row inmates undermines moral justification of capital punishment. The two moral justifications of capital punishment are retribution and deterrence of future criminal acts, and organ donation by death row inmates undermines both justifications.[2] These arguments are not strong enough, in my view, to prohibit death row inmates from willingly donating their organs for transplantation.

Retribution "may be made far more difficult to achieve as families and friends of victims watch as executed perpetrators are lauded in their final days by possible recipients and the media for their altruism in saving lives."[2] It seems unfair, at initial glance, that a person who committed a heinous crime would become a hero of some sort at the end. Consider the implications of this position: if the goal is to uphold retribution in capital punishment, then perhaps society should not allow "condemned prisoners to apologize or make amends for their crimes, to perform the simplest unselfish acts of kindness, to seek religion, or experience any form of spiritual growth or awakening."[7] Viewed in this way, retribution seems to be a weak justification for capital punishment. The same ethicists who claim that organ donation after execution will be seen as a heroic act contradict their other assertion that subtle coercion forces donation on the prisoners. Is such donation a willing, altruistic, laudable deed, or is it a coerced action? The logical inconsistency of the moral opposition to donation by death row inmates is evident.

The deterrence function of capital punishment is undermined when "social good is seen as issuing from the practice [of condemned prisoners donating organs]."[2] It seems highly unlikely that the perpetrator of a violent crime would contemplate, in advance of his evil deed, the potential benefit to society by the availability of organ donation. Furthermore, if deterrence is an important goal of capital punishment, then "execution preceded by extended torture" might be a better deterrent than "execution preceded by imprisonment," so advocates of deterrence might find torture to be morally superior to mere imprisonment.[8]

OPINION POLLS

In our liberal democracy, public acceptance of a policy or a practice is important. We were able to find three extensive opinion polls related to this topic, and all provided overwhelming support for the idea that condemned prisoners should be allowed to donate their organs for transplantation.[9,10] A month after Longo's editorial, MSNBC news organization found that 77.3% of 86,736 subjects responded "yes" to the question, "Should death row inmates be allowed to donate their organs?"[9] Another opinion poll conducted in conjunction with Longo's story asked, "Should a man who killed his wife and two children be allowed to donate his organs?"; nearly 90% of 588 voters responded "yes."[10] Clearly, the general public seems to see death row inmates like Longo as potentially acceptable donors for those who are in dire need of transplantable organs. [. . .]

SUMMARY

Given appropriate screening, no medical reason renders death row inmates unsuitable as organ donors. Individuals with past criminal records and those with unknown medical and social background are currently not excluded from organ donation, and many donors who were once considered marginal are now known to contribute safely to helping patients who are suffering from end-stage organ failure. Thus, there is no logical reason why condemned prisoners, after execution, cannot donate usable organs. Death row inmates willingly request it, the general public supports it, and potential recipients accept it. Should poorly grounded moral objections of a few people prevent the precious opportunities for those who might benefit from receiving those organs? Ultimately, opinions for or against donation after execution reflect the values of our society—are we more interested in retribution and deterrence, or in actually helping those who have no other options?

Con
Jay D. Pal, MD, PhD

Organ donation is a life-saving treatment for patients who suffer from advanced organ failure. [...] With the exception of living related kidney (and to a much smaller extent, liver) donors, most transplanted organs are obtained from cadaveric donors. As such, organ transplantation remains limited by the number of available donors. Despite the incidence of traumatic death in the United States, only 6,000 to 8,000 deceased donors are available annually, compared with 112,718 patients currently awaiting transplantation.[11] Approximately 18 individuals will die each day while awaiting a suitable organ donor.[12] Therefore, many novel attempts have been made to increase the potential donor pool. These have included donor registries, first-person consent, surrogate consent, and the use of prisoners as a source of organs. [...]

Transplant physicians are regularly confronted by the effects of an inadequate donor population on patients awaiting transplantation. However, deeper consideration of the use of prisoners as organ donors raises several concerns. These reservations can be grouped into three categories: legal, moral or ethical, and logistical. Thoughtful insight into these concerns will provide ample evidence that death row inmates are not suitable organ donors.

LEGAL ISSUES

Two basic tenets of organ transplantation as stated by the World Health Organization and the World Medical Association are that vital organs should only be removed from dead patients, and that living patients should not be killed for or by organ procurement. This dead-donor rule has been fundamental in the identification of potential organ donors since the 1950s. Accordingly, the accepted definition of death can be by (1) traditional cardiopulmonary criteria, which is the cessation of circulatory and respiratory functions, or (2) brain-death criteria, which is the irreversible cessation of brain function including brainstem activity (Uniform Declaration of Death Act of 1981). Although there has been recent discussion regarding the modification of the dead-donor rule in the case of patients with irrecoverable brain injury with remaining brainstem activity, the prevailing norm is that potential donors meet the currently accepted definitions of death.[13]

The concept of brain death provided the legal justification for organ procurement.[14] More recently, the declaration of brain death has been clarified and standardized.[15] The primary obstacle for organ donation from executed prisoners is that they do not die (brain death) on life support, as is typical for most organ donors. The most common method of execution in the United States is a three-drug protocol to cause sedation, then respiratory and circulatory arrest. After a waiting period of 10 to 15 minutes, the prisoner is examined for evidence of cardiac activity, and in its absence, declared dead. Any modification of the method of execution to decrease this waiting period may result in death occurring as a result of organ procurement, which places the surgeon in the role of executioner.

The second legal question to arise in the use of organs from death row inmates is the ability to consent. The concept of informed consent requires the ability to understand the procedure, as well as the autonomy to make a decision without coercion. Although there are some differences among states, all prisoners lose some component of citizenship rights at the time of conviction. Death row inmates, in particular, are expressly stripped of the right to make personal decisions. In most states, the prisoner becomes a ward of the state, or a property of the state, and therefore the state holds the legal authority to consent for the inmate. In every case regarding prisoner donation of organs, state prison boards have upheld this authority and denied inmate petitions. Furthermore, numerous legal reviews have provided arguments against the legality of organ donation from executed prisoners, citing lack of defined first-person consent, implied coercion, and an inherent conflict of interest.[16]

MORAL OR ETHICAL ISSUES

A far more problematic issue in the use of organs from death row inmates is the ethical dilemma of obtaining organs from patients who are being executed. Prisoners are subject to physically and psychologically stressful conditions that undoubtedly affect the decisions they make. Mr. Longo states that he "spend(s) 22 hours a day locked in a 6 foot by 8 foot box on Oregon's death row."[3] The Uniform Anatomical Gift Act requires that all organ donation be provided without coercion. However, prisoners are particularly vulnerable to both direct and implied coercion by virtue of their incarceration. This coercion may be subtle, without any explicit promise of reward for donation, but prisoners may "understand themselves to be making an implicit exchange for their generosity."[17]

The National Institutes of Health acknowledges this coercion in its rules regarding prisoner consent: "Prisoners may not be free to make a truly voluntary and uncoerced decision … the regulations require additional safeguards."[18]

Organ procurement in the setting of such coercion is often cited by bio-ethicists as a reason to avoid the use of executed prisoners as organ donors.[19] In addition, the American Society of Transplant Surgeons states that the use of organs from executed prisoners is unacceptable and that procurement under these circumstances violates the basic principles of transplantation, such as the need for free and willing donation of organs. […]

Given the numerous outstanding ethical issues regarding organ pro-curement from executed prisoners, the Organ Procurement and Transplant Network/United Network of Organ Sharing Ethics Committee generated a white paper that concluded: "The UNOS Ethics Committee has raised a small number of the many issues regarding organ donation from condemned prisoners. The Committee opposes any strategy or proposed statute regarding organ donation from condemned prisoners until all of the potential ethical concerns (coercion, method of execution, issues of informed consent) have been satisfactorily addressed."

LOGISTICAL ISSUES

A third argument against the feasibility of transplanting organs from prisoners is the logistical and practical difficulties in procuring and preserving organs after execution. The most common method of execution in the United States is lethal injection. Prisoners are typically sedated, paralyzed to induce respiratory arrest, then injected with potassium to induce cardiac arrest. After a waiting period of 10 to 15 minutes, the prisoner is examined for evidence of cardiac activity, and in its absence, declared dead. Because executions are performed in maximum security prisons and not in medical facilities, the prisoner would be dead for an extended period before the donor is transported to a hospital and organ procurement can be performed. Organ donation from brain-dead donors occurs with preservation of organs at the time of circulatory arrest. This allows preservation of graft function by immediately halting cellular respiration by instillation of cold preservation solution as systemic blood flow is interrupted. During DCD, circulatory death occurs in an environment (typically an operating room) where the procurement procedure can commence rapidly and organs can be placed in preservation solution within minutes. However, fewer organs are recoverable because of the delay in preservation. Highly metabolically active organs such as the heart and lungs are frequently not recoverable with DCD. In the setting of death in a prison environment, the extended delay to procurement would yield very few transplantable organs.

A possible solution would be to move the execution to a facility where organs can be recovered more rapidly, similar to DCD procedures. But that would require moving an inmate to a hospital before execution. The process of moving an inmate to an unsecured location would be difficult, given the uncertainty of the appeals process, protests, demonstrations, security requirements, and potential for escape. Also, many hospitals will likely be resistant to accepting prisoners for execution. Despite the potential financial benefit from providing a location for organ procurement, the public relations impact of becoming a center of execution would be detrimental. [...]

CONCLUSIONS

Although organ donation after prisoner execution will continue to be debated, it is helpful to consider how much benefit may actually be realized. In the first 9 months of 2011, 10,558 individuals donated organs in the United States. In contrast, 39 inmates were executed. The average age of executed prisoners is older than 50 years, and many suffer from chronic illnesses such as diabetes and hypertension. By conventional criteria such as age, medical conditions, and communicable disease, half of these prisoners would not be eligible donors. Therefore, the net increase in donors is less than one fifth of 1%. And given the DCD nature of these donations (with prolonged ischemic times), only kidneys are likely to be recoverable.

Given the contentious nature of this topic, we must evaluate the legal, moral, and logistical impediments to organ procurement from prisoners for the net gain of only 20 donors per year. Less controversial methods to increase the number of donor organs can be obtained by increasing public awareness of organ donation, creating donor registries, and improving organ yield from the eligible donors.

Concluding Remarks
Robert M. Sade, MD

Lin and Rich make a single but telling point in favor of allowing prisoners on death row to be organ donors: the primary focus of physicians should be on helping patients, in this case, patients with failing organs who need a replacement organ. They classify objections to allowing condemned prisoners to donate into two categories: practical obstacles and ethical or moral issues. They respond to several concerns in each category, indicating why they believe none is decisive. They also cite opinion polls asking whether condemned prisoners should be allowed to donate and report the results of a survey of waiting lung transplant recipients in their institution. All survey results strongly favor allowing donation.

Pal finds problems with allowing donation in three areas: legal, moral or ethical, and logistical. He discusses the 10- to 15-minute delay between lethal injection and pronouncement of death, which increases warm ischemic time, threatening the quality of recovered organs. He says that the situation of prisoners makes coercion unavoidable, but this claim rests largely on how one frames the meaning of coercion.[20]

[...] He also believes that the small number of potential donors under these circumstances, perhaps 20 a year, is not worth overcoming the many objections to the practice and could result in adverse publicity for organ donation.

We have not been told the reasons for parole boards denying condemned prisoners the option of voluntary organ donation, apparently the conclusion in all the cases of which we are aware. Legally, there is little question that prison authorities have the power to decide whether to allow organ donation. From an ethical viewpoint, however, the question is, should donation be denied a condemned prisoner who makes a voluntary request? For physicians, the idea of allowing donation draws support from the highest of physician's obligations, our paramount responsibility for the welfare of our patients. As a matter of law, the decision of whether organ donation by prisoners on death row should be permitted rests with prison authorities. As a matter of ethics, however, the question has not been settled, as this debate demonstrates. For physicians, our primary ethical responsibility—doing what is best for our patients, including the few whose lives would be saved by organs from executed prisoners—seems to place the burden of proof on those who would deny condemned prisoners the option of donation.

References

1. Longo C. Giving life after death row. *The New York Times*, March 5, 2011:WK12.
2. Caplan A. The use of prisoners as sources of organs—an ethically dubious practice. *Am J Bioeth.* 2011;11:1–5.
3. Tsai DF-C, Tsai M-K, Ko W-J. Organs by firing squad: the medical and moral implausibility of death penalty organ procurement. *Am J Bioeth.* 2011;11:11–3.
4. Council on Ethical and Judicial Affairs. Opinion 2.06, Capital Punishment. In: Code of Medical Ethics of the American Medical Association, 2010–2011 ed. Chicago: American Medical Association, 2010:23–32.
5. Potter NN. What it means to treat people as ends-in-themselves. *Am J Bioeth.* 2011;11:6–7.
6. Goldberg AM, Frader J. Prisoners as living organ donors: the case of the Scott sisters. *Am J Bioeth.* 2011;11:15–6.

7. Johnson LSM. The ethically dubious practice of thwarting the redemption of the condemned. *Am J Bioeth.* 2011;11:9–10.

8. Murphy P. Would donation undercut the morality of execution? *Am J Bioeth.* 2011;11:13–4.

9. http://health.newsvine.com/_question/2011/04/20/6504300-should-death-row-inmates-be-allowed-to-donate-their-organs.

10. Should man who killed wife and two children be allowed to donate his organs?: http://www.sodahead.com/united-states/should-man-who-killed-wife-and-two-children-be-allowed-to-donate-his-organs/question-1707899/. Accessed March 13, 2012.

11. Transplant trends. Richmond, VA: United Network for Organ Sharing. http://www.unos.org. Accessed March 13, 2012.

12. Health Resources and Services Administration. Organ Procurement and Transplantation Network. http://optn.transplant.hrsa.gov. Accessed March 13, 2012.

13. Truog RD, Miller FG. The dead donor rule and organ transplantation. *N Engl J Med.* 2008;359:674–5.

14. A definition of irreversible coma. Report of the Ad Hoc Committee of the Harvard Medical School to Examine the Definition of Brain Death. *JAMA.* 1968;205:337–40.

15. Quality Standards Subcommittee. Practice parameters: determining brain death in adults. St. Paul, MN: American Academy of Neurology, 1994. http://www.aan.com/professionals/practice/guidelines/pda/Brain_death_adults.pdf. Accessed March 13, 2012.

16. Hinkle W. Giving until it hurts: prisoners are not the answer to the national organ shortage. *Indiana Law Rev.* 2002;35: 593–619.

17. Youngner SJ, Arnold RM. Ethical, psychosocial, and public policy implications of procuring organs from non-heart-beating cadaver donors. *JAMA.* 1993;269:2769–74.

18. Research involving vulnerable populations, OER US Department of Health and Human Services, ed. Washington, DC: National Institutes of Health.

19. Hillman H. Harvesting organs from recently executed prisoners. Practice must be stopped. *BMJ* 2001;323:1254.

20. Wertheimer A. *Coercion.* Princeton, NJ: Princeton University Press; 1987:3–14.

Conflicts of Interest in Surgery

Robert M. Sade

> *It is asking more than human perfection to assume*
> *that a surgeon's judgment may not be influenced*
> *unconsciously by a pressing financial need.*
>
> —Edwin P. Lehman, MD (Surgery, 1950;28:595)

A conflict of interest (COI) is present when an individual has a primary responsibility that could be unduly influenced by a secondary interest. COIs can be found in every profession; they are widespread and occur frequently every day. In medicine, a physician's primary responsibility when caring for patients is to serve the interests of the patient. Secondary interests may be personal financial gain, personal nonfinancial gain (e.g., academic promotion, enhanced recognition and reputation), and interests of a third party, such as a group practice, partnership, hospital, or health-care insurance plan. Financial conflicts may arise from investments in or payments for services from pharmaceutical or device companies, reimbursement incentives, or gifts from industry.

Usually, COIs are quickly and easily resolved, so they may not even be recognized as COIs. For example, consider the case of a surgeon who could recommend either a low-revenue operation that is appropriate for the patient or a high-revenue operation that is at best a distant second choice; he is being considered for elevation to full partnership in his surgical group based in part on the income he generates. The surgeon is faced with a COI: The interests of the patient are best served by recommending the lower-revenue procedure, but the surgeon's career (the secondary interest) would be better served by recommending the higher-revenue procedure. It is unlikely that a surgeon would give a second thought to recommending the higher-revenue procedure. Like the many other COIs the surgeon faces every day, he probably would not even recognize that a COI is present because he resolves it so easily in the patient's favor.

When he is in a nonclinical role, such as a researcher or teacher, a physician's primary interest may not be what is best for the patient. For example, as a researcher, his primary responsibility is to contribute to the body of scientific knowledge by carrying out investigations and publishing results that add valid information. Secondary interests that could undermine his fidelity to the search for knowledge include incentives to falsify or fabricate data in order to produce a publishable paper or to make his grant application more competitive. In the role of teacher, a physician's primary interest is the accurate presentation of knowledge to students. Secondary interests in this setting could be saving time for other projects by preparing a lecture rapidly and sloppily or by being unavailable to provide guidance for students after class.

The presence of a COI is independent of the occurrence of impropriety. Questions of inappropriate behavior arise not when a COI is present but when it is resolved. A COI may produce harm to a patient, a research study, or a student if it is resolved in favor of a secondary interest rather than the primary interest. Among regulatory organizations, emphasis in recent years has shifted from recognizing the presence of a COI through disclosure requirements to managing its resolution. COIs in medicine received little attention until around the year 2000, following a series of sensational scandals in medical research (see chapter 24). These concerns have expanded to include clinical COIs as well, resulting in a new focus on developing policies to mitigate the harms that may result from them. Many medical organizations have developed policies regarding COIs and their management; for example, the Accreditation Council for Graduate Medical Education has promulgated rules governing the nature and content of presentations at meetings approved for continuing medical education credit,[1] and many hospitals and academic medical centers have developed their own policies limiting how their faculty and staff interact with industry representatives. The evolution of laws and regulations regarding relationships between physicians and industry is ongoing, as additional measures are being considered by Congress and many nongovernmental organizations. In response to this state of affairs, the Ethics Forum has sponsored debates on questions surrounding COIs and their management.

Chapters

Chapter 22 explores the question of whether small gifts from industry representatives to physicians are sufficiently harmful to patients to warrant restriction of access, as has been enforced by policy in many medical centers.[2] The arguments in favor of such restrictions rest on the claim that even small gifts influence people to favor certain companies or products because of the effect of reciprocity, a fundamental aspect of human behavior. There is also evidence that drug companies engage in marketing practices that mislead physicians in ways they often do not recognize. Patients may be harmed when physicians make substandard choices under the sway of this unconscious bias. The contrary view is that the harm that comes from supposed bias under the influence of industrial representatives is overblown and based on anecdotal information that is scientifically unsound, comparable in some ways to the witch-hunts of the sixteenth century. Collaborative relations between industry and medicine have been highly productive and ought to be protected rather than attacked.

In **chapter 23** the relation between industry and physicians who consult for industry is debated, specifically whether the financial link between the two should be cut.[3] According to one view, a few high-profile scandals have created the impression that fraud is rampant in the health-care industry, leading to the passage of laws intended to regulate physician COIs through mandatory disclosure of financial transactions. Disclosure alone is insufficient to protect against harmful effects of conflicts, however —management of COIs is required to ensure appropriate resolution of the conflict. An important method for accomplishing this might be through institutional oversight of individual consulting activities. From a different perspective, relations between industry and surgeons have been extremely productive, and this relationship should not be disrupted by overregulation. The best approach, instead, would be for physician leaders, legislators, and businesspeople to join in an effort to craft legislation that would regulate the financial relationships between physicians and industry in a way that protects productive collaboration. Given the developments of the past few years, it is argued, some form of regulation is certain, but its form and substance are hidden in the shadow of the regulatory environment's evolution.

Another highly controversial issue regarding COIs is the question of how much disclosure of conflicts should be required; this question is discussed in **chapter 24**, which departs from the usual format of these debates—it takes the form of a point–counterpoint discussion.[4] In one view, it is not enough to report the existence of a COI; full disclosure is needed and should include how long a relationship between a surgeon and industry has existed and how many dollars were exchanged. Underlying this position is the primary obligation to patients—we must protect them by ensuring that unbiased information reaches their physicians. Moreover, physicians should control their own destinies by anticipating the coming legislative regulation. The counterargument asserts that there is virtually no reliable evidence that the collaboration between industry and physicians poses any credible threat to the safety of patients; the real threat is the potential for interrupting the long-existing and highly productive industry–physician collaboration by increasing financial disclosure requirements.

References

1. Accreditation Council for Continuing Medical Education. Standards for Commercial Support: Standards to Ensure Independence in CME Activities. Chicago: Accreditation Council for Continuing Medical Education. http://www.accme.org/requirements/accreditation-requirements-cme-providers/standards-for-commercial-support. Accessed April 2, 2014.
2. Iserson KV, Cerfolio RJ, Sade RM. Politely refuse the pen and note pad: gifts from industry to physicians harm patients. *Ann Thorac Surg.* 2007;84(4);1077–84.
3. Immelt SJ, Gaudiani VA, Sade RM. Should the financial link between industry and physician consultants be severed? *Ann Thorac Surg.* 2011;92(3):781–7.
4. Murphy JP. Full disclosure—presentations and publications should include dollar amounts and duration of surgeon–industry relationships. *Ann Thorac Surg.* 2011;92(2):413–6; Sade RM. Ethics in cardiothoracic surgery: full disclosure—where is the evidence for nefarious conflicts of interest? *Ann Thorac Surg.* 2011;92(2):417–20.

22

Politely Refuse the Pen and Note Pad
GIFTS FROM INDUSTRY TO PHYSICIANS HARM PATIENTS
Kenneth V. Iserson, Robert James Cerfolio,
and Robert M. Sade*

Introduction
Robert M. Sade, MD

Drug companies use many methods to bring their products to the attention of physicians. Most of us are familiar with contacts between drug company representatives, formerly called detail men, stemming from the time when, as medical students, we were beneficiaries of the Eli Lilly Company's largesse: doctor's bag, stethoscope, hammer, and tuning fork. Since then, most of us have been offered many other small (sometimes big) gifts that are intended to gain our attention. Decades ago, no one saw much of a problem with this practice; rather, most saw it as a harmless, friendly gesture that led to valuable educational exchanges between detail men and physicians. In recent years, however, there has been a crescendo of warnings that such gifts are not harmless but endanger patients by binding us to the giver of the gift through the elemental human response to gifts: reciprocity, the need to give something back to the giver. Some worry that the impulse of reciprocity may lead us to prescribe products that are not quite right for a particular patient or prescribe an expensive drug in place of an effective drug that is much less expensive. Do we unwittingly endanger our patients by accepting gifts?

*Iserson KV, Cerfolio RJ, Sade RM. Politely refuse the pen and note pad: gifts from industry to physicians harm patients. *Ann Thorac Surg.* 2007;84(4);1077–84. Copyright Society of Thoracic Surgeons, republished here with permission.

THE CASE OF THE DETAILED SURGEON

Dr. John DeNile is always happy to see Cindy, a representative of the NovoCefalo Company, in his office. She is an articulate and attractive brunette who visits Dr. DeNile once every month or two with information that has recently become available about the various drugs produced by NovoCefalo. She always brings with her ball-point pens, note pads, Post-it pads, and other small gifts (most bearing the company's logo), which Dr. DeNile finds useful in his office. On this particular visit, Cindy provides Dr. DeNile with information about NovoCefalo's fourth generation cephalosporin, Cefprophylax. [...] Dr. DeNile is impressed with the spectrum and the safety of the drug. He has routinely used cefazolin for antibiotic prophylaxis for 48 hours after his open heart operations, in accordance with practice guidelines from the Society of Thoracic Surgeons and the Surgical Infection Society. After listening to the details Cindy has provided, he thinks that it is a good idea to switch to Cefprophylax.

Dr. DeNile uses Cefprophylax after every open heart operation, as he did cefazolin. Two months after changing antibiotics, he does an uncomplicated coronary artery bypass on 62-year-old John Luckless. Mr Luckless is doing quite well at his 2-week follow-up visit, but a month later, he reports that for the last several days he has not been urinating as much as he did previously, has noted that his urine is tinged pink, has vomited several times after meals, and has gained nearly 10 pounds.

These symptoms are of great concern to Dr. DeNile, and he orders laboratory tests; the blood urea nitrogen is 36 mg/dL and creatinine is 3.2 mg/dL. He consults a nephrologist colleague, who, after an appropriate workup, makes the diagnosis of interstitial nephritis, probably resulting from an allergic response to the antibiotic Mr Luckless received at the time of his operation. The patient's interstitial nephritis progresses and he is placed on dialysis. He is worked-up as a possible kidney transplant candidate and is placed on the kidney transplant waiting list.

Dr. DeNile is sure this is a rare complication of the antibiotic and continues using it. The nephrologist reports the allergic reaction to the company. Eight months later, Dr. DeNile receives notification from NovoCefalo and from the FDA that Cefprophylax has been withdrawn from the market because of a high incidence of kidney damage. He immediately switches back to cefazolin, his former routine prophylactic antibiotic.

At Cindy's next visit, she gives Dr. DeNile a small leather-bound date book with NovoCefalo's logo on the cover and the surgeon's name engraved below it. She has some very interesting information on the latest generation corticosteroid, which lacks the fluid retention side effect that has been so troubling with other corticosteroids. While she is talking, Dr. DeNile wonders whether the article he read recently on the effect of gifts on physician's prescribing patterns might apply to him and whether the small gifts Cindy always brings might have affected his decision to use the now withdrawn Cefprophylax. Although he believes the literature showing that even small gifts produce a sense of obligation to reciprocate and that most physicians are by gifts, he is certain that his dedication to his patients' welfare prevents any such influence on him. He turns his full attention back to Cindy's recitation of the new steroid's pharmacologic details.

Pro
Kenneth V. Iserson, MD, MBA

A battle is being waged to win the hearts and minds of the physicians who write 2.2 billion drug prescriptions annually in the United States. Given that virtually all these physicians accept some gifts from pharmaceutical or equipment manufacturers, and the case described demonstrates merely one tragic outcome, what new information might be imparted to change attitudes and behavior toward drug/medical device manufacturers' sales tactics? Perhaps what might be most useful is to look at the truth behind typical physician responses to such tactics.

The following are common responses physicians give when asked about why they accept gifts, in any form, from drug and medical device companies:

1. Why do you think that I accept gifts? And if I do, why do you think that would influenced my prescribing habits, which equipment I use, or what I recommend to my hospital or group to buy?

Nearly all of you accept gifts. We know from multiple studies that nearly all physicians accept gifts from the drug detailers whom they meet with an average of four times a month.[1] [...] Those gifts, worth billions of dollars, run the gamut from free pens, pads, and drug samples to high-priced meals, entertainment tickets, trips, and honoraria. In fact, gifts are one of the main reasons physicians meet with drug detailers.

It does influence you. These studies also show that physicians believe that company representatives present accurate drug information. And although physicians deny that gifts influenced their behavior, those who accepted drug samples preferentially and rapidly began prescribing the new drugs—often in lieu of equally effective or less-expensive generic drugs or previously used medications.[2] [...]

Even the smallest gifts influence you. Even the small tokens that physicians receive from pharmaceutical companies may make a large impact. As a prestigious physician group recently wrote in the *Journal of the American Medical Association,*

Most of the recommendations from medical and industry groups share key assumptions. The first is that small gifts do not significantly influence physician behavior. The second is that disclosure of financial conflicts is sufficient to satisfy the need to protect patients' interests. Although these two assumptions are widely accepted among physicians, compelling research findings using a variety of methods have called their validity into question.... Social science research demonstrates that the impulse to reciprocate for even small gifts is a powerful influence on people's behavior.[3] [...]

Receiving industry gifts compromises professionalism and your fiduciary duty to your patients. Part of the surgeon's professional role is to manage the patient's resources for his or her best interest. This so-called fiduciary duty means putting the patient's interests before personal benefit. Market incentives to surgeons and relationships between them and pharmaceutical companies and medical device manufacturers may compromise this duty. [...]

2. I'm smarter than they are; they can't fool me.

Devious marketing strategies. Drug detailing has been a major part of the pharmaceutical industry for more than a century. Although their methods have changed over time, the fact that they continue to spend large sums to promote drugs and devices to the physicians who control access shows that it is working.

"Devious" may seem like a harsh term to describe the industry's marketing strategies. Yet, as a result of a federal lawsuit over the marketing of gabapentin, we got a rare glimpse into the real, often deceitful, world of pharmaceutical promotion. The companies involved eventually admitted to violating federal regulations by promoting the drug for pain, psychiatric conditions, migraines, and other unapproved uses.[4] [...]

3. Why can't I spend a few minutes talking with the very pleasant (and pretty/handsome) drug rep? They have to make a living, too.

Ever see an ugly drug rep? "Detailing" is sending attractive company representatives (lobbyists) to meet with physicians in their offices or clinics to discuss (push) their newest drugs. These are individuals who are knowledgeable about the drugs they are selling, about how to best interact with physicians, and who have excellent sales techniques. [...]

How intense is drug detailing? It costs a great deal for you to receive the drug companies' largesse. The industry employs 80,000 to 100,000 drug company detailers, a ratio of 1 salesperson for every 5 office-based physicians and an increase of more than 100% from the approximately 42,000 employed in 1996. During 2003, drug manufacturers spent $22 billion on direct marketing to doctors in the United States alone. That amounts to about $25,000 per physician per year.[5] [...]

4. Why shouldn't I have someone to tell me about the newest drugs and devices? I don't have the time to read all the journals.

Admittedly, about 150,000 medical journals are now being published worldwide. No one can keep up with this deluge of information. However, there are good alternatives, such as the subscriber-supported, rather than advertiser-supported, Medical Letter and Thoracic Surgery Clinics.

5. Anyway, the reps don't know whether I prescribe their drugs or not.

Of course, they do! Most physicians don't realize that each week drug detailers receive detailed lists of every prescription written by every physician they visit.[6] Huge data-mining companies purchase information on the millions of prescriptions that physicians write each month and resell it to pharmaceutical manufacturers, who then distribute the information to their detailers. This information allows pharmaceutical reps to target individual doctors and to adjust their sales pitches until they find the one that works best. [...]

6. Are you claiming that I don't practice elegant, evidence-based medicine?

Elegant medicine is providing patients with the best result that has the lowest cost, the least discomfort, and the fewest and least-risky interventions. Evidence-based medicine is the integration of the best available clinically relevant research evidence with clinical expertise and patient values. [...]

7. Don't indigent patients need drug samples?

This is the most frequent defense physicians give for interacting with industry salespeople. It is best viewed by asking [two] separate questions:

[A] What drugs are given to physicians as samples? Sample medications given to physicians are the most costly gifts that pharmaceutical companies distribute. Although individual trips, medical equipment, grants, and consulting fees are more expensive, they are much less commonly dispersed. Samples are never generic and are seldom for inexpensive therapy.[7]

[B] What happens to these samples? Although the medical community likes to assert that drug samples are used for patients, either because they are indigent or for the convenience of being able to start the medication immediately, this often is not true. Physicians, their families, and office staff often use these samples. Many samples are stolen and resold.[8] [...]

8. Don't medical journals, medical societies, and fellowship programs need funds from the pharmaceutical and medical device industries to survive?

Journal publishers become anguished when anyone suggests that they eliminate drug and medical equipment advertising. In 2003, the pharmaceutical industry spent $448 million on advertising in medical journals, a relatively paltry amount given the $5.3 billion spent on detailing aimed at physicians and the $16.4 billion (market value) on providing free drug samples. (The real value of the sample drugs is estimated as $2 to $3 billion per year.)[9] [...]

9. Doesn't the pharmaceutical industry regulate itself? How about government regulations? Aren't there enough controls on pharmaceutical/equipment marketing to physicians to prevent abuses?

Aren't there industry and medical association guidelines? The PhRMA adopted voluntary ethical guidelines in 1990, and slightly revised them in 2002. Those guidelines prohibit gifts worth more than $100. [...]

The American Medical Association's (AMA) Council on Ethical and Judicial Affairs developed a policy on gifts to physicians from industry in 1990. They conformed to the same standard of allowing gifts only if they "primarily entail a benefit to patients and should not be of substantial value" (less than $100).[10] [...]

What guidelines does the US government have? In April 2003, the Office of the Inspector General (OIG) for the US Department of Health and Human Services issued final federal guidelines for physician-pharmaceutical industry relations, including the gray areas that they said had a "significant potential for abuse": funding for education, research and consulting, as well as gifts and gratuities.[11] [...]

10. It doesn't really matter what I do. The drug companies are switching tactics.

Pharmaceutical industry advertising increasingly targets consumers directly through the media and the Internet, which is often difficult to counter. Physician-directed advertising is also changing with the times and with companies' need to comply with federal guidelines to avoid prosecution. The pharmaceutical and medical equipment industries are increasingly targeting physician-customers using electronic media, including Web sites, e-mail, Web-based "surveys," instant messaging, and personal digital assistant programs.

Given this onslaught, what individual practitioners do matters enormously. We serve as role models for colleagues and trainees, and as examples to our patients. Compromising our values for any reason diminishes our self worth and our professionalism.

To know what to do, we need only ask ourselves. Are we adequately protecting our patients' interests?

Con
Robert James Cerfolio, MD

The history of the relationship between industry and medicine is long and productive. It is marked by many great achievements. Millions of Americans and patients all around the world have benefited greatly from this partnership. The facts are clear. Many more patients have benefited from this partnership than have the pockets of doctors or members of industry. A plethora of examples illustrate just how well this relationship works and how it has helped a large number of patients. [...]

The interaction between industry and physicians takes place on many different levels [...] [One] type of interaction occurs mostly at academic centers and involves research projects or studies. These types of interactions can involve large dollar amounts and are more problematic. Once again, strict rules and regulations exist on both sides and help promulgate rules to protect both sides. The specific rules vary for each academic hospital and for each drug company but can be easily viewed at the Web sites of each university or industry. Yet, it has been this latter relationship that has been the focus of great debate and controversy lately. We will focus our discussion on this second type of interaction.

Any relationship between two large, diverse groups that are composed of many different individuals gives rise, unfortunately, to negative events as well as positive. The negative events often gain quick overnight national attention. A complicated issue becomes compressed into a perfunctory 10-second sound bite by the media. Irrational exuberance often follows, sometimes leading to sweeping legal changes. One or two egregious cases that receive national attention can quickly and permanently overshadow the thousands of previous positive stories that go untold. [...]

In 1988, a news report suggested misconduct at a Harvard-affiliated hospital in an industry-supported clinical study. The immediate response from the Harvard administration, as it has to be in today's legal climate, was to tighten its academic-industry research rules and regulations, even though not all of the facts behind the case had been fully discovered or evaluated.[12] Similarly, the National Institutes of Health (NIH) mandated that their 20,000 employees sell all of their investments in stocks and bonds in any health-related industry.[13] These types of internal changes at many academic institutions illustrate the climate that exists within these centers. [...]

This debate, for which no true scientific data exist to support either side, is as much about the promulgation of laws and the protection of academic institutions from lawsuits as it is about the protection of physicians' morals or patients' rights. Because no prospective randomized data support either side in this debate, decisions must be based on common sense and experience.

[...] [T]he supporting literature offered by Kenneth Iserson [...] was all retrospective and subjective. There is no prospective data that industry and greed have led to increased mortality secondary to compromised ethics by physicians or industry members. In fact, the death rate in industry-sponsored research has held constant over the past decade, even though the level of involvement between industry and academia has significantly increased.[14] Thus, the only objective evidence available implies the opposite conclusion.

In an amusing but tragically accurate article [...], Thomas P. Stossel equates the witch-hunts of the 16th century to the call by the Journal of the American Medical Association (JAMA) and the NIH to outlaw all industry from their society. Stossel shows the similarities between the hysteria of the two events: lack of logic, absence of data, and subsequent actions out of fear and ignorance. Stossel writes:

> The witch hunters of "The Hammer" and of the JAMA paper propose extreme remedies that promise great but practically unattainable rewards. The Hammer recommended torture to elicit confessions from witches and severe punishments following convictions ... the JAMA authors want all commercial contributions removed from academic health centers. The JAMA article badly states "that a system review of the medical literature on industry gifting ... found that an overwhelming majority of industry interactions had negative results on patient care" Although the sources it cites explicitly say "No study used patient outcome measures," the JAMA article reminds us that industry marketing influenced the prescribing habits of physicians ... but it repeatedly neglects documented evidence that physicians fail to prescribe appropriate drugs according to evidence-based guidelines.... The Hammer predicted that eliminating witches would cleanse the world of ills.... But witches burned and the problems persisted. The JAMA article says that abolishing the commercial interface in academic health centers will lower the cost of drugs by encouraging prescriptions of cheaper ones. Since physicians not in academic centers write by far the most prescriptions the basis of this hypothetical cost savings is unclear. Even stranger is the idea that companies would sponsor research of no direct benefit to them.... They wield the hammer of a new witch hunt.[15]

The facts and data that supported burning witches at the stake are strikingly similar to the facts and data presented on the malevolent effect that industry has on physicians. There exist no data for either, only hysteria.

What does common sense tells us about this issue? How many of us really believe that the daily decisions we make to treat our patients are swayed by the company's logo on the pen in our pocket? Do we truly believe that the care of our patients is affected or subconsciously altered because a drug company sponsored a lunch that we attended earlier in the day or last week? If we answer no, it is possible that we are completely blind to the unconscious effect the drug companies are having on our free will? However, if we receive a cash bonus each time we place a certain type of cardiac valve or chest wall prosthetic in a patient's chest are we sure we are not biased toward using that company's product?

Common sense guides us in our answers to these questions. In my experience, members of industry often supply me with important peered-reviewed scientific articles and educational pamphlets. They are well informed and provide sound educational information to me and my residents and fellows. Regulations and restrictions already in place help monitor our interaction and keep us both honest and ethical. These rules and regulation have been specifically cited earlier in this article and are found in every academic university in the United States (although each center's rules slightly vary). In addition, each industry has specific guidelines for its employees as well.

There are, however, obvious differences between us. Our main objective during our training (a long road that entails 12 grueling years of education and training after college) is to learn how to best care for the sick. The main objective of members of industry is to make money for their companies. This difference uniquely positions us to handle our interaction with members of industry and to ensure it remains responsible and ethical. This is not to imply that members of industry do not want physicians to provide outstanding patient care; we all know that the vast majority of them do—in fact, I have never meet a single one who did not. They know that the optimal way for them to maximize their profits is to provide us with products that help us improve the care of our patients. [...]

A healthy interaction is a critical pathway towards achieving the best medicine, medical equipment, and care that our patients deserve. If we eliminate our contact with our friends and colleagues from industry; that is, if we "refuse the pen and notepad," the repercussions on future research and development would be severe. Most importantly, the impact on our patients would be profound. Our health care system, which is already financially strapped, is ill positioned now more than ever to avoid all contacts with industry. President Bush recently called for further reduction in the federal funding of cancer research. Industry and physicians need one another to further improve patient care. Thus, a relationship between us is needed on all levels. But further refinements and education of these existing laws and regulations are needed to ensure that the relationship remains appropriate, honest, and open to peer review.

So, "refuse the pen and notepad"? Of course not. We should accept them and be willing to discuss our knowledge with local members of industry. We should be able to learn from them as well as allow them to learn from us. Together, we can share each other's expertise and strength and together develop better medicines and medical devices for our patients. We should maintain an amicable relationship, but ensure it is appropriate and is carefully regulated by sensible rules that are open and subject to review. Our patients have reaped the benefits of this relationship in the past and they deserve to continue to enjoy the fruits of a healthy physician-industry relationship in the future.

Concluding Remarks
Robert M. Sade, MD

[...] Industry, physicians, and patients have benefited from physicians' inter-actions with drug and device representatives for decades, as Cerfolio has summarized, and at least some harm has been done, as Iserson has docu-mented. The possibility that the benefit-harm ratio has diminished or per-haps even reversed, producing a net harm, raises important ethical issues. The principle at the core of medical ethics is this: we, as physicians, owe our first allegiance to our patients. There is no question, therefore, that we should do whatever is necessary to protect the interests of our patients. Iserson alerts us to the harm he sees being done to patients and urges us, as individuals, to maintain our professionalism. He stops short, however, of recommend-ing banning drug representative interactions with physicians, as others have. For example, Stanford, Pennsylvania, and Yale Universities, among others, have pioneered a policy of excluding drug representatives entirely from their academic medical center campuses.[16] The extent to which this policy has pro-tected patients has yet to be demonstrated.

We might consider following their example, but before we go beyond Iserson's hortatory conclusion and take more severe measures, we must rec-ognize that the evidence impelling us in that direction is not strong in any scientific sense. In science, we have a generally accepted standard of valid-ity: the probability that a proposition is not true is less than 5%, or $p < 0.05$. In the law, decisions are made under several standards of evidence, depend-ing on the nature of the charge: preponderance, clear and convincing, and beyond reasonable doubt. The preponderance of evidence on the effects on physicians of gifts from industry favors harm over benefit, in my view, but the truth of this conclusion is far from beyond a reasonable doubt.

There will be a wide spectrum of views on whether the evidence is clear and convincing. It seems simple enough merely to do as Iserson sug-gests: maintain sensitivity to potential ill effects of gifts and do not compro-mise professional values. Others have suggested far more draconian responses to the information we have on the effects of gifts from industry on physicians, as I have noted. An important question arising from the exchange between Iserson and Cerfolio is this: How strong must be the evidence of harm to patients before we should be willing to undertake such drastic measures as locking drug and device representatives out of our teaching hospitals?

References

1. Wazana A. Physicians and the pharmaceutical industry. Is a gift ever just a gift? *JAMA*. 2000;283:373–80.

2. Harder B. Pushing drugs: how medical marketing influences doctors and patients. *Science News* 2005;168(5):75–76. www.sciencenews.org/articles/20050730/bob10.asp. Accessed October 16, 2006.

3. Brennan TA, Rothman DJ, Blank L, et al. Health industry practices that create conflicts of interest. *JAMA*. 2006;295:429–33.

4. Steinman MA, Bero LA, Chren MM, Landefeld CS. Narrative review: the promotion of gabapentin: an analysis of internal industry documents. *Ann Intern Med.* 2006;145:284–93.

5. Center for Policy Alternatives, Prescription Drug Marketing 2004. www.stateaction.org/issues/issue.cfm/issue/PrescriptionDrugMarketing.xml. Accessed October 16, 2006.

6. Brownlee S, Lenzer J. Spin doctored: how drug companies keep tabs on physicians. *Slate*, May 31, 2005.

7. Grant DC, Iserson KV. Who's buying lunch: are gifts to surgeons from industry bad for patients? *Thorac Surg Clin.* 2005;15:533–42.

8. Westfall JM, McCabe J, Nicholas RA. Personal use of drug samples by physicians and office staff. *JAMA*. 1997;278:141–3.

9. Scherer FM. The pharmaceutical industry—prices and progress. *N Engl J Med.* 2004;351:927–32.

10. American Medical Association's (AMA) Council on Ethical and Judicial Affairs: E-8.061 Gifts to physicians from industry. Chicago: American Medical Association; adopted December 1990; updated June 1998.

11. US Department of Health and Human Services, Office of Inspector General: Compliance program guidance for pharmaceutical manufacturers. *Federal Register* 2003;68: 23731–43.

12. Presidents and Fellows of Harvard College. Policy on conflicts of interest and commitment. Cambridge, MA: Harvard University. http://www.hms.harvard.edu/integrity.conf.html.

13. Steinbeck R. Financial conflicts of interest and the NIH. *N Engl J Med.* 2004;350:327–30.

14. Montaner JS, O'Shaughnessy MV, Schechter MT. Industry-sponsored clinical research: a double-edged sword. *Lancet* 2001;358:1893–5.

15. Stossel TP. Witch Hunt. *Wall Street Journal.* February 2006.

16. Croasdale M. Some medical schools say no to drug reps' free lunch: Stanford, Yale and the University of Pennsylvania have adopted policies to create a brighter line between medicine and marketing. *AMNews.* October 9, 2006. http://www.ama-assn.org/amednews/site/free/prl21009.htm. Accessed March 16, 2006.

23

Should the Financial Link Between Industry and Physician Consultants Be Severed?

Stephen J. Immelt, Vincent A. Gaudiani,
and Robert M. Sade*

Introduction
Robert M. Sade, MD

Conflicts of interest come about when one must choose between two or more options that are incompatible. In medicine, they usually relate to choices between serving the interests of patients directly or indirectly versus serving one's own interests, which might be career related or financial. A particularly controversial area lies in the relations between physicians and pharmaceutical or device companies. For cardiothoracic surgeons, the most frequent interactions are with device companies.

The high level of public attention to such Conflicts of interest has led the drug and device industries and medical specialty societies, including The Society of Thoracic Surgeons and American Association for Thoracic Surgery, to develop guidelines for physician-industry interactions.[1] The guidelines generally are not intended to eliminate Conflicts of interest, which is impossible, but to "manage" them. To Congress, however, self-imposed management is not enough. Scandalous payments of millions of dollars have received front-page coverage. [...]

Senator Charles Grassley of Iowa has been the bulldog behind Senate investigations, and introduced a bill that requires all health care–related companies to report publicly all payments to physicians: the Physician Payments Sunshine Act. The provisions of this bill were included in the new health care

*Immelt SJ, Gaudiani VA, Sade RM. Should the financial link between industry and physician consultants be severed? *Ann Thorac Surg.* 2011 Sep;92(3):781–7. Copyright Society of Thoracic Surgeons, republished here with permission.

reform law [...].[2] In the view of Congress, medical centers may not be capable of managing industry payments to physicians, so it seems altogether possible that Congress will eventually enact laws that will entirely sever the financial link between industry and physicians. At the least, we are in a regulatory atmosphere that seems headed toward ever-increasing restrictions on such financial interactions.

In a point-counterpoint discussion [...], an argument for institutional oversight of physician-industry financial interactions was made by Stephen Immelt, an attorney who focuses primarily on complex enforcement litigation [...]. Taking exception to Immelt's views, Vincent Gaudiani, a cardiothoracic surgeon who has had long-time interests in quality assurance in cardiac surgery and in relations between physicians and industry, argues that institutional oversight is inadequate and collaboration between physicians, health care institutions, industry, and Congressional leaders is needed to legislate rationality into a chaotic area.

Pro
Stephen J. Immelt, JD

CONFLICTS OF INTEREST: THE CASE FOR INSTITUTIONAL OVERSIGHT OF INDIVIDUAL CONSULTING ACTIVITY

Twenty years ago, health care fraud and abuse was viewed as the province of shady doctors and crooks engaged in clear and obvious fraud such as billing for nonexistent patients. At the same time, there existed a web of financial relationships between physicians and providers and a range of suppliers such as pharmaceutical and device companies. Extravagant entertaining and gifts were common, as were a range of other payment relationships. These relationships took place outside the public eye, and the participants viewed them as standard business practices, not a form of corruption or a conflict of interest. This was, in essence, a black box.

Here we are in 2010, with meetings generally at an airport hotel, a deli platter for lunch, and increasing insistence that physicians document their consulting activities to the level of a lawyer. Yet still questions linger. What happened?

One explanation is that the health care sector, including the medical profession, lost control over the narrative. Using two key federal statutes—the Anti-Kickback Act (AKA) and the False Claims Act—a group of determined prosecutors sought to pry the lid off that black box. What they found was not a pretty picture. To be sure, that did not happen in one step. They started with clinical laboratories, then moved to dialysis providers, hospitals, and academic medicine, then hit the mother lode in pharmaceuticals, an effort that has been expanded in recent years to include devices.[3] Some observers have applauded this development. After all, the AKA is a criminal statute, so these must have been corrupt practices.[4]

The problem is that the AKA can be construed quite broadly through the so-called "one purpose" test, and the huge penalties, which can include exclusion from participation in all governmental health care programs, can make it ruinous to contest the theories. That is not to imply that there were no bad facts in these cases. There were. But the format of these settlements had the effect of casting the issues in extremely broad terms. And the narrative that emerged from these many proceedings was that the health care system suffered from rampant fraud, particularly with respect to the financial relationships.

Another consequence of these various enforcement efforts was to expose the scope and scale of the financial dealings. Putting aside any notion of corruption, there has been increasing discomfort with those appearances. This has been particularly true as more information has emerged about the details of the collaboration between industry and the profession in areas like medical education, publications, and treatment standards. But the inflammatory labels applied to these activities do not capture the nuances and good faith efforts to develop and communicate useful scientific information.

Although the "corruption" model continues to play a primary role in driving the mainstream narrative, there has been a recognition that corruption cannot explain all the areas of concern. Increasingly, the discussion has been cast in terms of conflicts of interest. The American Medical Association, Pharmaceutical Research Manufacturers of America (PhRMA), and Advanced Medical Technology Association (AdvaMed) codes all speak in terms of good ethical practice.

A focus on conflicts of interest has brought an interesting dimension to the discussion. The classic legal paradigm for dealing with conflicts of interest is disclosure and consent. Acting on that model, we have seen a series of legislative initiatives at the state level focused on disclosure, and the approach of a federal disclosure requirement. And recent settlements in orthopedic and pharmaceutical cases have mandated public posting of the company's financial dealings with physicians and customers.

But does disclosure solve the problem?

The 2009 Institute of Medicine (IOM) study [...] suggests not.[5] The IOM study posits that the goal of conflict of interest policies is to protect the integrity of professional judgment, not just to remediate problems after they occur. Defining a conflict of interest broadly as "a set of circumstances that creates a risk that professional judgment on actions regarding a primary interest [e.g. patient care] will be unduly influenced by a secondary interest," the IOM cautions that failure to adopt a more robust approach to such conflicts may ultimately erode public trust in health care providers. Although the IOM views the identification of conflicts as a crucial undertaking, it considers disclosure to be merely a preliminary step, not a solution. Why is disclosure insufficient? One problem is that patients may not be in a position to analyze the relevance of a disclosed relationship, nor feel comfortable raising it with someone who they are trusting with their care. More importantly, the IOM canvasses the psychological and medical literature and develops an intriguing case for the proposition that unconscious bias plays a much stronger role in decision making than any of us may be prepared to acknowledge. In this regard, such bias poses a larger threat than corruption, and one that disclosure cannot address or mitigate. Thus, as the IOM sees it, there must not only be a system for disclosing conflicts but a way to manage them.

Unfortunately, the IOM report does not identify a clear way forward beyond identifying the need for stronger standards and active management. Yet without effective attention to these issues, the pressure for external regulation will increase, driven by a "corruption" narrative that may seek to reduce further or eliminate financial relationships without regard to any corresponding benefits. One available option that warrants consideration might be to insist that consultant activity be directed through the institutions that employ physicians—namely, academic medical centers and practice organizations—as opposed to being viewed as the independent province of those physicians. Most institutions, and virtually all academic medical centers, already have conflict of interest policies and, more importantly, a mechanism for managing the conflicts. Ensuring that institutions are in a position to manage these relationship would help blunt both the influence and appearance of the payments, and also ensure compliance in other areas such as National Institutes of Health regulations, Bayh-Dole, and policies dealing with the ownership and transfer of intellectual property.

Admittedly, a shift toward institutional funding would work against the interests of private practice physicians, many of whom have been active and productive consultants. But the IOM study challenges the assumption that the public interest in unbiased decision making can be ensured simply by broader disclosure. Even presuming complete good faith, there is only so much an individual physician consultant can do. Certainly, the relationship can be disclosed, but how can that relationship be managed? The burden arguably should be on those entrusted with making professional judgments to demonstrate that the possible bias attendant to a financial relationship can be managed and ameliorated in a meaningful way. Perhaps it may be possible to develop a model for third party oversight of individual consulting arrangements, but until that happens, the institutional approach would seem a better option for ensuring that the public supports industry collaboration and avoiding another round of embarrassing enforcement actions.

Con
Vincent A. Gaudiani, MD

HOW SHOULD PHYSICIANS INTERACT WITH THE
HEALTH CARE INDUSTRY?

Corrupt practices have infiltrated an otherwise enormously fruitful relationship between physicians and big business. These practices have lead two states to pass legislation that substantially changes how business and physicians interact. In this essay, we examine whether severing all financial relationships between individual physicians and big business will reduce corruption and improve patient care. This idea is incorrect for reasons we outline, but this relationship does need grooming. We recommend that physician leaders join with legislators and businessmen to craft template legislation to regulate this important relationship. Unless we come together to decide upon optimal pro forma rules, we will continue to get a mishmash of State laws that will serve all parties poorly.

BACKGROUND

Open heart surgery began with collaboration between big business and visionary surgeons. As many of you know, just after World War II, John Gibbon, a young Philadelphia surgeon, was struggling to develop a cardiopulmonary bypass machine. He enlisted the help of Tom Watson, the founder of IBM, and the result of that collaboration was the beginning of our craft. [...] A few years later, Lowell Edwards, a successful aeronautical engineer, challenged Albert Starr to collaborate on a total artificial heart. [...] The result of that encounter is a company that is still at the forefront of valve replacement technology. Starr and Edwards had barely begun when they encountered Tom Fogarty. Fogarty had already patented the embolectomy catheter that would save thousands of lives and limbs and started the era of less invasive surgery even before the era of large incision surgery had hit its stride. These pioneers and others lit the tinder that would not only save millions of lives, but would create, in less than a lifetime, a huge and vibrant health care industry that is the envy of the world.

Now, less than a half century later, industry and physicians have formed increasingly complex relationships to solve increasingly complex clinical problems. For instance, consider the elaborate partnership required to introduce percutaneous aortic valve prostheses into the United States. There are scientific, ethical, regulatory, training, proctoring, and manufacturing issues that can only be solved by committed physicians and businessmen working together. Physicians contribute their time and expertise, and business contributes millions of investors' dollars and their own special knowledge. [...]

THE PROBLEM

Such efforts as these occurring through all the specialties and with both device and pharmaceutical companies could not occur without a ration of the vices that flesh is heir to. These are as common to us as speech itself and deeply a part of our nature: it is the corruption of greed, kickbacks, misrepresentation, and cronyism that have always been the camp followers of legitimate enterprise, be it legal, political, religious, medical, or commercial. Some forms of it are clearly illegal, and all are distasteful. Those who would sever the financial relationship between physicians and industry argue that there have been numerous scandals in which doctors were paid kickbacks to use a certain device or drug. More generally, they argue that physician prescribing behavior is influenced by sales visits and small gifts from industry and that many follow-up studies, educational dinners, and speaking fees are sub rosa bribes to encourage use of a particular drug or device. [...]

SOME INFERENCES

Given these observations, we can make certain inferences. First, Western democracies have thrived by encouraging private enterprise, and private enterprise requires that businesses create and maintain customers. The customer relationship in every business is complex and interactive, particularly in medicine, because the businessmen and the physicians each have special skills required to create new products and teach their proper use. In addition, most of the contact between industry and physicians has not only been moral, but has also produced health, wealth, and employment for millions of people. We should be wary of outlawing whole classes of business relationships unless they are pervasively immoral.

The term "conflict of interest" is omnipresent in discussions such as this, but it is widely misused by all sides. It is the job of all professionals, preachers, lawyers, and doctors to skillfully negotiate these conflicts. What is really at stake here is immoral conduct. We must define it clearly, and punish it appropriately, as I will suggest with a few recommendations at the end of this essay.

Some believe that all business arrangements between physicians and industry should be mediated by an academic institution or hospital. That belief is deeply ironic because the most damaging behavior between business and medicine occurs at the institutional level, not with individual doctors. You will learn the sad facts when you read The New York Times,[6] Marcia Angell's book on big pharma, or her article in the New York Review of Books.[7] [...] These and many other recent works document serious malfeasance among physicians, their official institutions, and the business community. They are final proof that all relationships involving money and power require rules and laws to minimize corruption. The key question is what form they should take to minimize our vices without trampling the relationships that have brought us so far. [. . .]

SOME FRAMEWORKS OF A SOLUTION

The crux of the problem is to define a framework for interaction between business and medicine that encourages valuable collaboration, deemphasizes the normal jostle and the imperfections of capitalist interchange, and punishes what is immoral and what is dangerous for patients. So let us begin the discussion of how we should relate with a few observations:

First, business will always be business. No rules will make it otherwise. Most major health care companies recognize that in the long run, ethical behavior best serves shareholders' interest. [. . .] Some marketing is just hype, but some of it is genuinely useful education. These businesses should foster their brands and offer their newest products. None of this is corrupt, in my view. Perhaps medical students and physicians need courses to help them to analyze the difference between valuable information and lipstick, both of which are inevitable in a society such as ours.

Second, a business cannot be a business unless it has customers. Peter Drucker, the original management consultant, once said that the purpose of a business is to create customers, and that is a deep truth about the construction of our society.[8] We physicians are one group of customers served by business. Patients are another. At every level, our society depends on moral contact between customers and businesses. Therefore, I respectfully propose that we avoid legislation that interferes unduly with this fundamental American relationship. We must aim to regulate these important relationships to achieve better care, not impair them because they might become corrupt.

Third, physicians must act in the best interest of the patients they care for. This is an absolute. Physicians simply cannot choose inferior or unnecessary therapies because they have a strong customer relationship with a business. [. . .]

Fourth, all major research centers must demand freedom from industrial interference in the research mechanism. That doesn't require laws; it requires that all such institutions demand academic freedom.

Fifth, we should concentrate on structuring relationships between business and individual physicians that will bear fruit for patients and, for the moment, ignore the many other classes of problems between society and health care businesses. [. . .]

Finally, any rules we create must account for the variety of ways physicians interact with the business world. We are consultants, teachers, inventors, and investors. Each of these roles must be addressed, and I believe they must be addressed directly between physicians and business. [. . .]

Fortunately, we have an ethical framework to start the process of making safe venue for physicians and business to continue creating products and procedures without endangering patients. It is an excellent start, but it is a long way from a robust template of rules that might be incorporated into various State laws. That should be our goal.

To achieve this goal, I respectfully suggest that our major Societies convene a meeting with leaders from AdvaMed, distinguished health care attorneys, and interested legislators [...] to craft optimal legislation to set the standard for robust, moral interchange between physicians and business. [...]

At about the same time that Dr. Gibbon was struggling to develop cardiopulmonary bypass, Peter Drucker had just finished his landmark study, The Concept of the Corporation.[9] He wrote, "The central problem of all modern society is not whether we want Big Business but what we want of it, and what organization of Big Business and of the society it serves is best equipped to realize our wishes and demands." This is the fundamental problem we face as we try to decide how and under what constraints physicians and the health care industry should interact. Together we must weed the garden that has produced so much health and wealth.

Concluding Remarks
Robert M. Sade, MD

[...] Relations between industry and physicians have a checkered history. As recently as the 1950s and 1960s, contacts between industry representatives and physicians were seen in a strongly positive light; drug representatives were viewed as important sources of information for physicians. That light has dimmed considerably in recent decades, to near extinction. Since the turn of this century, frank condemnation of such contacts has become prominent in both the medical literature and the lay press.

The number of articles in the medical literature dealing with conflicts of interest in health care professionals' relations with industry has grown over the past 15 years (Figure 23.1).[10] No paper on this topic was published until one appeared in 1987. Thereafter, the number of articles per year grew slowly, remaining in the range of 10 to 15 through the 1990s. In 2000, the number jumped to the range of 35 to 70 papers per year, stimulated at least in part by several high-profile scandals in medical research. This plateau has been sustained through 2010.

Most published articles during this period have been critical of interactions between industry and health care professionals, and many propose regulation, some draconian, of physician-industry interactions. Yet, there is a small but eloquent and persuasive literature arguing that the seriousness of these problems has been overblown.

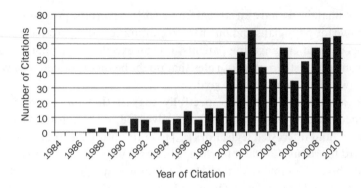

FIGURE 23.1 Health-care professionals' conflicts of interest related to industry: number of citations per year in PubMed. The numbers were derived from a PubMed search using the search term "conflict of interest industry," with limitations to English language and core clinical journals. Adapted from Sade RM. Dangerous liaisons? Industry relations with health professionals. *J Law Med Ethics*. 2009;37:398–400.

In a widely cited paper in the *New England Journal of Medicine*, Thomas Stossel asserts that none of the justifications for regulating physician-industry interactions hold up under close inspection.[11] In countering several types of arguments for regulation, for example, he points out that no data exist showing that research misbehavior is more common in studies that are sponsored by industry than in those that are not. There is also no evidence that financial interactions are disproportionately associated with fabrication of data, nor is there any credible evidence that industry consultants are biased positively toward the companies for which they consult. No data supports claims of a low quality of research done under commercial sponsorship. Moreover, there is no evidence that public trust in the health care enterprise has suffered because of high-profile scandals involving physician-industrial interactions. To the contrary, Stossel says, a great deal of damage can be done by excessive regulation arising from overreaction to adverse events, by erecting barriers between academic and industrial entities with a history of highly productive collaboration in the past.

In addition to Stossel's observations, a recent editorial in these pages points out that there is little to no evidence that patients are harmed by conflicts of interest arising from physician-industry interactions, but there is much evidence that such interactions have resulted in great benefit.[12] Evidence or lack of it, however, does not drive public policy; rather, the impetus for change comes mostly from anecdote, publicity, and the perceptions they generate. It seems likely that policy making that is designed to rectify perceptions of wrongdoing in relations between physicians and industry will not be deflected by rational arguments, such as Stossel's, which point to greater harm than benefit of such policies. It seems nearly certain that further regulation is in the future of industry-sponsored biomedical research. Regulation of physician-industry interactions seems highly likely to develop over the next few years through a political process of compromise and accommodation among our health care institutions, accrediting agencies, and lawmakers. What is uncertain is the form and substance of future regulations. All sides in the many debates surrounding these issues hope to influence the political process, guaranteeing that we will be hearing much more about this issue in the coming years.

References

1. Mack MJ, Sade RM, for the American Association for Thoracic Surgery Ethics Committee and the Society of Thoracic Surgeons Standards and Ethics Committee. Relations between cardiothoracic surgeons and industry. *Ann Thorac Surg.* 2009;87:1334–6.
2. Transparency Reports and Reporting of Physician Ownership or Investment Interests. Social Security Act 1128G 42 U.S.C. §1320a-7h (2010). http://www.ssa.gov/OP_Home/ssact/title11/1128G.htm#ft116. Accessed July 13, 2011.
3. Kalb PE. Health care fraud and abuse. *JAMA.* 1999;282:1163–8.
4. Libby RT. *The Criminalization of Medicine: America's War on Doctors.* Santa Barbara, CA: Praeger; 2007.
5. Institute of Medicine. Conflict of interest in medical research, education and practice. Washington, DC: National Academy of Sciences, 2009. http://www.iom.edu/reports/2009/conflict-of-interest-in-medical-research-education-and-practice.aspx. Accessed December 2, 2010.
6. Harris G, Carey B. Researchers fail to reveal full drug pay. *The New York Times.* June 8, 2008. http://www.nytimes.com/2008/06/08/us/08conflict.html?ex=1370664000&en=a8295c43acc64e60&ei=5124&partner=permalink&exprod=permalink. Accessed December 14, 2010.
7. Angell M. Drug companies and doctors: a story of corruption. *New York Review of Books.* January 15, 2009.
8. Drucker P. *The Practice of Management.* New York: Harper-Business, 1954; reissue ed., 1993.
9. Drucker P. *Concept of the Corporation.* New York: John Day; 1946.
10. Sade RM. Dangerous liaisons? Industry relations with health professionals. *J Law Med Ethics.* 2009;37:398–400.
11. Stossel TP. Regulating academic-industrial research relationships—solving problems or stifling progress? *N Engl J Med.* 2005;353:1060–5.
12. Sade RM. Counterpoint: full disclosure—where is the evidence for nefarious conflicts of interest? *Ann Thorac Surg.* 2011;92:417–20.

24

Full Disclosure—Should Presentations and Publications Include Dollar Amounts and Duration of Surgeon-Industry Relationships?

J. Peter Murphy and Robert M. Sade*

Point: Presentations and Publications Should Include Dollar Amounts and Duration of Surgeon-Industry Relationships

J. Peter Murphy, MD

Much has been written regarding relationships between practicing physicians, the pharmaceutical industry, and device manufacturers and their interface with the medical and ethical duties we have to our patients. As medical fiduciaries, we are obligated to discharge our responsibilities of trust openly and ethically. It has been suggested that even such trivial items as pens and notepads should be refused, as the acceptance of such items might "endanger patients" through a sense of "reciprocity, the need to give something back to the giver," and thereby compromise faithful execution of our duties.[1]

The primary issue with such concerns is whether such trivial gifts or items of far greater value generate conflicts of interest and thereby might result in compromised decision making and possible harm to patients with resultant erosion of doctor-patient relationships. The Institute of Medicine (IOM) defines conflict of interest as "circumstances that create a risk that professional judgments or actions regarding a primary interest will be unduly influenced by a secondary interest."[2]

Those "secondary interests" noted by the IOM may include items such as professional appointments, academic advancement, lucrative consulting

---

*Murphy JP, Sade RM. Ethics in cardiothoracic surgery. Point: Full disclosure—presentations and publications should include dollar amounts and duration of surgeon–industry relationships. Counterpoint: Full disclosure—where is the evidence for nefarious conflicts of interest? *Ann Thorac Surg.* 2011;92(2):413–20.

contracts, stock ownership and options, speaker fees, and even the lowly pen and notepad. The issue at play in the present debate deals with effective and appropriate management of these conflicts and attempting to resolve the question of whether true "full disclosure" and complete transparency will be beneficial in the quest for optimal conflict management, and thereby protect us from accusations of intellectual dishonesty and moral compromise.

While it might seem intuitively obvious that "secondary interests" could possibly unduly influence physician behavior and judgments, evidence based on tightly controlled studies is lacking, and even the IOM recognizes that these issues have not and cannot be analyzed by controlled trials. Data are available, but are primarily based upon observational studies and social science analysis.[3] There is solid evidence from social science research that "financial motives distort judgment," "self-serving bias is unintentional" and "unconscious," and that it can be "recognizable, but only in others." Based on these observations, many major academic centers (Yale, Harvard, and Stanford, among others) have taken a proactive position in this regard, and prohibit contact between industry representatives and medical students and residents in training, but, curiously, have less restrictive guidelines affecting full-time faculty.

With the preceding as background, it would seem logical and consistent to analyze and review the expectations of and guidance given to those with the highest level of potential conflict of interest, that being those physicians who have contractual/financial relationships (consulting, speaker, or product development), ownership positions (stock or stock options), or potential royalty revenues (based upon intellectual property rights) with device manufacturers or pharmaceutical companies, who also present or publish data pertaining to the efficacy and performance of those companies' drugs or devices. A recent joint position statement from the American Association for Thoracic Surgery (AATS) and the Society of Thoracic Surgeons (STS) specified that "disclosure" is required,[4] but the meaning of "disclose" is not defined, bringing to mind a very famous Presidential speculation on "what the meaning of the word 'is' is."

Presently, despite the aforementioned AATS/STS position paper, disclosure continues for the most part to consist of a bland acknowledgment that a "financial relationship" exists, but a more complete disclosure regarding precise dollar amounts involved and the duration of the relationship is absent. Interestingly, the Journal of Thoracic and Cardiovascular Surgery editorial staff requires that they be informed as to the dollar amount, but this information is not presented with published papers. It would be informative to learn the extent to which the editorial staff reflects on this information and why they have chosen not to fully disclose it with publication. Can disclosure absent these critical details truly be considered "full disclosure?" Certainly not.

It is important to acknowledge the advancements and benefits our profession and thereby our patients have derived from medical professionals working with device manufacturers on innovative and revolutionary products and with pharmaceutical companies to create life-enhancing drugs. Clearly, many such devices and medications have developed only because of such collaboration, and, unquestionably, full compensation for physicians involved in this manner should not be prohibited or be considered undesirable. Conflict does not arise solely from the work and compensation related to product or drug invention or development, but rather from the advocacy and analysis of the performance or outcomes related to the specific device or drug. There should be no issue with physicians deriving income based upon their unique expertise, but we should have the intellectual honesty to recognize the need for full transparency regarding the extent of the relationships when expounding on the efficacy or preferability of a device, product, or drug. [...]

Without full and absolute transparency regarding these potential conflicts, we are in danger of losing the trust that the public has in our profession. The key point is to proactively preserve our professional integrity and reputations rather than attempt to retroactively restore our stature after it has been compromised by embarrassing exposure of financial conflicts. The IOM reflects on the extent of needed information in disclosure: "The disclosure of financial relationships can be effective only if it provides sufficient information for others to use in assessing a relationship and judge the severity of the conflict." [...]

Unfortunately, the lay press has picked up on this issue, and one can cite many egregious examples of unethical behavior seemingly stemming from the vast sums involved. A recent example from The Wall Street Journal noted that "Medtronic paid the surgeon accused of falsifying study nearly $800,00."[5] In this case, a tenured professor of orthopedics at a prestigious Midwestern university was forced to resign his appointment after being accused of falsifying data regarding the efficacy of a Medtronic bone growth drug and having failed to acknowledge the extent of his consulting fees to the university and to the publishing journal (Journal of Bone and Joint Surgery).[6] If this journal had known upon submission of the article the extent of potential financial conflict, the editors might have vetted the data differently or more thoroughly before publication and thereby avoided this professionally humiliating and destructive circumstance.

I have already acknowledged that data utilized to support my opinions have not been derived from randomized, controlled trials, but to dismiss them solely upon this criterion seems irrational. Furthermore, how could one ever construct such a trial? It is rational that we attempt to manage conflicts of interest internally, and certainly if we do not, the Federal government will become even more intrusive than it is presently. In fact, if one argues that our current standards are acceptable, and no changes are necessary or appropriate, consider the following two points.

First, the Physician Payment Sunshine Act was signed into law as a significant component of the Patient Protection and Affordable Care Act of 2010 (PPACA). Under the provisions of this law, device manufacturers, drug makers, and others will be required to track any payments or gifts of $10 or more made to physicians or academic medical centers, and the federal government will store, collate, and disseminate this information to the public through an electronic database beginning in 2013. Interestingly, this act signed March 23, 2010, does require full financial disclosure, but puts no limits on financial relationships. [...]

Second, inevitably our patients will demand more information as they become increasingly aware of and more sophisticated regarding the extent of physician/industry relationships. Guy Chisolm [...] recently related that polling of 2,300 Clinic patients dealing with this specific topic generated a response rate of greater than 50%. Most respondents suggested that more information with greater specificity regarding the details of the relationships was desirable and important to them (personal communication). [...]

If the government is going to mandate it and our patients already want it, what is the legitimate argument against transparency and precise details regarding financial relationships? The first would seem to be that it is personally intrusive and is an unnecessary invasion of privacy. Those who express discomfort with the prospect of full reporting (dollars and duration) seem to validate the feeling that a problem does exist. [...]

The second argument against full disclosure relates to the costs and difficulties involved with collating and reporting the data. Obviously, consulting and speaker's fees that result in the issuance of 1099 forms will not be problematic as these are submitted to the recipient and to the Internal Revenue Service by the involved corporation on an annual basis. Equity and royalty positions might be somewhat more difficult, but certainly should not create insurmountable challenges. [...]

The issue of full transparency and full disclosure of potential conflicts of interest comes down to managing fiduciary obligations and preserving our trust with our patients. We must also acknowledge that full disclosure does not mitigate the potential for bias. It does, however, provide program committees, editorial staffs, and the listening and reading medical professionals important information that can be used in their analysis of data and positions presented and advocated. Conflicts do and will exist, and it is important that we manage them properly, for if we do not, they will undermine the reputation and stature of our profession, and erode the bond between ourselves and our patients. [...]

There has been pushback to the above positions, however, and recently a newly organized professional organization—the Association of Clinical

Researchers and Educators (ACRE)—suggested that "the push to police financial relationships has gone too far" and will "impede physician-industry collaboration."[7] Thomas Stossel, MD, a Harvard professor of medicine, stated that critics of current conditions "aim to bring about a conflict-of-interest police state." Transparency and full disclosure might be challenging and discomforting, but it certainly is not draconian and is not in any way a prohibition to collaboration and the future development of relationships between physicians and industry.

The ideas and suggestions advocated herein are by no means new or unique. Jerome Kassirer, MD, has articulated these views for years, and most explicitly in his book "On the Take."[8]

Among his observations are these: Most physicians who are close to industry swear that they are not and could not be influenced by a financial conflict of interest, yet this posture ignores what we know about human nature and the powerful influence of money. Dr. Kassirer further opines on the issue of disclosure: although disclosure is not a particularly high standard, and has flaws, it is better than no disclosure at all. Addressing the "precise meaning of disclosure," he states that there should be a requirement for full, detailed disclosure in legible handouts at all teaching events of the type (drug or devices), dollar amounts, and duration of the lecturer that relate to the subject at hand.

Although these statements are based on his opinion and observational studies rather than on randomized studies, they are precise in their intent and are reflective of an increasingly recognized and accepted ethical position. The possibility of any randomized trials resolving the debate seems remote and impractical.

We should leave the parsing of the "precise meaning of disclosure" to the professionals with legal degrees. We should "fully disclose" because not only is it right and honorable, but also it is inescapable as our government has legislated it and our patients will soon have access to it. We need to clearly stake out our position and plan of action before the public reporting coming in 2013. This is a "no brainer," and the time for action is now.

Counterpoint: Where Is the Evidence for Nefarious Conflicts of Interest?
Robert M. Sade, MD

Recent years have seen increasing focus on relations between physicians and industry, particularly pharmaceutical and device companies, and the conflicts of interest (COIs) that might arise from them.[9] Specific abuses of such relationships have often garnered national attention through scholarly journals and public communications media.

[...] The AATS and STS official journals, The Annals of Thoracic Surgery (*ATS*) and Journal of Thoracic and Cardiovascular Surgery (JTCVS), respectively, have specified the details of industry relationships that must be disclosed before a paper will be published. If a conflict is disclosed, ATS places a text box on the title page of the published article: "Dr. X discloses that he/she has a financial relationship with company Y." No additional details are provided.[10] The JTCVS disclosure statement requires reporting not only the name of the company with which a conflict exists and the nature of the relationship, but also the dollar amount received by the author—other details, such as the duration of the relationship, are omitted.[11]

The published disclosures of COIs for these annual meetings and journal publications include neither dollar amounts nor duration of the reported relationships.

SHOULD FULL DISCLOSURE INCLUDE DOLLAR AMOUNTS AND RELATIONSHIP DURATION?

Cardiothoracic surgeons are familiar with the requirements of disclosure of COIs in presentations and in publications, as they are ubiquitous in presentations at meetings and papers in journals. In answer to the question of whether increased levels of disclosure are needed, J. Peter Murphy responds in the affirmative [...] and argues that we should add dollar amounts and duration of relationships to current disclosure requirements. [...] Disclosures of conflicts are rarely verified, making their accuracy unreliable; listeners and readers are often unable to identify biased information because of their lack of expertise; and attention may be distracted from bias by implying that the disclosure itself diminishes the speaker's or author's bias.[12] Moreover, the plethora of disclosures at conferences and in publications may dull sensitivity and interest in them by virtue of frequent repetition, inuring receivers of the information to the relevance of disclosures.[13]

Much anecdotal information has been published about biased presentations and publications. Yet, the gravity of problems related to inaccurate, unbalanced, or prejudicial presentations is poorly understood owing to the paucity of systematic investigations of the frequency and impact of such presentations.

ARGUMENTS AGAINST DISCLOSURE OF RELATIONSHIP DURATION AND PAYMENTS

Murphy makes several observations with which we agree: COIs are not related only to money, but also to non-financial considerations such as career advancement and academic achievement; the collaboration between industry and physicians has been highly productive and beneficial for patients in the past; some, but not all, financial interactions between industry and physicians are unseemly or worse; hard evidence for the existence or severity of the problem is in short supply; and, finally, the status quo is unsatisfactory.

In making the case for increasing disclosure requirements to include dollar amounts and duration of relationships, however, Murphy cites what he understands to be the two "legitimate" arguments against such a requirement: it is an intrusive, gratuitous invasion of privacy, and collecting the data and reporting it are difficult and costly. These are legitimate arguments, but they seem of minor importance compared with two much more important counterpoints to the case for requiring more detail in disclosures: the real danger of slowing if not interrupting the highly productive research and innovation that has come from physician-industry collaboration over the last half-century, and the nearly complete absence of reliable evidence that this collaboration or any other interactions between physicians and industry poses a serious threat to patient safety.

PRODUCTIVE RESEARCH AND INNOVATION

To appreciate the progress that has been made through physician-industry collaboration, one need only mention the pump oxygenator developed by John Gibbon collaborating with engineer Thomas Watson of IBM, the cardiac valve prosthesis developed by Albert Starr working with engineer Lowell Edwards (resulting in the creation of the highly successful Edwards Laboratories), and external, then implantable, pacemakers developed by Dr. C. Walton Lillehei jointly with engineer Earl Bakken, creator of Medtronic. These pairs represent collaboration between heart surgeons and commercial engineers, each of which led to a major advance in heart surgery. Many other highly productive alliances could be cited in other surgical specialties, such as orthopedics and neurosurgery.

The contributions to human welfare by cooperative work between physicians and industry—both pharmaceutical and device companies—have been enormous. In the last few decades, fully half of the reduction in deaths due to coronary artery disease can be attributed to collaborations that have led to improvements in evidence-based therapies.[14] Indeed, such advances would not have been possible without merging the knowledge and skills of businessmen, engineers, and technical experts in industry with the clinical expertise of physicians, whose knowledge of clinical needs and the ways in which drugs and devices interact with the human body is indispensable to biomedical innovation. The higher the barriers that are erected between the creative minds of industry and of medicine, the less innovation and improvement of human health are likely to occur. Admittedly, there is little clear and convincing evidence that physician-industry collaboration has been harmed by current disclosure requirements, but given the amply proved benefits of such alliances and the absence of scientific evidence that they cause harm, the burden of proof rests on those who wish to impose additional regulation.

ABSENCE OF EVIDENCE

The facts underlying the national debate on relations between industry and physicians are seen to be meager when stripped of assumptions grounded in intuition and unsupported assertions. Murphy clearly documents much negative publicity in the media, some emanating from Congress, about disturbingly high levels of payment from industry to some physicians. Beyond that, very little hard evidence indicates that physician COIs vis-à-vis industry pose a serious threat to health care. Nearly all of the experimental research underlying this concern comes from the psychology and sociology literature, from which physician behavior is projected from investigations carried out in non-medical contexts. Most of the remaining evidence comes from surveys of the views and experiences of physicians, residents, and patients. Both of these data sources have low probative value.

The ranking and relative value of evidence types has been investigated and described by several groups, such as the US Preventive Services Task Force (USPSTF)[15] and the Grading of Recommendations Assessment, Development and Evaluation (GRADE) Working Group.[16] Rankings of the relative value of different kinds of evidence may be helpful in thinking about the question at hand. All of the evidence supporting the need for a high level of scrutiny and regulation of physician-industry relations falls into code D, quality of evidence is very low, suggesting that existing data are far from dispositive of this issue. Moreover, the lowest of five ranks on the USPSTF effectiveness of evidence scale is authoritative statement: "Opinions of respected authorities, based on clinical experience, descriptive studies, or reports of expert committees."[17] We ought to exercise extreme caution in using currently available information, all of which is of low quality, to make important policy decisions.

Murphy agrees that the data supporting his position is weak and points to the difficulty of carrying out randomized controlled trials in this area, implying that the only alternative to anecdotes, surveys, expert opinions, and extrapolations from experiments in unrelated fields is a randomized controlled trial. There are many other kinds of evidence, however, such as non-randomized prospective and retrospective studies of various types. In fact, one particular study that is both feasible and relevant to the debate has not been done. It is related to the critical central issue, the reason why anyone cares about physicians' COI: the possibility that COIs cause harm to patients. Harm to patients should be the primary outcome measure in studies of the concerns about COI, disclosures, and conflict management. Yet, no study, retrospective or prospective, has been carried out to examine the effects of physicians' COIs on the outcomes of patient care. In the absence of this critical information, no rational policy to regulate physician-industry relations is possible.

One of the most widely cited and exhaustively researched papers on investigations of the effects of relations between physicians and the pharmaceutical industry was published in 2000 and states this about the outcomes of such relations: "No study used patient outcome measures."[18] To fill in that information for subsequent years, this writer undertook an extensive search of the biomedical literature and was able to find only a single paper that addressed, albeit indirectly, COI and clinical outcomes. It is a meta-analysis of patient outcomes after autologous chondrocyte implantation, comparing commercially funded with independently funded studies.[19] The authors found no difference in patient outcomes between the two groups. Although this evidence is from meta-analysis, and therefore of only intermediate quality, it does not support a need for intensified regulation of physician-industry relations.

Until we have well-designed and executed studies of physician-industry COI that use the outcomes of patient care as the primary outcome measure, we will not be able to weigh the benefits to patients (known and documented medical innovation and improved health outcomes) against the harms (as yet undocumented compromise of patient care outcomes caused by physicians' biases in prescribing and using drugs and devices due to COI). Without such studies, we cannot create rational policy and law on physician-industry relations—that is, we cannot rationally decide whether optimal health care can be achieved most reliably by strengthening disclosure requirements, as Murphy suggests, or by encouraging collaboration between physicians and industry by breaking down barriers rather than building them. To this writer, the latter, although politically unpopular, seems the more reasonable course.

References

1. Iserson KV, Cerfolio RJ, Sade RM. Politely refuse the pen and note pad: gifts from industry to physicians harm patients. *Ann Thorac Surg*. 2007;84:1077–84.
2. Institute of Medicine. *Conflict of Interest in Medical Research, Education, and Practice*. Washington, DC: National Academies Press; 2009.
3. Dana J, Loewenstein G. A social science perspective on gifts to physician from industry. *JAMA*. 2003;290:252–5.
4. Mack MJ, Sade RM, and American Association for Thoracic Surgery Ethics Committee and The Society of Thoracic Surgeons Standards and Ethics Committee. Relations between cardiothoracic surgeons and industry. *Ann Thorac Surg*. 2009;87:1334–6.
5. Armstrong D, Burton TM. Medtronic paid the surgeon accused of falsifying study nearly $800,000. *The Wall Street Journal*. June 18, 2009. http://online.wsj.com/article/SB124527830694724953.html. Accessed December 30, 2010.

6. Kumar K. Surgeon accused of lying quits Washington University. *St Louis Post-Dispatch*. August 10, 2009. http://www.allbusiness.com/education-training/education-administration-university/12701347-1.html. Accessed December 30, 2010.

7. O'Reilly KB. Industry gift bans slammed for overreaching. *Am Med News*. 2009;52:19. http://www.ama-assn.org/amednews/2009/08/10/prl20810.htm. Accessed December 30, 2010.

8. Kassirer JP. *On the Take: How Medicine's Complicity with Big Business Can Endanger your Health*. New York: Oxford University Press; 2005.

9. Sade RM. Dangerous liaisons? Industry relations with health professionals. *J Law Med Ethics*. 2009;37:398–400.

10. *Annals of Thoracic Surgery*, conditions for publication form. http://ats.ctsnetjournals.org/misc/pubconditions.shtml. Accessed December 30, 2010.

11. *Journal of Thoracic and Cardiovascular Surgery*, disclosure statement. http://www.editorialmanager.com/jtcvs/. Accessed December 30, 2010.

12. Brennan TA, Rothman DJ, Blank L, et al. Health industry practices that create conflicts of interest: a policy proposal for academic medical centers. *JAMA*. 2006;295:429–33.

13. Cain DM, Loewenstein G, Moore DA. The dirt on coming clean: perverse effects of disclosing conflicts of interest. *J Legal Studies*. 2005;34:1–25.

14. Ford ES, Ajani UA, Croft JB, et al. Explaining the decrease in U.S. deaths from coronary disease, 1980–2000. *N Engl J Med*. 2007;356:2388–98.

15. US Preventive Services Task Force. Rockville, MD: USPSTF Program Office. http://www.uspreventiveservicestaskforce.org/. Accessed December 30, 2010.

16. Grading of Recommendations Assessment, Development and Evaluation (GRADE) Working Group. http://www.gradeworkinggroup.org/about_us.htm. Accessed December 30, 2010.

17. West S, King V, Carey TS, et al. Appendix C. Systems to rate the strength of scientific evidence. Evidence Reports/ Technology Assessments No. 47. Rockville, MD: Agency for Healthcare Research and Quality; 2002. http://www.ncbi.nlm.nih.gov/books/NBK33882/. Accessed December 30, 2010.

18. Wazana A. Gifts to physicians from the pharmaceutical industry. *JAMA*. 2000;283:2655–8.

19. Lubowitz JH, Appleby D, Centeno JM, Woolf SK, Reid JB. The relationship between the outcome of studies of autologous chondrocyte implantation and the presence of commercial funding. *Am J Sports Med*. 2007;35:1809–16.

20. Essential evidence plus: Levels of evidence. http://www.essentialevidenceplus.com/product/ebm_loe.cfm?show.grade#. Accessed December 29, 2010.

SECTION 7

Ethical Issues in Health-Care Policy

Robert M. Sade

No oppression is so heavy or lasting as that which is inflicted by the perversion and exorbitance of legal authority.

—Joseph Addison (1672–1719)

Coercion may prevent many transgressions; but it robs even actions which are legal of a part of their beauty. Freedom may lead to many transgressions, but it lends even to vices a less ignoble form.

—Wilhelm von Humboldt (1767–1835)

The etymological root of the word "policy" is the Greek *polis* (city) and *politeia* (citizenship), modified through Old French and Middle English to its current meaning: a course of action adopted by a government (e.g., federal regulations, executive orders), business (media communications, government relations), or individuals. Hospitals commonly separate policies into two categories: administrative (e.g., reporting medical errors to a risk-management office; a weather-emergency plan) and clinical (e.g., use of abbreviations in medical records and management of end-of-life care).

Medical ethics provides a basis for choosing among two or more competing options: good versus bad, right versus wrong, better versus worse. We generally think of surgical ethics as guides for behaviors that affect our relationships with patients and others in professional settings; however, it also applies in a broader sense to development of policies that affect medical practice. The role of physicians as policymakers encompasses a wide range, from making policies within one's own practice, over which one has a great deal of control, to voting at the national level, casting a single vote among millions. Between those ends of the policymaking spectrum are activities such as working on committees or task forces that develop or recommend policies in hospitals or state and national specialty societies. Policies above the personal level may change the way physicians relate to patients or may affect other professional activities. For these reasons, policies related to health care at all levels are rich with ethical implications for surgeons.

The Ethics Forum has sponsored discussions and debates focusing on ethical aspects of policy issues that are involved with surgical practice; these particular issues were chosen because of their currency and interest to surgeons. The debates address policies at several levels: surgical tourism at the international level, rationing of expensive therapies at the national level, regionalization of surgical care at the state level, and, at the local level, bans on smoking tobacco products in hospitals. These discussions and debates are intended to help surgeons think about the implications of broad policies for their professional and personal lives, how they could or should attempt to influence policy development, and how they might respond professionally to policies that affect their patients and their surgical practices.

Chapters

In most sectors of the US economy, individuals choose to spend their resources on goods and services, guided by their personal values, preferences, and available funds. This form of personal choice and responsibility does not hold in the health-care sector because individuals pay for their care at a steep discount: Only 10% of health-care purchases are paid with personal funds; the remaining 90% are paid by someone else in the form of health-care insurance, government programs, charities, or hospital cost-shifting, among others. Because most health care is purchased by someone other than the patient, the payor has substantial responsibility for determining what health-care goods and services will be purchased. Thus the question of whether expensive treatments with limited benefit to the patient should be allowed becomes a matter of public concern. **Chapter 25** describes the case of a patient with life-threatening leukemia who also has severe heart failure that can be treated with a left ventricular assist device (LVAD) at great cost.[1] The question of rationing expensive treatments, exemplified by this case, is debated by a surgeon highly experienced with the devices and a former state governor cum professor of public policy.

Regionalization is a public policy that mandates referral of patients with certain conditions to specialized centers that treat a high volume of such patients. The rationale is that high-volume centers generally have better outcomes for certain conditions than lower-volume centers. Some countries, such as Canada and the United Kingdom, use regionalization for certain surgical procedures, but this has not been done in the United States except on a relatively small scale, for example in the Veterans Health Administration hospital system. The debate over whether regionalization should be public policy in the United States has been ongoing for over three decades without resolution. In **chapter 26**, staunch advocates on opposite sides debate the question of whether existing data justify imposing regionalization of coronary artery bypass graft surgery.[2]

While there is little doubt that smoking tobacco products is harmful to health, it is not so clear that the passage of laws to prohibit smoking in public places is justified. Most of the public discussion has focused on the potential gains from passing such laws, but little has been said about what might be lost. **Chapter 27** begins with a vignette about a surgeon who has become a state legislator and is faced with vetting a bill that proposes a law prohibiting smoking in public places.[3] He has heard arguments on both sides of the question and now must decide whether to vote for sending the bill to the full legislature for final action or to kill the bill in committee. The question is debated by a thoracic surgeon who has been a staunch antismoking advocate and a philosopher who believes that insufficient grounds support such laws.

The national campaign against smoking has recently extended beyond prohibiting the use of tobacco products in public places to a more direct attack on smokers: denial of employment to physicians who smoke. An increasing number of medical centers, such as the Cleveland Clinic, which pioneered this policy in 2007, the Geisinger Health System, and the University of Pennsylvania Health System, have adopted such policies, including use of routine urine tests to detect nicotine metabolites toward enforcement of the policy. In **chapter 28**, a supporter of such employment policies argues that medical centers have an obligation to promote healthy activities and provide a healthy environment for employees, among others.[4] Opposing this position, another surgeon cites the hypocrisy of excluding smokers while hiring individuals who harm themselves in other ways, for instance, by overeating, driving recklessly, and using alcohol. Surgeons generally object strongly to the use of tobacco products, but does a hiring ban go a step too far?

References

1. McCarthy P, Lamm R, Sade R. Medical ethics collides with public policy: LVAD for a patient with leukemia. *Ann Thorac Surg.* 2005;80(3):793–8.
2. Nallamothu B, Eagle K, Ferraris V, Sade R. Should coronary artery bypass grafting be regionalized? *Ann Thorac Surg.* 2005;80(5):1572–81.

3. Dresler C, Cherry M, Sade RM. Should smoking tobacco products in public places be legally banned? *Ann Thorac Surg*. 2008;86:699–707.

4. Jones JW, Novick W, Sade RM. Should a medical center deny employment to a physician because he smokes tobacco products? *Ann Thorac Surg*. 2014;98(3):799–805.

25

Medical Ethics Collides with Public Policy

LVAD FOR A PATIENT WITH LEUKEMIA

Patrick M. McCarthy, Richard D. Lamm, and Robert M. Sade*

Introduction

Robert M. Sade, MD

There is a general perception that too much money is being spent on health care, and that costs are rising too rapidly. One source of the problem is believed by some to be the widespread use of expensive technologies, and this logically leads to a potential solution: get physicians to stop using such technologies. Obvious targets are cardiothoracic surgeons who have access to a substantial number of expensive technologies and a substantial number of patients to use them on.

To highlight some of the issues underlying the question of whether utilizing such technologies is justified, a case was constructed to illustrate the use of an expensive technology in a marginal clinical situation: a left ventricular assist device (LVAD) implanted in an older man with leukemia and an uncertain prognosis. To argue the question of whether or not the procedure was warranted, we recruited two outstanding proponents of differing views: Dr. Patrick McCarthy, a cardiac surgeon who has broad experience with LVADs, and former Governor Richard Lamm of Colorado, one of the few public figures audacious enough to use the word "rationing" publicly. [...] The case that served as the focal point of their discussion is detailed as follows.

---

*McCarthy P, Lamm R, Sade R. Medical ethics collides with public policy: LVAD for a patient with leukemia. *Ann Thorac Surg.* 2005;80(3):793–8. Copyright Society of Thoracic Surgeons, republished here with permission.

CASE

A 62-year-old male carpenter, Mr. I. Sandy Wood, noticed that he was tiring much earlier in the day than he had just a few weeks before, and that the frequent small cuts he received at work bled much longer than in the past. His family doctor ordered a battery of laboratory tests that revealed acute myelogenous leukemia. Echocardiogram at that time was normal, with a left ventricular ejection fraction of 63%. He was told that the chance of ultimately curing his acute myelogenous leukemia with appropriate chemotherapy was about 40%, and that nearly all relapses occur within 2 years of treatment. He underwent a full course of chemotherapy [...]. Aside from nausea and fatigue during chemotherapy, he did well.

Five months after the end of chemotherapy, Mr. Wood noticed increasing shortness of breath, generalized weakness, and ankle edema. An echocardiogram demonstrated a left ventricular ejection fraction of 19% and cardiac catheterization showed mild obstruction (25%) of the left anterior descending artery. Endomyocardial biopsy showed damage consistent with idarubicin-induced cardiomyopathy. Medical management included appropriate doses of an ACE inhibitor, beta-blocker, loop diuretic, spironolactone, and digoxin.

Despite intensive outpatient management, his dyspnea and edema continued to worsen, and he became dyspneic at rest. He was hospitalized 3 times during a 4-month period, requiring intravenous inotropic support and high-dose intravenous diuretics. During his third hospitalization, he failed to respond to intravenous drug therapy, and a repeat echocardiogram demonstrated an ejection fraction of 10%. He was deemed not to be a candidate for heart transplantation because of his recently active leukemia. Because he appeared unlikely to survive for more than a few weeks, he was evaluated as a candidate for support with a left ventricular assist device (LVAD) as destination therapy, was found to meet the criteria for support, and underwent placement of a HeartMate LVAD.

His postoperative course was initially uncomplicated. On the second postoperative day, the patient became febrile and was found to have septicemia with staphylococcal pneumonia. He was treated with intravenous antibiotics for 4 weeks. His septicemia cleared immediately and his pneumonia gradually improved. His LVAD flows stayed in the range of 6 to 7 L/min and he was discharged from the hospital in good condition on postoperative day 46. His health insurance company paid the discounted cost of the hospitalization and physicians' fees, totaling $210,000. The company also agreed to pay the costs of any needed hospitalizations, estimated to be in the range of $105,000 a year. At that time, it was estimated that the LVAD gave him a 40% to 50% chance of surviving 2 years if his acute myelogenous leukemia did not relapse.

Ten months after implantation of the LVAD, Mr. Wood was feeling well and walking 2 miles a day; his acute myelogenous leukemia was still in remission, now 2 years after treatment began, and therefore it was probably cured.

Pro
Patrick M. McCarthy, MD

The debate about the use of left ventricular assist devices (LVADs) for destination therapy has been with us for many years. An undercurrent has circulated, sometimes highly visible as in the opinion from Governor Lamm, that we will create another dialysis program, another costly burden on a burgeoning health budget under loose control.

The hypothetical case report [...] crystallizes our thinking on the issues. Rather than consider the medical wisdom of treating a cancer patient with an LVAD, let's take a fresh look at the "bigger issue" (not bigger to the patient and his family however!). How much will the United States LVAD program cost, and is it "worth it"?

First, the vast majority of the readers of this article will have to admit to a serious conflict of interest. We took an oath to treat the sick according to our ability and judgment. Nothing in the Hippocratic Oath speaks to cost of therapy, rationing, or withholding available therapy because society cannot afford it. This has brought us trouble before. Coronary artery bypass was controversial when introduced because it was expensive. However, it is part of our sworn duty as physicians to offer treatment, and fortunately millions of patients are alive after having heart surgery who now thank us for it.

Let's be clear about how much money is at stake. The Institute of Medicine projected that 50,000 United States patients per year were potential destination therapy LVAD recipients.[1] If each LVAD (with batteries, support equipment, and so forth) cost $100,000, that would cost $5 billion. If hospitalization, surgery, intensive care unit stay, and so forth cost another $100,000, that would add another $5 billion, or $10 billion total. The $200,000 cost per patient is very similar to the Randomized Evaluation of Mechanical Assistance in Treatment of Chronic Heart Failure (REMATCH) cost ($210,187).[2]

The REMATCH experience taught us more about patient eligibility too. For each patient placed in the trial, almost 50 were screened.[3] Medical comorbidities are frequent contraindications to destination therapy (i.e., diabetes with secondary complications, prior stroke with residual deficits, chronic renal failure, and elderly frail patients to name a few). Psychosocial issues may also be a problem, such as medical noncompliance and drug or alcohol abuse. Also, some patients just don't want destination therapy; they've "had enough." These factors rarely weigh heavily in the decision to use other implantable devices, such as pacemakers or implantable cardiac defibrillators, but because LVADs still require daily care and maintenance, these are important factors that limit the spread of current LVAD use. Perhaps 10,000 patients per year would be more reasonable, which translates to $2 billion per year. Finally, the surgeons and cardiologists cull even more of the potential patient population. The medical team weighs the morbidity and mortality of the operation and the potential for LVAD infection, emboli, and device failure versus the expected gain in quality and length of life. Even though the HeartMate device is Food and Drug Administration approved and reimbursed by the Centers for Medicare and Medicaid Services (albeit at a low level), the true number of implants is much less than 1,000 per year, or $200 million in health care expenditures. Also, consider that this is money returning to our economy.

This adds to the healthcare bill though, and the accelerating rise in healthcare spending relative to inflation. But we are not alone. Our spending on prison populations increased from $9 billion to $49 billion between 1982 and 1999, a 444% jump.[4]

Also, is $10 billion too much to pay for all potential LVAD patients? Advertising and promotions for cigarettes and tobacco products in 2001 cost $11.2 billion.[5]

Which would be money better spent? Perhaps a more conservative cost of LVADs would be more appropriate, such as $2 billion for 10,000 patients. After all, United States revenue at McDonalds in 2003 rose to its highest level ever, $6 billion, due to numerous factors including Americans spending on the new McGriddle breakfast sandwich. The most conservative spending on LVADs, $200 million, perhaps, is reasonable to save a thousand lives. To put this in perspective, we spent $213 million just at the box-office on "Austin Powers in Goldmember."[6] Is it unreasonable to suggest that patients should help pay part of the $100,000 for this life-saving device? In 2001, the average retail selling price of a new vehicle was $25,800. The Transportation Department reports there are 107 million United States households with an average of 1.9 cars, but only 1.8 drivers.[7] For the first time there are more vehicles than people to drive them.

Governor Lamm has written: "To avert a collapse of the system, citizens and policy makers must come to grips with the fact that they cannot do everything for everyone."[8] He was referring to regulation of the healthcare system. But as a former policy maker, as our government deepens its deficit spending to try to protect everyone from everything, is he equally outraged by the revived $10 billion dollars per year spending on a missile defense system (i.e., Star Wars)? Finally, if the policy makers and citizens didn't want us to use these devices, then why did they invest hundreds of millions of dollars through the National Institutes of Health to help us develop them?

These are difficult questions and there are no easy answers. How we as a society spend our money in relative terms is an issue most cardiac surgeons ponder only rarely. If I had been asked to see the patient described in this report, I probably would have acted as those clinicians did. I would have tried to relieve his suffering, improve his quality of life, and hopefully prolonged his life. Those collective actions by thousands of physicians, motivated by an oath we swore when we took this job, have led to the rise in healthcare spending. One last question: Is that such a bad thing? It seems there are worse ways to spend your money.

Con
Richard D. Lamm, LLB, CPA

Decisions evaluating LVAD support in stage D chronic end-stage heart failure patients cannot be made in a vacuum. Let me suggest a proposed procedure that we should go through to truly evaluate the practicability of such a technology. [...] [W]hen we fund health care with commonly collected funds, everything we do prevents us from doing something else. As General George Marshall said during WW II, "When deciding what to do, one is also deciding what not to do."

You can't build a modern health care system an individual at a time, and you can't adequately evaluate an individual technology in isolation of all other needs of the funder's system. The sum total of our ethical choices, an individual at a time, has given us an unethical health care system. We see the trees but not the forests. Left ventricular assist devices compared with what? [...]

Unavoidably, there is a conflict between individual goods and societal goods. No person sees his or her health care in context with the other health needs of society. Just as every driver in a traffic jam pleads "not guilty," so also no patient ever sees his or her health care as "too expensive." But someone must set limits. We cannot simultaneously optimize the health of the individual and the health of a group.

Medical research into increasingly marginal health care such as the LVAD is crowding out many of the other needs of society. We are developing more and more high-cost, low-benefit medical technology in a society that offers health care to fewer and fewer people at a higher and higher cost. [...]

Public policy is a different world from that of the medical bedside. Medical ethics can educate and enlighten, but they cannot control public decision making. Medical ethics are useful and hold important information but not the full picture that must be considered by third party payers. The only way third party payers have of saying yes, is saying no somewhere else.

Making optimum social policy is "terra incognito" that must be mapped anew. [...]

In a world of limited resources, you cannot explore the best use of your resources, the so-called "opportunity costs" of each dollar unless you set priorities on what you can afford. We must start a community dialogue about how we can put our health care dollars to the highest and best use. It is an inevitable dialogue and we ought to make a virtue out of necessity. [...]

If we are really going to take the World Health Organization's comprehensive definition of health (complete physical, mental, and social well being) seriously, public policy must panoramically consider the entire public policy landscape. As the Canadian study "The Determinants of Care" found: "For more than half a century the understanding that there is much more to health than health care has been largely ignored, despite the fact that increased spending on the formal health care system is no longer having a corresponding positive impact on overall population health."[9] [...]

Our current system maximizes demands for medical services paid for with pooled resources within a system that insulates patients from the cost. People usually buy health care with free or deeply discounted dollars. No system, public or private, can allow people to consume as worried patients and fund as parsimonious taxpayers or rate payers. Someone must judge whether or not an intervention is a fair and reasonable expenditure of the group's limited funds.

No common pool of funds collected by third party payers can ultimately ignore the law of diminishing returns. If every American would get all the "beneficial" health care demanded by current medical ethics and practice, it would create an unethical society in which medical care trumps too many other important social goods. Medical ethics provide no mechanism to weigh and balance individual health needs with other social or group needs. However elegantly reasoned, medical ethics cannot control the practical allocation of pooled funds. [...]

For a state or nation to cover all its citizens with modern medicine, it must (1) subsidize those who cannot afford coverage, (2) avoid "free riders" by compelling all citizens to pay something into the system, and (3) set limits on what health care is covered. Limits are painful but inevitable if we are to avoid crowding out all other social spending.

We need a new moral vision for health care that allows us to evaluate cases like the LVAD; I set forth what I see to be the essential elements of that new vision:

1. A nation's health goal can never be, nor should it be, to fund the sum total of all its citizens' individual needs. Thus, the legislature should not be limited to or controlled by the ethics of the physician-patient relationship. That relationship is important, but not exclusive. [...]

2. Public policy should concern itself more with extending the health care floor than raising the research ceiling. Public policy makers must care about the health of the total society as passionately as health provider's care about an individual's health.

3. Group funds, public or private, should maximize the health of the group. It is the duty of those distributing pooled money to optimize the health of all those in the pool. The doctor-patient relationship may be the most important relationship in health care, but it is not the only relationship. Doctors are patient advocates, but they are imperfect agents to maximize the health of a group of patients or a nation.

4. When people pool funds, they cannot maximize the amount of beneficial treatment to each member of that pool, and cost has to be a consideration when distributing those funds. We optimize the health of a group by sub-optimizing the treatment of the individual.

5. Oregon set up a system that prioritizes health care and uses limited public monies to fund the most health-producing priorities for the maximum number of insured. Not only is the Oregon health plan ethical, it is unethical for a state not to have a system of priorities. Likewise, those in health plans who distribute pooled resources have an independent ethical duty to prioritize and budget those funds to maximize the total health of the group. [. . .]

6. We must recognize that the problems of the uninsured and the problems of cost containment are not separate problems, but inextricably intertwined and must be solved together.

7. We must go substantially beyond "eliminating waste and inefficiency" into the unpopular issues of life, death, and cost-benefit thinking. One of the toughest issues of the future is: "What beneficial medicine can we ethically avoid funding?" What may have been unthinkable under assumptions of infinite resources becomes thinkable in the tradeoff world of finite resources. Many concepts must be reconsidered and re-debated. Does not a society owe a greater moral duty to a 10-year old than a 90-year old? Shouldn't a patient's smoking and drinking habits be laid on the scale for high cost rescue procedures?

8. Life is precious but it cannot be priceless. Death is always a loss, but now it is often a publicly subsidized event. There will always be "10 leading causes of death" no matter how brilliant our medicine. The threat to biologic life cannot highjack a disproportionate share of finite resources needed elsewhere for the quality of life. People have a "right to die," but it is a negative right against interference, not a positive right to a state-subsidized LVAD for such marginal

improvement. The postponement of death is an important value, but it must take its place among other health values.

9. We do not necessarily maximize health by maximizing health care. Society must better analyze and study the determinants of health for a state and for the nation. The most important question for Congress to debate is not prescription drugs for the elderly, but "How do we keep a nation healthy?" What factors produce health? In this we have the benefit of a number of other countries in which the subject has been considered.

10. Goethe warned, "If you are going to live in your father's house, you must rebuild it." We have not adequately structured the house of health care. We have overbuilt and over-furnished the first floor, but most of the rest of the structure remains not only unfinished but also unframed. There is more than one level of ethical analysis in health policy, there are multiple levels. A legislator, a health plan, and a family member have different moral duties and a different moral geography than a doctor. We need different levels of ethical analysis corresponding to the various levels of moral obligation.

11. All modern health care must be based first on self-responsibility. We are our own best "doctor," and we cannot expect society to cure the consequences of all our self-imposed illnesses.

We have to rebuild the house of health care by rethinking the moral duties of each level of the health care organization. The foundation of the house of health care is self-responsibility. The first floor is the ethics and duties of the doctor-patient relationship; the second floor is the ethics and duties of the health insurance plan whose financial and moral obligation is to the total group whose premiums made up the money under their control. The third floor of health care is the state and the nation. Neither the second nor the third floor of health care can give the Hippocratic Oath a blank check. We need new ethical analysis to determine the role of the health plan for government and better evaluate their fiduciary duty in the funding of health care. All three levels of analysis are necessarily related but not coterminous, and rationing is unavoidable on the top two floors. Only when we have a system that considers all the social needs and sets priorities can we know whether or not if LVAD support fits into those priorities.

Concluding Remarks
Robert M. Sade, MD

Dr. McCarthy and Governor Lamm have reached different conclusions about whether Mr. Wood's should have received his LVAD: yes, I would have done the same thing, says one, but you can't know whether he should or not, replies the other. It may seem strange, therefore, to recognize that they may both be correct.

How can two very different conclusions be compatible and correct? They can be because they are reached through two different sets of guiding principles. Dr. McCarthy's perspective is that of a physician working within an ethical context that we, as physicians, can easily understand: our first priority must be to serve the best interests of our patients. Governor Lamm, on the other hand, is a social scientist who necessarily takes the broad view of society as a whole. He accepts that physicians are ethically bound to do their best to serve the needs of their patients, arguing, for that very reason, that physicians are in a poor position to be the decision makers for allocation of commonly held resources. [...]

Governor Lamm's metaphor (i.e., the house of health care) powerfully conveys the diversity of ethical obligations incumbent upon the many players in health care. [...] Priorities must be set for how these limited common funds should be spent, as they are insufficient to satisfy all needs and wants. [...] Those who wish to advance the cause of free choice in health care will want to maximize the funds available to the foundation and to the first floor and, as much as possible, to control tightly the expenditures at levels two and three. The Health Savings Accounts enacted by Congress and signed into law by President Bush in December 2003 are a step in that direction, giving individual patients far more control over their health care dollars than they have had in the past, thereby increasing the self-responsibility of individuals for both their own health and their own health care.

A tension exists today between commentators who wish to reinforce the paramount obligation of physicians to the welfare of their patients, which they see as *sine qua non* of a salutary healing relationship,[10] and bioethicists who wish to redirect the focus of physicians toward social welfare, which they see as a higher obligation emanating from a purported basic right to health care.[11] One consequence of such a realignment of ethical obligations is likely to be the co-option of physicians as agents of society, helping to control health care costs by bedside rationing of such technologies as LVADs.

Dr. McCarthy and Governor Lamm disagree about the need for constraints on the use of expensive technologies, such as LVAD for a patient with leukemia, but they are in agreement on an important underlying ethical principle: physicians are obligated to do the best they can for their patients. Regardless of the outcome of the debate on limiting the use of high technology, physicians should resist the siren call to "social responsibility" and continue to advocate whatever is medically best for the patients we advise and treat. If certain technologies should not be used, it is the responsibility of insurance companies, government agencies, or sociopolitical units such as states (perhaps using an Oregon-like method) to set the limits. We physicians can and should help to develop rationing policies by participating on

310 The Ethics of Surgery

hospital committees, speaking at public hearings, or consulting with insurance companies and government agencies, but we should never ration technology at the bedsides of our patients. In an important sense, both McCarthy and Lamm are right.

References

1. Hanna KE, Manning FJ, Bouxsein P, Pope A, eds. *Innovation and Invention in Medical Devices: Workshop Summary*, 1st ed. Washington, DC: National Academy Press; 2001.
2. Oz MC, Gelijns AC, Miller L, et al. Left ventricular assist devices as permanent heart failure therapy: the price of progress. *Ann Surg.* 2003;238;577–85.
3. Rose EA, Gelijns AC, Moskowitz AJ, et al. Long-term mechanical left ventricular assistance for end-stage heart failure. *N Engl J Med.* 2001;345:1435–43.
4. Wickham D. ABA report offers wise Rx for ailing U.S. penal system. *USA Today.* June 29, 2004:A13.
5. Tobacco Industry Marketing. Fact sheet. TIPS. Atlanta: Centers for Disease Control and Prevention. http://www.cdc.gov/tobacco/factsheets/Tobacco_Industry_Marketing_Factsheet.htm. Accessed February 2004.
6. BoxofficeGuru.com. All-Time Domestic Blockbusters. http://boxofficeguru.com/blockbusters.htm. Accessed July 5, 2004.
7. Americans' love affair with cars, trucks and SUVs continues. *USA Today.* http://www.usatoday.com/news/nation/2003-08-30-outnumbered-cars_x.htm. Accessed: August 30, 2003.
8. Lamm RD. High-tech health care and society's ability to pay. *Health Finance Manage.* 1990;44(9):20–24, 26, 28–30.
9. The determinants of health. CIAR Publication No. 5. Toronto: Canadian Institute for Advanced Research; August 1991:4.
10. Levinsky NG. The doctor's master. *N Engl J Med.* 1984;311(24):1573–5.
11. Buchanan A, Brock D, Daniels N, Wikler D. *From Chance to Choice: Genetics and Justice.* New York: Cambridge University Press; 2001.

26

Should Coronary Artery Bypass Grafting Be Regionalized?

Brahmajee K. Nallamothu, Kim A. Eagle,
Victor A. Ferraris, and Robert M. Sade*

Introduction
Robert M. Sade, MD

Several studies have shown that cardiac care centers that provide a high volume of cardiac services, particularly coronary artery bypass grafting (CABG), have better outcomes than those with low volumes. Some analysts have used these data to suggest that patients in need of care for coronary artery disease would be best served if they were referred only to those centers that treat a large number of these patients. They reason that regionalizing coronary artery disease treatment will result in fewer deaths, because low volume–high mortality programs would be deleted and may have additional advantages in efficiencies of scale.

Those who oppose regionalization claim that the data justifying regionalization are seriously flawed. Reliable measurement of outcomes requires accurate risk stratification; technologies for accomplishing this are being developed and used, but are far from perfect. Moreover, although it is true that many studies show a relationship between volume and outcome, a few well-designed recent studies have not found such a relationship.

In the unregulated referral system that now exists in this country, regionalization already occurs informally; primary care physicians are more likely to refer their patients to centers with good results, and many large-volume centers achieved their dominant status by virtue of good outcomes. Formal

*Nallamothu B, Eagle K, Ferraris V, Sade R. Should coronary artery bypass grafting be regionalized? *Ann Thorac Surg.* 2005;80(5):1572–81. Copyright Society of Thoracic Surgeons, republished here with permission.

regionalization already exists in other countries, such as Canada and Great Britain, and it exists on a small scale in this country (e.g., in the VA hospital system). Many have suggested formal regionalization of CABG in the United States on grounds of achieving better outcomes and gaining efficiency, whereas others object on the grounds of inadequate supportive data. Do currently available data justify regionalization of CABG?

The cases for opposing points of view (i.e., for and against regionalization) are made herein by scholars with deep and persistent interest in this question.

Pro

Brahmajee K. Nallamothu, MD, MPH and Kim A. Eagle, MD

A quarter of a century has passed since Luft and colleagues first published their seminal article on the hospital volume–outcome effect.[1] In that study, the investigators found a strong and consistent association between higher hospital volume and lower in-hospital mortality for several high-risk procedures, including CABG, using a national administrative database of nearly 1,500 hospitals. Numerous additional reports have confirmed this association across a variety of procedures, populations, and clinical settings.

Despite compelling evidence supporting the existence of a hospital volume–outcome effect, little has been done during the intervening 25 years to ensure minimum volume requirements for high-risk procedures in the United States. Traditional arguments against the regionalization of high-risk procedures to higher volume hospitals through volume-based referral have relied on two fundamental lines of reasoning: (1) analyses supporting the hospital volume–outcome relationship are flawed, and (2) the design of the United States health care system prohibits its practical application.[2]

In this article, we briefly review the evidence supporting the existence of a hospital volume–outcome effect for CABG and address common fears that are typically mentioned when regionalization is discussed. We conclude by proposing a practical strategy for initiating CABG regionalization within the current environment of the United States health care system.

EVIDENCE SUPPORTING THE HOSPITAL VOLUME–OUTCOME EFFECT

Nearly 300 studies have examined the hospital volume–outcome effect in various medical conditions and procedures with CABG being one of the more thoroughly studied procedures. Most published studies have reported statistically significant associations between hospital volume and outcomes favoring higher–volume hospitals. Only a small number of studies have not demonstrated a hospital volume–outcome effect in CABG. In general, these "null" analyses were performed in specific patient populations (e.g., the Veterans Affairs health care system) or under circumstances in which hospital volume did not vary widely. In the largest study to date, Birkmeyer and colleagues analyzed Medicare data in over 900,000 patients undergoing CABG and demonstrated a 20% reduction in 30–day mortality for hospitals with the highest volume (> 849 annual cases) when compared with those with the lowest volume (< 230 annual cases).[3]

EVIDENCE SUPPORTING REGIONALIZATION: MOVING
BEYOND THE FEARS

Critics of regionalization strategies have raised both methodological and practical concerns regarding earlier hospital volume–outcome studies and their implications for regionalization:

¤ *Fear No. 1: Most studies are outdated and use administrative data sources.* The concern is that studies do not reflect recent advancements in surgical technique, anesthesia, and perioperative medical therapy, or they inadequately adjust for important confounding variables. Some have also focused exclusively on Medicare patients, a group that is generally older and at higher risk for complications.

However, recent data from the New York Cardiac Surgery Reporting System (CSRS) and The Society for Thoracic Surgery (STS) National Cardiac Database continue to support the existence of a hospital volume–outcome effect in CABG.[4] [...]

¤ *Fear No. 2: There is inconsistency of statistical analyses in earlier reports.* Studies have varied broadly in their methodological modeling of the hospital volume–outcome effect.[5] [...]

Yet more recent analyses have largely addressed these methodological concerns. Both contemporary studies from the New York CSRS and the STS National Cardiac Database have used complex statistical techniques (i.e., adjusting for surgeon volume and use of a hierarchical modeling), and they have reconfirmed significant associations between hospital volume and surgical mortality. [...]

¤ *Fear No. 3: Hospital volume is an imperfect proxy for quality.* This concern is undeniable. There are certainly some low-volume programs that may have acceptable risk-adjusted mortality rates for CABG when compared with hospitals that have higher–volume programs. However, an unfortunate reality is that policy, like clinical decisions based on randomized clinical trials, needs to be based on aggregated or "averaged" data. [...]

Furthermore, hospital volume has been correlated with quality measures such as postoperative renal failure or prolonged mechanical ventilation in addition to short-term mortality.[4] [...]

- *Fear No. 4: There is insufficient data for setting a specific volume threshold.* As mentioned earlier, studies have varied widely in their use of specific thresholds during statistical analyses.[6] [...]
- *Fear No. 5: The hospital volume–outcome effect is small in CABG and not worth the effort.* When compared with other high-risk procedures, such as operations for pancreatic or esophageal cancer, the absolute risk difference in surgical mortality between very high-volume and very low-volume hospitals for CABG is relatively small at between 1% and 2%.[3] However, the large number of CABG procedures performed each year in comparison with these other procedures makes it likely to have a broader impact in regard to avoiding deaths. [...]
- *Fear No. 6: Regionalization will limit access and be impractical for a large number of patients due to geographic location.* Previous studies have suggested that physical access would not be substantially restricted if very low-volume programs were closed as most patients live within reasonable distances of high-volume hospitals.[7] In addition, existing data suggest that although a substantial number of health referral regions (i.e., tertiary-care catchment areas) do not have a single high-volume hospital for CABG, the number of annual population-based rates for surgeries performed in these areas could support a high-volume hospital if smaller surgical programs were combined.[8] Despite these facts, we recognize that there will continue to be geographically isolated communities that need to be excluded from any strategy for CABG regionalization.
- *Fear No. 7: The quality of care and financial viability of smaller hospitals will be threatened.* This is an important and valid fear. The performance of CABG at a hospital is tied to a large number of cardiovascular-related services including PCI, cardiac catheterization, and noninvasive cardiovascular services. [...] Lost revenue from eliminating CABG and related services may reduce the hospital's ability to provide other less lucrative but necessary care to its community. Although this fear is a compelling argument, it must be balanced against the strong evidence supporting the potential benefits of regionalization for patients undergoing major surgery such as CABG.

RECOMMENDATIONS FOR REGIONALIZATION IN THE UNITED STATES

With several legitimate fears still existing, how can regionalization possibly occur? We believe that the availability of empirical data highlighting the limitations of CABG regionalization should be used to guide policy, not to eliminate any attempts toward regionalization. We support a strategy that uses volume-based standards in addition to other criteria for hospital referrals with CABG. The alternative, which would be waiting for the "ideal" study to be performed, is inadequate in our view. Accordingly, we suggest the following strategies for regionalization:

1. Eliminate very low-volume programs at hospitals with an average annual cardiac surgery volume of less than 100. This would include the total number of CABG procedures and other adult open-heart procedures, with exceptions made for hospitals that serve geographically–isolated communities. The evidence is too strong and consistent that hospitals with such low numbers of cases have poor outcomes when compared with higher–volume centers. [. . .]
2. For hospitals with annual cardiac surgery volumes above 100 cases, additional criteria, such as the use of risk-adjusted mortality rates, should be used to assess hospital quality. When annual cardiac surgery volumes are between 100 to 250 annual cases, strong consideration should be made for referring high-risk patients such as the elderly (> 65 years old) or complex procedures like concomitant valve replacement to higher–volume hospitals.[9] [. . .]
3. Initiate a nationwide, mandatory reporting system for CABG in order to collect outcomes data on quality and processes of care at individual programs. This could be piggybacked onto the established framework of the current STS National Cardiac Database. With this we would encourage participation in regional collaborative networks targeting key quality opportunities and providing a forum for continuous quality improvement strategies. [. . .]
4. Begin formal assessments of the appropriateness of CABG at individual programs. We believe no volume-based regionalization strategy can be properly implemented without concurrently evaluating appropriateness. Without this precaution, the incentive to do inappropriate cases may be too great for providers and hospitals wishing to meet strict volume criteria. [. . .]

We believe the last two points are critical. As regionalization is implemented in small steps, the process of collecting and refining data to modify structural changes in the strategy is needed. As procedures "mature" and transform over time, the importance of the hospital volume–outcome effect may change. Although this strategy for regionalization may not completely address all the fears previously raised, we believe that it is a fair and equitable plan that can be transitioned into the current health care system. [. . .]

FUTURE ISSUES

Techniques for coronary revascularization are advancing rapidly in the United States. In particular, recent evidence supporting the use of PCI in acute coronary syndromes and ST segment elevation myocardial infarction is compelling. The impact of eliminating very low-volume CABG programs on the availability of PCI in the general population will need to be evaluated. In addition, advances in medical therapy and PCI may be contributing to diminishing population-based rates for overall CABG. How regionalization will influence cardiac surgical training programs and the physician workforce, given the declining use of CABG, will need to be assessed. We also believe that continued research into why volume is so strongly associated with better outcomes is needed. If key system-level characteristics are identified, these processes of care can hopefully be disseminated across more hospitals. Finally, the impact of regionalization on cost needs to be better understood. [...]

CONCLUSIONS

Evidence supporting the hospital volume–outcome effect in CABG is persuasive. Although several studies have cautioned us on the importance of cautiously interpreting the data, these studies should not be used to justify avoidance of regionalization. Instead, we should use the data to inform and direct our policy decisions to create a rational and effective system of regionalization. This is particularly important as diminishing CABG volumes may create larger numbers of very–low volume CABG programs. For the nearly 500,000 patients undergoing CABG each year in the United States, the implications of regionalization are enormous. Given its potential benefits, we should not wait to collect data for yet another 25 years before considering its implementation.

Con
Victor A. Ferraris, MD, PhD

WHAT IS REGIONALIZATION?

Regionalization of health care resources is the selective referral of patients to regional centers. Health care payers have jumped on the concept of regionalization to attempt lowering the spiraling health care costs. There are at least two unique features of the United States health care system: (1) the ability of patients to seek medical care from whomever they want (i.e., access), and (2) the expectation that access to health care will be readily available at a local level (i.e., availability). Regionalization infringes on these two principles. To understand regionalization, it is necessary to talk about provider volume, health care costs, and quality of care. All of these concepts are wrapped up in discussions of regionalization of health care resources.

EXAMPLES OF REGIONALIZATION OF HEALTH CARE

There is absolutely no evidence that deliberately concentrating procedures in the hands of regional providers will actually improve outcomes. In fact, the opposite may be true. The hypothesis that regionalization based on some criteria (either provider volume or cost) results in better outcomes has not been tested in a randomized trial or in any rigorous way. [. . .]

Regionalization of trauma care is an important component of most statewide trauma systems. On the surface it may seem that regionalization of trauma resources would focus care in high-volume hospitals and result in a drop in mortality. Many other factors undoubtedly influence improved outcome from major trauma, including better treatment algorithms (Advanced Cardiac Life Support protocols), improved response times, and focused training of physicians. A review of the National Trauma Databank in the United States found no positive relationship between outcome and treatment of severe trauma in high-volume centers.[10]

Another example of regionalization of resources is the localization of cardiac care in regionalized centers in the Department of Veterans Affairs (VA) health care system. Petersen and co–authors found underuse of indicated angiography in patients with acute myocardial infarction in the VA system.[11] This rate of underuse was greater than that of similar non-VA Medicare patients. [. . .]

REGIONALIZATION BASED ON PROVIDER VOLUME

Almost by default, the concept of regionalization springs from multiple investigations that find better outcomes from high-volume providers (both hospitals and surgeons). Among health care planners it is almost axiomatic that high-volume providers will have better outcomes [. . .]. Health care payers are quick to embrace this concept. [. . .]

Provider (either hospital or physician) volume is a structural variable. Structural variables are those that reflect the setting or system in which care is delivered. Structural variables are different than process variables that describe the care that patients actually receive. The disadvantages of using structural variables as indicators of quality include: (1) inability to evaluate outcomes by randomized trials, (2) other confounding variables are more important in determining outcomes, and (3) structural variables are not readily actionable (e.g., a small hospital cannot readily increase its volume). The advantages of using structural variables include: (1) expediency, which is easily measured, (2) structural variables are inexpensive to measure, and (3) association exists between hospital volume and outcomes in most reports. It is easy to see why health care payers chose structural variables as surrogates of quality, because simply put, it is easier.

More than 88 studies examined the relationship between provider volume and outcome [...]. A higher–volume, better outcome association was observed in three fourths of the studies. At least 10 of these large studies addressed the notion that hospitals performing small numbers of CABG operations have higher operative mortality. Interestingly, in the three studies done more recently (since 1996) there was no clear relationship between outcome and volume.[12] In two separate studies done on some of the same patients in the New York State cardiac surgery database, completely opposite results were obtained. The Institute of Medicine summarized the relationship between higher–volume and better outcome [...] and concluded that "volume per se does not lead to better outcome."[12] The dilemma is that some low-volume providers have excellent outcomes, whereas some high-volume providers have poor outcomes. [...]

It is simplistic to suggest that hospital volume is a principle surrogate of outcome and much more sophistication is required to sort out this relationship. Several published studies reveal the inadequacy of the volume–outcome relationship. Peterson and co–authors reviewed the STS National Cardiac Database to evaluate the relationship of CABG volume to outcome. They found almost no potential benefit in closing low-volume centers.[4] [...]

Halm and co–workers performed an exhaustive review of the literature on the volume–outcome relationship.[13] They observed an association between high–volume and better outcomes across a wide range of procedures. They also observed multiple methodological shortcomings in most of the studies dealing with the volume–outcome relationship. Even when a significant association exists, volume did not predict outcome well for individual hospitals or physicians. [...] Even advocates of regionalization of health care resources concede that the best indicator of provider outcome is uncertain and provider volume alone should not be used as a means to direct referral of patients.[8] [...]

REGIONALIZATION BASED ON COST SAVINGS

Why is regionalization of health care touted as a cost saving measure? There is no good answer. In the United States, the Leapfrog Group (Washington, DC) and other consortiums of health care payers are concerned about the spiraling increase in health care costs, and ultimately the cost that corporations must pay to provide health care to their employees. [...] Menke and Wray suggest that most empirical estimates of the cost implications of regionalization suffer from methodological shortcomings.[14] He outlines the various factors that must be taken into account before an accurate assessment of cost benefit from regionalization can be assessed. The remarkable thing is that no one has done this assessment, yet regionalization is viewed as cost beneficial. Regionalization is just as likely to result in increased costs as it is to result in decreased health care costs.

WHAT REGIONALIZATION IS NOT

In the current health care climate, it is important to understand what regionalization does not imply. What regionalization is not is the concentration of patients with a particular medical illness, such as diabetes or hypertension, in centers that only treat high volumes of these medical illnesses. Why are medical illnesses excluded from talks about regionalization? Procedures such as CABG, esophagectomy, and aortic aneurysm repair are big ticket items and cost far more than giving a shot of insulin to a diabetic. Furthermore, very little data is available on quality of care for common medical illnesses. [...]

Make no mistake that regionalization of health care resources is about money and the potential for saving health care dollars. Proponents of regionalization advocate, quite rightly, that there is nothing wrong with using cost savings as a driver for regionalization, yet no clear cut cost savings has ever been observed from any form of regionalization.

UNINTENDED CONSEQUENCES OF REGIONALIZATION

Regionalization of health care resources is an untested concept that may have the opposite effects to those anticipated. Crawford and co–workers pointed out that a policy of regionalized referrals for CABG may have several adverse effects on health care, including increased cost, decreased patient satisfaction, and reduced availability of surgical services in remote or rural locations.[15] [...] [E]nforced referrals of CABG patients to high-volume providers may actually increase operative mortality, which is an undesirable consequence of regionalization.

Advocates of regionalization point to the potential number of lives saved by artificially forcing referrals to high-volume providers. They attempt to intervene and influence the natural market forces that are expected to result in patients migrating to the best places regardless of the volume of cases done. The very clear impression is that patients should have their CABG done by high-volume providers.[16] In the past, market forces shifted patients to places where they get good outcomes regardless of the volume of the provider. After all, high-volume providers were once low-volume providers and only achieved their high-volume status by providing excellent care and obtaining high-quality outcomes. [...]

Several authors speculated on the consequences of directed referral of patients. There are likely to be adverse effects on the health care systems from these directed referrals. [...]

ARE THERE ALTERNATIVES TO REGIONALIZATION?

The Leapfrog Group [...] is a consortium of health care purchasers formed "to initiate breakthrough improvements in the safety, quality, and affordability of health care for Americans" [...]. The Leapfrog Group practices "evidence-based hospital referral." Based largely on an estimate of patient lives saved by referral to high-volume providers, the Leapfrog Group recommended payment premiums to hospitals that performed more than 500 CABG procedures per year.[17] Because of concerns about rural health care, the Leapfrog Group's standards only apply to urban settings. [...] Birkmeyer and Dimick reviewed the potential effects of applying these new Leapfrog Group standards to a typical CABG population.[18] They found that standards comprised of process of care or direct outcome measures would be more effective than those based on volume alone in improving outcomes for CABG. For CABG and PCI, standards based on risk-adjusted mortality rates would save at least five times more lives than those based on volume criteria alone. [...]

Corporations and health care payers embrace provider volume as an indicator of outcome because of expediency. Hospital or physician volume is an inexpensive and easily measured structural variable that is readily understood by the consumer and the payer. [...] There is little doubt that a comparison among providers using risk stratification methods is better than using volume to judge quality. Using quality indicators like the STS database risk-adjustment scheme can improve quality of care by low-volume providers.[19] [...]

Quality improvement projects, either in-house or in collaboration with high-volume providers, would improve outcomes to a level at which directed referrals away from low-volume providers would not be necessary. Sollano and coworkers reanalyzed the CABG mortality from the New York State database between 1990 and 1995.[20] They found that the previously observed volume–outcome relationship disappeared after the implementation of a statewide quality improvement program. [...] Clinical guidelines, quality improvement projects, provider education, and collaborative interactions between high-volume and low-volume providers are just a few interventions that do not involve regionalization but are likely to improve quality for low-volume providers.

Should we as health care professionals and scientists give in to the expediency of measuring provider volume and embracing regionalization when we know that there are better measures of outcome and better ways to improve quality? [...] The unproven concept of regionalization may become a non issue when providers address outcomes using risk adjustment and process of care variables in an open transparent way aimed at self improvement and enhancing high-quality care. [...] There is almost certainly a better alternative. It remains for us as a profession to lead and not to follow, to embrace transparent risk-adjusted outcome analysis proactively, and to work interactively with payers to reach a common goal of high-quality care. Regionalization is not the first place to start.

Concluding Remarks
Robert M. Sade, MD

A fundamental ethical principle is central to this discussion: the paramount obligation of physicians is to serve the medical interests of their patients.

Flowing from this principle is the imperative to make the health care of patients as safe as possible. Would regionalization of CABG move us toward or away from that goal? The preceding discussions suggest that the available data do not provide an unambiguous answer.

To understand how the principle of fidelity to the patient's interests can guide our thinking about this question, let us assume much clearer data than we have now. The assumptions, for the sake of discussion, are that programs and surgeons performing a high volume of CABG procedures have significantly lower mortality rates than low-volume programs and low-volume surgeons. Assume further that patients are indifferent to how far they must travel for their cardiac care and that family physicians referring the patients have no preferences for where the surgery is done or who will do it. The case then seems to be closed: regionalizing CABG so that all patients needing the procedure are referred to high-volume, low-mortality programs will best serve our patients.

But is the case really closed? Perhaps not, for there is a hidden assumption in this scenario, namely that the universe of CABG programs and surgeons and their respective capabilities to provide safe operations is immutable. This assumption is false. High-volume programs can become complacent and lose their competitive edge; high-volume surgeons grow old, their skills diminish, and their knowledge may become outdated. Low-volume programs want to thrive, so they strive for efficiency and patient friendliness; low-volume surgeons strive for better results and other means of increasing referrals. Thus, high volume may become low, and low volume may become high.

Studies of volume–outcome relationships provide a snapshot, yet health care, like every other human activity, is dynamic. The slow ebb and flow in which large programs shrink and small programs grow is driven by quality, cost, accessibility, and many other factors. Even if there were a causal relationship between high volume and low mortality, we have no way of knowing in advance which large programs have peaked and are moving down the mortality rate scale and which small programs are dynamically moving up the scale. [. . .] [A]t the local level, competition is based to a great extent on quality of care, which includes subjective factors (such as patient satisfaction) and objective information (such as mortality rates). These rates are known at least roughly by referring physicians, whether or not the actual data are published. So it may be that in the long run, the interests of patients will be best served by allowing physicians and patients to decide, thousands of times every day, where the patient's cardiac care will be provided and by whom. Such freedom of choice may be the surest way to foster excellent care for the largest number of patients for the long term.

We know of no studies that examine the flux of CABG volume in surgical programs and practices over time. Therefore, even if the assumptions in the "closed case" previously described were true, there still would be no useful data with which to compare the benefits and harms of regionalizing CABG with those of freedom of choice in the CABG market. The short term would favor the lower mortality rates of regionalization, but the price would be freezing the dynamism of the current unregulated market for CABG. The long term may well favor the current dynamic system, as low-volume, low-mortality programs grow bigger and become the new high-volume, low-mortality programs.

For physicians, the ethical dilemma in the debate on regionalization, it appears, turns on the question of how to best serve the interests of patients (i.e., with a static referral system based on today's snapshot of CABG results or with a dynamic system that more easily allows future change?). Unfortunately, we cannot weigh the evidence for and against the alternatives, because reliable data do not exist. Volume itself does not lead to good outcomes, as both discussants have agreed; it is a proxy measure for other factors that affect care. [...]

Like most robust debates, this one has left us with more questions than answers. If an immediate decision is urgently needed, we must choose between the alternatives on the basis of philosophical beliefs about how the best outcomes are likely to be achieved (i.e., from a centralized, orderly command-and-control system or from an untidy free market system). If we judge that the situation is not urgent, then we can wait for reliable and valid data generated by measures of quality of care more accurate and specific than volume to guide a well-grounded decision.

References

1. Luft HS, Bunker JP, Enthoven AC. Should operations be regionalized? The empirical relation between surgical volume and mortality. *N Engl J Med.* 1979;301:1364–9.
2. Russell TR. Invited commentary: volume standards for high-risk operations: an American College of Surgeons' view. *Surgery* 2001;130:423–4.
3. Birkmeyer JD, Siewers AE, Finlayson EV, et al. Hospital volume and surgical mortality in the United States. *N Engl J Med.* 2002;346:1128–37.

4. Peterson ED, Coombs LP, DeLong ER, Haan CK, Ferguson TB. Procedural volume as a marker of quality for CABG surgery. *JAMA*. 2004;291:195–201.

5. Shahian DM, Normand SL. The volume–outcome relationship: from Luft to Leapfrog. *Ann Thorac Surg*. 2003;75:1048–58.

6. Shahian DM. Improving cardiac surgery quality—volume, outcome, process? *JAMA*. 2004;291:246–8.

7. Grumbach K, Anderson GM, Luft HS, Roos LL, Brook R. Regionalization of cardiac surgery in the United States and Canada: geographic access, choice, and outcomes. *JAMA*. 1995;274:1282–8.

8. Dimick JB, Finlayson SR, Birkmeyer JD. Regional availability of high-volume hospitals for major surgery. *Health Aff* (Millwood) 2004(Suppl. Web Exclusive):VAR45–53.

9. Nallamothu BK, Saint S, Hofer TP, Vijan S, Eagle KA, Bernstein SJ. Impact of patient risk on the hospital volume–outcome relationship in coronary artery bypass grafting. *Arch Intern Med*. 2005;165:333–7.

10. Glance LG, Osler TM, Dick A, Mukamel D. The relation between trauma center outcome and volume in the National Trauma Databank. *J Trauma*. 2004;56:682–90.

11. Petersen LA, Normand SL, Leape LL, McNeil BJ. Regionalization and the underuse of angiography in the Veterans Affairs Health Care System as compared with a fee-for-service system. *N Engl J Med*. 2003;348:2209–17.

12. Nallamothu BK, Saint S, Ramsey SD, Hofer TP, Vijan S, Eagle KA. The role of hospital volume in coronary artery bypass grafting: is more always better? *J Am Coll Cardiol*. 2001;38:1923–30.

13. Halm EA, Lee C, Chassin MR. Is volume related to outcome in health care? A systematic review and methodologic critique of the literature. *Ann Intern Med*. 2002;137:511–520.

14. Menke TJ, Wray NP. When does regionalization of expensive medical care save money? *Health Serv Manage Res*. 2001;14:116–24.

15. Crawford FA, Anderson RP, Clark RE, et al. Volume requirements for cardiac surgery credentialing: a critical examination. The Ad Hoc Committee on Cardiac Surgery Credentialing of the Society of Thoracic Surgeons. *Ann Thorac Surg*. 1996;61:12–6.

16. Birkmeyer JD. High-risk surgery—follow the crowd. *JAMA*. 2000;283:1191–3.

17. Dudley RA, Johansen KL, Brand R, Rennie DJ, Milstein A. Selective referral to high-volume hospitals: estimating potentially avoidable deaths. *JAMA*. 2000;283:1159–66.

18. Birkmeyer JD, Dimick JB. Potential benefits of the new Leapfrog standards: effect of process and outcomes measures. *Surgery*. 2004;135:569–75.

19. Ferguson TB Jr, Peterson ED, Coombs LP, et al. Use of continuous quality improvement to increase use of process measures in patients undergoing coronary artery bypass graft surgery: a randomized controlled trial. *JAMA*. 2003;290:49–56.

20. Sollano JA, Gelijns AC, Moskowitz AJ, et al. Volume–outcome relationships in cardiovascular operations: New York state, 1990–1995. *J Thorac Cardiovasc Surg*. 1999;117:419–428; discussion 428–30.

27

A Clash of Rights

SHOULD SMOKING TOBACCO PRODUCTS IN PUBLIC PLACES
BE LEGALLY BANNED?

Carolyn M. Dresler, Mark J. Cherry,
and Robert M. Sade*

Introduction
Robert M. Sade, MD

There is little question that smoking tobacco products is an important con-
tributor to the development of many kinds of cancer, as well as to morbidity
through its effects on lungs, blood vessels, and other vital organs and processes. Virtually all thoracic surgeons advise their patients who smoke to
stop smoking because of the risks it poses to health, both short-term and
long-term. Yet, it is a valid question to ask whether or not or to what extent
these medical facts constitute justification of coercive action against smokers
through enactment of laws.

There seems to be strong sentiment among thoracic surgeons in support
of such laws, probably driven largely by their personal experiences with the
pathology that smoking visits on those who are exposed to it. They are not as
vocal, however, about the need for laws to control other destructive habits, such
as eating too much (obesity is also a major cause of morbidity) or drinking too
much (prohibition of alcohol early in the last century was not notably successful in reducing the damage caused by drinking, and was eventually repealed).

Much discussion in the popular media and medical literature has focused
on what might be gained by legal prohibition of smoking in public places,
but relatively little discussion has focused on what might be lost by enacting
such laws. To put the arguments of both sides of this issue on the table for our

---

*Dresler C, Cherry M, Sade RM. Should smoking tobacco products in public places be legally
banned? *Ann Thorac Surg.* 2008;86:699–707. Copyright Society of Thoracic Surgeons, republished
here with permission.

inspection and thoughtful consideration, we present the case of a conflicted legislator who is also a thoracic surgeon.

THE CASE OF THE AMBIVALENT SURGEON

Dr. Thomas Brady, a thoracic surgeon, has never had strong political inclinations, but he is very concerned that politicians seem to have little appreciation of the complexities of the contemporary health care system. In a moment of what he would have considered lunacy when he was younger, he decided to run for public office. He took his campaign seriously and worked hard, but realistically, he had little hope of winning. To his considerable surprise, however, he awoke on the first Wednesday of November to find himself elected to membership in his state's House of Representatives. [...]

Ever since his earliest days of training as a surgeon, he has known of the many dangers of cigarette smoking. The cancers of the lungs, head and neck, and bladder caused by smoking disturb him, as do the effects of smoking on lung function and blood flow, especially to the heart and brain. Secondhand smoke, he is convinced, damages people who don't smoke at all, especially those who live with or are otherwise in close proximity to someone who smokes. [...]

A bill is filed in the House and it is assigned to the Medical Affairs Committee on which Dr. Brady serves. At the committee's hearing on the bill, they listen to several proponents testify on the need for a law to protect the health of the public. Smokers may damage themselves, if they so choose, but they have no right to damage others by exposing them to ambient tobacco smoke. A much smaller number of opponents argue that it is legislative overreaching and paternalism to use the force of law to protect people from damage they can easily avoid on their own. Decisions by private business owners, they say, will allow people to make their own judgments about protecting their health, and the free choices of proprietors and customers, taken in aggregate, will arrive at the correct balance between the pleasures of smoking and its dangers to smokers and those around them.

Dr. Brady understands the arguments of both sides and is uncertain whether he should vote for the bill, sending it to the House for final action, or vote against it, effectively killing it within the committee. He asks two of his friends, a thoracic surgeon and a philosopher, to help him think through the issues.

Pro
Carolyn Dresler, MD, MPA

Dr. Brady is puzzled on how to proceed with his vote and is wondering where to seek advice to help him make his decision. Some basic topics should first be reviewed that are relevant, and this will provide some background for solving Dr. Brady's dilemma.

First of all, a review of the science should be made so that it is clearly understood. The recent 2006 United States' Surgeon General report states that the health consequences of involuntary exposure to tobacco smoke result in four key conclusions:[1]

1. Secondhand smoke causes premature death and disease in children and in adults who do not smoke.
2. Children exposed to secondhand smoke are at an increased risk for sudden infant death syndrome, acute respiratory infections, ear problems, and more severe asthma. Smoking by parents causes respiratory symptoms and slows lung growth in their children.
3. Exposure of adults to secondhand smoke has immediate adverse effects on the cardiovascular system and causes coronary heart disease and lung cancer.
4. The scientific evidence indicates that there is no risk-free level of exposure to secondhand smoke.

Secondhand smoke, or involuntary exposure to tobacco smoke—this terminology is used to emphasize that it is an undesired or involuntary exposure to tobacco smoke—is unsafe at any level for everyone. This is explicitly clear with solid, scientific evidence. Solid science has also demonstrated several factors: that secondhand smoke bans do increase smoking cessation efforts among smokers, the bans do create more "smoke-free homes," as people are educated about the dangers to loved ones from secondhand smoke, and the bans do not drive businesses to close with loss of profits, as this has been proven to be true around the world nationwide down to cities, from Ireland to El Paso, Texas. Studies have demonstrated that people who do not smoke, but work in smoking environments have higher levels of tobacco metabolites than nonsmokers who work in nonsmoking environments, thus clearly demonstrating the exposure and consequent potential health effects from working in a smoky environment.[2] Therefore, the science is clear. However, oddly, science is probably not the issue in this discussion.

As an elected official, it is Dr. Brady's responsibility to review or create laws and regulations (or both) that provide for an orderly, yet functional society. The United States often adds a caveat to this mandate that we do not interfere too much and that we value our individual independence! [...]

What are we owed by our society and what do we owe it? "What" or "who" is our "society" anyway? One could say that our "society" is the group of people with whom we interact. They are the school teachers who teach our children, the people in the grocery store that supply our food, our bankers, the people who staff our hospitals, and our families. Because we are a complex society, our society also includes the people who grow our food, those who ship our food, those who make or sell our clothes, our bus drivers, or for some of us, our housekeepers or our babysitters. [...]

What do those people, that is, all of those "other people" owe us. What is meant by "owe" in this case? One could say that they don't owe anyone else anything. Actually, they do. They owe others the respect of their person and of their ability to exist and prosper within our society. As an obvious example: they are not allowed to kill another person. We, as a society, have decided that killing one another is not allowed. Another example, our society owes individual adults the right to vote, that is, an adult individual has the ability to decide on what the rules and regulations are to be by which we all live. Each person is a part of the society that has decided that one can not be killed by another member of the society. Each person helps decide the penalty for breaking these rules, because each person can vote. To follow this example, as a member of United States society, each adult has the right to due process of law, that one's being or belongings will not be illegally searched or seized. These are all legally protected "rights" and it is the duty of the governing bodies, whom adults of the society have elected or [who have] been appointed, to provide each of us with these legally protected "rights."

So far, the discussion has reviewed what the society owes each of us, but what does each person owe their society? Depending on how one looks at this question, it is an easier one to answer. Each person owes society their ability and willingness to follow the rules that govern us all equally. We will treat fellow members of our society with all the respect that we claim for ourselves.

All of this to this point is very basic, we know all of this already, but how can this help Dr. Brady make his decision? Actually, a few key words and concepts have been sprinkled into this dialogue; what are they and how can they help us find the answer for Dr. Brady?

First, what are legally protected rights and human rights? They are different, very different, yet one often derives from the other. Human rights are the highest order of "rights" and they supersede any "legally protected" rights. Remember, legally protected rights, such as one person cannot be killed by their neighbor, result from laws passed by our elected representatives. Human rights have a very well-delineated description; in legal terminology, these describe what our behavior should be to others in our society, and in addition, what our group or society has a duty to provide to us individually. One of those rights is the right to life, and this human right, in the example of murder, has been codified as a legally protected ability to claim one's life. Conversely, our society has the duty to provide each of us, as individuals in our society, these human rights, and thus, the enforcement of the laws that punish the murderer.

For the purposes of this brief discussion, the legal documents that were created after World War II and the Nuremberg trials will be acknowledged as the impetus in the development of modern human rights discourse.

However, three main documents resulted: (1) the United Nations' Charter, (2) the International Convention on Civil and Political Rights, and (3) the International Convention on Economic, Social, and Cultural Rights.[3] These three documents have formed the core of international human rights declarations. The vast majority of countries have chosen to codify these human rights into national law that make them into legally protected rights.

The International Covenant on Economic, Social, and Cultural Rights discusses human rights, such as the right to work, the right to choose who to marry, the right to health, and with this, the right to a healthy environment. Both the Convention on Civil and Political Rights and the Convention on Economic, Cultural, and Social Rights delineate human rights, that is, rights that accrue to us as individuals that we have the responsibility to claim, and our society has the duty to provide. We, as individuals in our society have a right to health and the right to a healthy environment. We have the right to claim for ourselves this healthy environment, which is called having the agency to claim our duly owed human right, and our society has the duty to provide that healthy environment.

Some have argued that certain public health measures are examples of a coercive political authority. However, there are public health measures that are allowable even though they could be construed as coercive. Such interventions that serve to benefit the greater whole are allowed to restrict certain "freedoms" of the individual. Such public health interventions are allowable if they are based on three constructs:

1. the magnitude of the problem: greater than 50% of all children in the United States are still exposed to secondhand smoke and 1 in 4 American children between 3 to 19 years of age live in a household with a smoker;
2. logical construct: secondhand smoke causes significant morbidity and mortality with a strong and solid scientific base;
3. legal construct: the right to health; the right to a healthy environment is part of our human rights that needs to be codified into our society's laws.

With such constraints, it is not likely that public health interventions will become insidious.

We have, as individual members of our society, the right, the human right, to a healthy environment. We have this human right because we are a member of our society, our group of people. Our elected representatives have the duty to provide that healthy environment. [...]

As a society, we owe its members the right to a healthy environment, and as individuals we must have the agency to claim this right. Dr. Brady, as our representative, must vote to provide a healthy environment to his society, his constituents, to the best of his ability, because it is the duty of the government to provide such human rights. When such a law is passed that provides a healthy environment, then we have incorporated what is considered a human right into a legally protected right. Human rights trump legally protected rights; they are from a higher order. Our government should move to incorporate our human right to a healthy environment by legally protecting us with a comprehensive smoke-free law.

Con
Mark J. Cherry, PhD

Public health has become the very willing agent of coercive political authority. The power vested in the public health community has become increasingly significant. Its judgment is sought on nearly all aspects of life, from appropriate births and deaths, diets and sexual behaviors, to methods of child rearing and permissible lifestyle choices. Public health expertise serves as the basis of expert testimony in courts of law and [...] it is widely sought in the framing of governmental policy. Because the concern for "health" has become a pervasive aspect of modern culture, Dr. Brady's unease with the proposed smoking ban reflects the circumstance that such agency has the potential to be particularly insidious.

Witness the growing popularity of banning smoking from all so-called "public" venues, including privately owned facilities, such as businesses, bars, and restaurants. Such bans have become popular among state and local governments, with the hope of anti-smoking advocates that "100% of Americans will live in smoke-free jurisdictions within a few years";[4] smoking bans of various forms exist in California, Hong Kong, Singapore, France, Ireland, and elsewhere worldwide. [...]

In contrast to such well-intentioned assertions, this article argues that legislative smoking bans can not be justified either in terms of private good or public good. To justify a smoking ban in terms of private good, the state must overturn longstanding legal and moral considerations that highlight individual autonomy and individual authority of persons over themselves. The weight of this moral and jurisprudential tradition establishes persons as in authority over themselves and as the presumed authoritative judge of their own interests. To justify a smoking ban in terms of the "public good," the state would need to demonstrate that accidental exposure to secondhand smoke in public places significantly increases actual personal risk above the level of background health risks that routinely exist in public. Otherwise, smoking bans simply enact a facile, hyperbolic, and discriminatory solution to what is a very complex moral and scientific issue.

PRIVATE GOODS

Environmental tobacco smoke, that is, secondhand smoke, in bars, restaurants, and other indoor venues is typically characterized as "involuntary" exposure. Note the recent United States Surgeon General's report on "The Health Consequences of Involuntary Exposure to Tobacco Smoke."[1] The rhetorical force of this depiction is that nonsmoking patrons and employees are forced into breathing secondhand tobacco smoke, a purported harm, which somehow violates their rights. At least with regard to businesses, bars, restaurants, and other private venues that the public freely choose to patronize, this characterization is inaccurate. Although such establishments are the usual target of legislative public smoking bans, these are not genuinely public places; rather, they are privately owned and operated businesses that the public freely chooses to frequent.

Consider bars and restaurants that permit smoking. Patrons who choose to enter thereby volunteer to breathe the internal air, including ambient viral and bacterial loads (e.g., influenza spread by the sneezing individual next to you), bad breath, body odor, smelly food, flower pollens, nauseating perfumes and scented candles, and present levels of tobacco smoke. Those who do not wish to inhale the establishment's internal air may leave; each is free to seek establishments with a personally acceptable (by whatever criteria) internal atmosphere. Whereas employers are typically at liberty to craft no-smoking policies, employees who chose to work in smoking establishments have consented to such risks; each person is free to seek a profession with types and levels of risk that one finds acceptable. [...]

In general, one may permissibly engage in more or less risky activities, such as joining the military or the police, working on oil rigs, climbing mountains, donating a kidney or liver segment while alive,[5] parachuting out of airplanes, undergoing elective plastic surgery, engaging in promiscuous sex, piercing body parts, having oneself tattooed, and so forth, setting life and health at risk for national patriotism, career advancement, monetary profit, recreational or altruistic interests, personal pleasure, or to enhance one's attractiveness to potential sexual partners. [...] Persons may thus grant permission to be touched or used in ways that (absent their permission) could profoundly harm them (e.g., kidney donation vs assault, or free love vs rape). [...] Such moral and legal considerations constitute, for example, one of the central justifications of the practice of informed consent in medicine.[6] [...]

Advocates of smoking bans often rationalize that "... the general public accepts smoke-free bars and restaurants and that such smoke-free laws will not cause their targets to lose money."[7] Conclusive empirical data is needed to document such contentious claims, as many businesses continue to maintain that anti-smoking laws drive away customers and reduce profits. [...]

Furthermore, not all important interests are health-directed or profit-minded. Consider a good old-fashioned, Texas bar owner, Billy Bob, a Bible-belt Christian, who combines his interests in profits with other personal interests, such as sermonizing, hunting, drinking, and smoking. In addition to bourbon and single-malt whisky, patrons are offered the opportunity to listen to the occasional sermon, admire the preserved animal heads lining the walls, and purchase cigars and cigarettes for the pleasurable activity of smoking with friends and colleagues. The sign outside his door reads: "Smoke if you wish, but blasphemers and animal rights activists will be shown to the door." Billy Bob realizes that his facility stands out as different from the more "up-scale" bars, like the La Grenouille Qui Danse, a nonsmoking wine-tasting bar up the street. [...] No one is forced to enter his establishment, and no one is hindered from leaving. He offers a choice of lifestyle, social risks, and freedom of association with others of similar tastes and interests. It is his venture capital or his private property at stake; his business is open to success or failure based on the free choices of others. [...]

PUBLIC GOODS

"The comprehensive body of research documenting the serious adverse health effects of passive smoking provides a powerful rationale for prohibiting smoking in all public places. The time has come to clean the air."[7] So concludes yet another advocate of smoking bans, but let us honestly consider the case of public risks and the element of accidental exposure to environmental tobacco smoke in the overall level of social risk.

Consider just a few sources of indoor air pollution in public places. According to the American Lung Association, radon, which is a tasteless, colorless, odorless gas, naturally occurring in the environment as a product of decaying uranium that becomes trapped in well-insulated buildings, is the likely cause of approximately 21,000 annual lung cancer deaths.[8] [...]

Consider some sources of public outdoor air pollution. Ozone, the central component of most ground-level smog, is formed when hydrocarbons and oxides of nitrogen react with volatile organic compounds in sunlight. Ozone is considered a powerful oxidizing agent that can damage lung tissue.[9] Sources of hydrocarbons and nitrogen oxides include automobile emissions, electric utilities, refineries, waste storage, recycling, and chemical solvents. [...]

Consider other risks to life and health in the public space. According to the National Highway Traffic Safety Administration, there were some 42,636 automobile traffic fatalities and 2,788,000 injuries in the United States in 2004.[10] Approximately 76 million individuals contract food-borne illnesses, leading to some 325,000 hospitalizations and more than 5,000 deaths each year in the United States, with salmonella, listeria, and toxoplasma each responsible for more than 1,500 deaths each year.[11] [...]

The actual health risk of accidental exposure to environmental tobacco must be appreciated in light of the overall level of background public risks. Given this lengthy, but incomplete, list of health risks to which individuals are exposed daily, it is arbitrary to hold smoking to a significantly higher standard than we hold other types of pollution or hazards to the "public health." [...]

Governments lack legitimate authority to restrict individual freedom to smoke in public places unless the risk to others is greater than the normal background risks that persons assume simply by going about their daily lives. Persons consent to many background risks as they venture into the public space, but not to all risks. For example, highway drivers consent to the usual risks of driving (e.g., the slipperiness of a wet road, possible automobile failure, and so forth), but not to all risks (e.g., the risk that others are driving under the influence of heroin).

Similarly, persons consent to many health risks, but not usually to the risk of picking up a highly contagious and crippling or deadly disease, which can be passed on to others through casual public contact. [...]

Such an argument likely justifies compulsory vaccination for diseases, such as polio and smallpox, which are dangerous and highly contagious through casual contact. It might even justify quarantine for persons with highly infectious and dangerous diseases. The risks associated with such diseases are significantly greater than the background risks that one generally assumes in daily life. [...]

To bring these reflections to bear on smoking bans: it is fairly straightforward to step out of the way of most environmental tobacco smoke (e.g., ceasing to patronize a smoking permitted bar) and to avoid most truly involuntary environmental tobacco smoke (e.g., moving to a different bench at a public park). Perhaps with sufficient data regarding environmental hazards, pollution levels, and other background public risk factors, such reflections might support a sliding scale for the standard of proof necessary to justify a smoking ban in truly public locations, considering both risk level and ease of avoidance. In areas with very little pollution, involuntary exposure to environmental tobacco smoke in public places might significantly increase individual health risks above local background risk levels. However, in many other locales such truly involuntary exposure will likely constitute only a very small element of one's daily overall level of health risk. [...]

To return to the point-counterpoint discussion, Dr. Brady's decision against legislative smoking bans ought to be made in recognition of the limits of moral political authority—much to the frustration of many public health advocates. Morally permissible legislation does not extend to the coercive imposition of paternalistic regulations on free citizens, as if they were mere children. Smoking bans that target restaurants, bars and other private establishments, seek to overturn a longstanding moral and jurisprudential tradition that highlights the authority of persons over themselves to make their own judgments regarding acceptable costs and benefits, risks and pleasures. Smokers enjoy the taste and smell of fine tobacco, and smoking provides stress relief and other benefits; those who frequent smoking establishments evidently prefer these opportunities, pleasures, and other benefits to different opportunities with fewer tobacco-associated risks. [...] In addition, Dr. Brady ought to appreciate that smoking bans in truly public places simply pick out one small element of overall health risk for social approbation, civil liability, and political criminalization, and therefore constitute biased and unjust discrimination. It may be easier, less expensive, and more politically expedient coercively to ban smoking rather than to encourage the reduction of other much more substantial sources of public pollution, or to persuade individuals to engage in less risky behavior, but such factors do not change the strongly paternalistic and discriminatory character of legislative smoking bans.

Concluding Remarks
Robert M. Sade, MD

Our fictional legislator, Dr. Brady, has received the advice he sought. He suspected that his cardiothoracic surgeon friend would advise in favor of the bill banning smoking in public places and that his philosopher friend would advise him to reject the bill. He was correct on both counts. [...]

Each essayist fails to address key points made by the other. Dr. Dresler does not consider the distinction between public places that are privately owned and those that are held in common. She does not explain why international declarations are superior to the national law cited by Dr. Cherry. She does not justify the requirement for laws focused on mitigating the harms caused by secondhand smoke when there are so many other agents that may, singly or in aggregate, cause even greater harm. Dr. Cherry speaks only of state and federal law and does not mention international conventions and declarations, which assert that health and a healthy environment are basic human rights that take precedence over national laws. He does not explain why national law should override international conventions.

Comments made by thoracic surgeons at our meetings and in other public forums nearly uniformly support legal prohibition of smoking in public places. This attitude is easy to understand, because we all have seen firsthand the devastation inflicted by the diseases caused by smoking. [...] When considering the arguments advanced by Drs Dresler and Cherry, we should put aside the biases that arise from our personal experiences. We should instead dispassionately consider not only what we as individuals and as a society have to gain but also what we have to lose by passing laws that go beyond the hortatory messages we have been giving to our patients and to the public for decades. [...]

References

1. United States Department of Health and Human Services. *The Health Consequences of Involuntary Exposure to Tobacco Smoke: A Report of the Surgeon General— Executive Summary*. Atlanta: Centers for Disease Control and Prevention, Coordinating Center for Health Promotion, National Center for Chronic Disease Prevention and Health Promotion, Office on Smoking and Health; 2006.
2. Stark MJ, Rohde K, Maher JE, et al. The impact of clean indoor air exemptions and preemption policies on the prevalence of a tobacco-specific lung carcinogen among non-smoking bar and restaurant workers. *Am J Public Health*. 2007;97:1457–63.
3. International human rights laws. Geneva: Office of the High Commissioner for Human Rights, United Nations. http://www.ohchr.org/english/law/index.htm. Accessed November 2007.
4. Griffith M. Smoking bans cover half of all Americans. *Seattle Times*. January 21, 2007.
5. Cherry MJ. *Kidney For Sale by Owner: Human Organs, Transplantation, and the Market*. Washington, DC: Georgetown University Press; 2005.
6. Engelhardt HT, Cherry MJ. Informed consent in Texas: theory and practice. *J Med Philos*. 2004;29:237–52.
7. Eisner MD. Banning smoking in public places: time to clear the air. *JAMA*. 2006;296:1778–9.
8. American Lung Association. Radon fact sheet. Chicago: American Lung Association. www.lungusa.org. Accessed January 31, 2007.
9. American Lung Association. Annotated bibliography of recent studies of the health effects of ozone air pollution 1997–2001. Chicago: American Lung Association. www.lungusa.org. Accessed January 31, 2007.
10. National Highway Traffic Safety Administration. Traffic safety facts 2004. Washington, DC: National Highway Traffic Safety Administration, 2005. www.nhtsa.dot.gov. Accessed January 31, 2007.
11. Mead PS, Slutsker L, Dietz V, et al. Food-related illness and death in the United States. *Emerg Infect Dis*. 1999;5:607–25.

28

Should a Medical Center Deny Employment to a Physician Because He Smokes Tobacco Products?

James W. Jones, William M. Novick,
and Robert M. Sade*

Introduction
Robert M. Sade, MD

A growing number of health care institutions are adopting a policy of denying employment to smokers, based on urine testing for the presence of nicotine and nicotine metabolites.[1] [...]

These policies are controversial. Arguments favoring them include a social obligation of medical centers to promote healthy activities, an obligation to provide a healthy environment for employees, and not supporting a habit that is addictive and lethal. Moreover, smokers add considerable cost to the institution's bottom line, because of their higher health care expenses and costs in lost productivity.

Arguments against denial of employment to tobacco users include the hypocrisy of banning smokers, while continuing to hire those who are obese, have a record of reckless driving, and use alcohol. Also, such policies are paternalistic: it's none of the hospital's business what its employees do when they are not at work.

Thoracic surgeons as a group strongly oppose tobacco use, but a hiring ban changes the game: should surgeons oppose or support a hiring ban of smokers? [...]

---

*Jones JW, Novick W, Sade RM. Should a medical center deny employment to a physician because he smokes tobacco products? *Ann Thorac Surg.* 2014;98(3). Copyright Society of Thoracic Surgeons, republished here with permission.

THE CASE OF THE PERPLEXED PRESIDENT

Dr. Nicholas Ateene is the president of University Physicians, the group practice that comprises all physicians who work in the University Hospital. The hospital's Executive Director has asked him to review a policy the hospital will implement in a few months. The hospital campus has been smoke-free for several years, and under the new policy, the hospital will not hire any job applicants who currently smoke tobacco products. The executive director is requesting that University Physicians adopt a similar policy for physician applicants. Dr. Ateene asks two of his colleagues, Dr. James Jones and Dr. William Novick, for their advice about how he should respond to this request.

Pro
James W. Jones, MD, PhD. MHA

I was surprised when I heard this topic was going to be debated because the ethical answer is so obviously clear. Next, I was saddened by such a deficiency of professional self-regulation that institutional regulation again was necessary. The ethics of the topic will be discussed on an ethical basis, a societal basis, an institutional basis, and on a professional basis.

Everyone knows smoking is harmful but to be a difference something needs to make a statistically significant difference. Smoking clearly qualifies as an major threat to health. According to the Centers for Disease Prevention (CDC) data, the top four causes of death in America (about one and a half million deaths combined)—heart disease, malignancy, chronic respiratory disease, cerebrovascular disease—are smoking related.[2] Lung cancer—one of the least desirable cancers, smoking's signature sickness—is increased twenty fold in smokers.

Further CDC calculates 443,000 deaths in 2010 resulted from smoking related diseases. These are from protracted conditions requiring continuing sometimes debilitating therapies. Consider for a moment, the total amount of suffering of those dying and in those recovering from the scourges of smoking associated diseases.

The question is: Can smoking be considered a moral failure? Smoking violates the virtue of prudence which is the ability to personally self-govern and professionally to wisely advise others. Engelhardt defines prudence succinctly as: soundness of judgment to achieve a positive balance of benefits over harms.[3] This definition clearly echoes and emphasizes the most important concept in surgical therapeutic decision making—"the risk/benefit ratio." Is a proposed benefit of an action worth the risk it entails? If not, the action violates prudence and is reckless at best and most likely foolish.

The benefits are meager indeed when compared to the risks. Nicotine is an acetylcholine receptor agonist which briefly enhances mood. It promotes alertness, calmness, and relaxation as it opens the door for the reaper. Smoking violates the virtue of prudence.

Rights include rights of three principals: the patient, the surgeon, and the institution. The patient has the right to be treated by a knowledgeable competent surgeon and to have his or her health valued more than the surgeon's interests.[4]

The surgeon has the right to be rewarded financially for clinical work and has all other non-professional rights and duties of the public. Professional rights have strict limitations because of the assumption of a fiduciary role. Physician behavioral freedoms end where fiduciary obligations begin.

Medical institutions operate more in accordance with duties than rights. Its rights are those of a business. Aside from meeting substantial regulatory compliance, a medical institution has the right to maintain its health-promoting image to secure the trust of patients. All institutions, medical and non-medical, have the right to "employer branding" their products and services. Since tobacco smoking is causal for the majority of diseases treated by the Cleveland Clinic and smokers carry a recognizable odor of their habit, why should they permit smokers to be caregivers?

Dr. Paul Terpeluk, director of Occupational Medicine at the Cleveland Clinic updated me about their employee non-smoking policy. The policy was initiated in 2007 [...] and the policy is regarded as very successful for several reasons. Three thousand surgeons and forty thousand employees work there and none can smoke. The health-promoting image of the Clinic is not weakened which is vital to an important heath care institution. And the rate of smoking in the county where the clinic is located has declined double the average elsewhere. The basis legitimizing their right to institute the policy was the desire to have healthier employees for the business of medical care.

Physicians are overwhelmingly chosen as the source of information and encouragement for patients adopting healthier lifestyles.[5] This ethical obligation is at risk when physicians have adopted the unhealthy lifestyles they should be recommending that patients stop. The compromise occurs because our beliefs often adjust to defend our behavior.

The STOP study (Smoking: The Opinions of Physicians) examined the interactions of several thousand physicians with patients about smoking.[6] Physician smokers considered beneficial stress relief from smoking was a major barrier to cessation and were less likely to counsel against smoking. And, amazingly, one-third of physician smokers did not believe that smoking was a health hazard.

The harm principle has broad legal standing for limiting behavioral autonomy to prevent one from harming others. First articulated by John Stuart Mill: "... the sole end for which mankind are warranted, individually or collectively, in interfering with the liberty of action, of any of their number, is self-protection."[7] Equally, one's right to liberty ends when it imposes on another's rights—especially when the imposition induces observable harm. As data showing harm to others accumulated from public smoking, it was banned.

American Medical Association in publication H-490-917 entitled, "Physician Responsibilities for Tobacco Cessation" supports and advocates measures by physicians to: ... quit smoking and to urge colleagues to quit; inquiring of all patients at each visit about their smoking habits; and at every visit, counseling those who smoke to quit using tobacco in any form. It supports the concept that hospitals, among others, be primary sites for educating the public about the harmful effects of tobacco.

According to the American Association of Thoracic Surgery's and the Society of Thoracic Surgeon's combined Code of Ethics, article 1.4: "Members should use their best efforts to protect patients from harm by recommending and providing care that maximizes anticipated benefits and minimizes potential harms."[8]

Ethics are defined by logical examination of the societal mores in which we are immersed. Currently personal illness is a societal responsibility from medical insurance and obligations of medical institutions to provide care regardless of payment probability. Illness not physicians drives medical cost. Loss of heath drives illness and health is frequently behaviorally controlled.

In American society, cost of medical care is approaching a tipping point of no return. The Affordable [...] Care Act [ACA] is a financial tsunami which is fiscally unsound. The Office of the Actuary for the Centers for Medicare and Medicaid Services projects the 2014 National Medical Expenditures, after the [ACA] actualizes, are over $3.1 trillion. The government will pay half or $1.55 trillion. The 2012 total direct governmental revenue was 2.5 trillion.

Chronic disease is the deadly killer and there is no greater promoter of chronic disease than smoking. The answer to the ballooning cost of medical care is not to provide more medical treatments; it is to avoid needing expensive care; the only answer is prevention.

The arguments against refusing to hire smokers lack validity. "It is callous—and contradictory—for health care institutions devoted to caring for patients regardless of the causes of their illness to refuse to employ smokers."[9] That argument erroneously equates the relationship of the institution with patients and employees; the ethics are very different: one is a fiduciary relationship and the other is an employer/employee relationship.

The claim that the policy of excluding smokers is discriminatory because more smokers are poor and minorities is not a legitimate claim because the demographics of health care employees differs from the general population; nurses commonly are smokers. Correlation is not always confirmation. Being qualified for employment at the Cleveland Clinic requires the same for all groups: They must give up smoking. Societies are improved by increasing top down standards and diminished by reducing bottom up standards.

Make no mistake: we are our profession's keepers. There is no higher calling than our fiduciary role in providing exemplary medical care to our fellow human beings. Emotional, religious, legal, financial, and occupational problems take a backseat when the health of us or our loved ones is seriously threatened. To default, even minimally, from that calling is at best a moral error and we should thank [...] the Cleveland Clinic.

Con
William M. Novick, MD

Is it ethical for a hospital to deny employment to a physician who smokes tobacco products? This is the essence of the current debate. We are not discussing the negative impact smoking has on the individual. The position of those in favor of such a ban regarding employment is based upon a number of assertions:

1. Tobacco usage contributes to 20% of all annual deaths in the United States
2. Physicians should be role models for our patients, and therefor practice a healthy life-style, which includes no use of tobacco products
3. Hospitals should practice what they preach, i.e., healthy life-styles in their employee's
4. Health care systems and practitioners should strive to decrease health care expenditures, i.e., decreasing use of tobacco products would decrease costs
5. companies in the US can set the standards for employment in their institution.

[...]

OTHER UNHEALTHY LIFE-STYLES THAT CONTRIBUTE TO THE ANNUAL DEATHS IN THE US

Obesity contributes to 15% of all annual deaths in the US and 35.7% of all adults in the US were considered obese in 2010 [10,11,12,13]. Smoking of tobacco products is estimated to occur in approximately 19% of the adult population in the US, just over half the number of obese individuals. The estimated contribution to the annual death rate in the US for alcohol consumption is 80,000 [...].[14] Fatalities from traffic accidents were estimated to cause 35,000 deaths in 2012 and the protective effects of seat-belts, driving at the speed limit and not having consumed significant amounts of alcohol, are all well known to decrease fatalities in traffic accidents.[15] [...]

The debate over whether or not obesity actually contributes 400,000 deaths annually is another political maneuver specifically designed to keep tobacco smoking at the top of the list of causative agents and to preserve funding.[16] [...]

DOCTORS SHOULD SERVE AS ROLE MODELS FOR THEIR PATIENTS BY PRACTICING HEALTHY LIFE-STYLES

While this is certainly a laudable goal, doctors are just as human as the next person. Smoking among physicians has decreased from 18.8% to just over 3% between the 70's and 1991.[17] [...] It would appear that the decrease in the percentage of physicians who smoke has leveled out over the last 20 years. However, when one examines other unhealthy life-styles among physicians, we find that 42% are overweight or obese, 35% exercise less than 30 minutes once per week (if at all) and alcohol intake up to 2 drinks per day is common (men 18.9%, women 11.3%). Where do we stop with this idea of physicians being role models for healthy life-styles? [...]

Hospitals Should Practice What They Preach, Healthy Life-Styles[...] hospitals in the US are institutions where the treatment of disease occurs. To suggest that they have somehow undergone a metamorphosis into preventative treatment centers alone is disingenuous at best.[18] Cleveland Clinic advertises on its web-page that it has a Wellness Institute, yet within the different options are those offering treatment plans for smoking cessation.[19] By offering of such a program, the clinic promulgates the hypocrisy of not allowing new employees to smoke. Why is it that they offer to help others stop smoking and yet are so callous to not help potential employees? [...]

A COMPANY IN THE UNITED STATES HAS THE RIGHT TO SET STANDARDS FOR HIRING PEOPLE

Although companies do have the right to set standards for individuals they hire, they must do so within the legal limits of state and federal laws in the United States. Currently, there are 29 states which have enacted laws protecting smokers from what state legislators viewed as a form of workplace discrimination.[20] [...]

Discrimination in the workplace is not a new concept in the US. The Equal Employment Opportunity Act was signed into law by President R.M. Nixon in 1972. At the signing ceremony, Nixon stated, "One of the basic principles in our way of life in America has always been that individuals would be free to pursue the work of their own choice, and to advance in that work subject only to consideration of their individual qualifications, talents and energies."[21] Where in this statement or in this law does it allow for discrimination against individuals who smoke in the privacy of their own homes, cigar lounges or golf games? What exactly is the point of this highly discriminating action by a few hospitals? Physician smoking is at an all-time low, yet by self-admission, over 40% of physicians are overweight or obese. What is more evident to casual observers: a doctor who smokes, but they never see smoking or an obese physician that is clearly seen by all? The economics of a few smokers (2% or less) regarding health care expenditures compared to the economics of overweight physicians clearly is not the issue. The issue is one of marketing. Those hospitals that can claim a 100% smoker free staff stand to gain in the eyes of the public [. . .].

ETHICAL? IS IT LEGAL?

The United States was founded upon the principles of individual rights and, over the years since our founding, we have consistently reviewed our society and added laws to protect those who are discriminated against, regardless of the issue. The three pieces of paper that make the foundation of our government; the Declaration of Independence, the Constitution and the Bill of Rights, all uphold our rights to independent choice and decision without the fear of discrimination. The requirement for blood and urine tests for legal products used in the privacy of our own homes, which do not impact one's ability to practice their specialty, is very close to violating the Fourth Amendment as an illegal search and seizure.[22] Currently, 29 states have enacted laws specifically preventing discrimination on the basis of an individual being a smoker. It is important that the other 21 follow suit before this act of discrimination gains any more ground. The overt paternalism in this edict is not that different from the "nanny-state" of New York City where Mayor Bloomberg recently pushed a plan to prevent the purchase of "big sized" soda beverages[23]. [. . .] We are not a culture or society that responds well to having our choices made for us by the government, as exemplified by the 60% of New York City residents who opposed Bloomberg's proposal.[24] [. . .]

SUMMARY

Smoking among physicians is at an all-time low, indicating that we as health-care providers, for the most part, practice what we preach. The hypocrisy of preventing those remaining physicians who smoke from practicing at a particular health care institution that provides care for individuals who suffer the consequences of smoking is obvious. We should accept these colleagues who continue to smoke and provide them with the necessary support to quit. The hard, paternalistic position of some institutions seems in principle to violate the very ideals on which this country was founded and is actually against the law in the majority of states. Let us embrace our roles as physicians and help our colleagues who smoke rather than discriminate against them and ostracize them from our society.

Concluding Remarks
Robert M. Sade, MD

Both essayists were asked to advise the hypothetical Dr. Ateene on how he should respond to a request to adopt a policy of not hiring any physician applicant who smokes tobacco products. Jones is clear in advising him to adopt such a policy, while Novick is similarly clear in advising him not to do so. Each makes a strong case in support of his position.

In arguing their viewpoints, however, both also are blowing smoke at their audience in the form of irrelevant or misleading discussions. For example, Jones goes to some length in describing smoking as a moral failure of individuals, but the issue was not the morality of individuals' smoking; rather, it was the ethics of institutional policy making. Novick mistakenly equates coercive law with corporate policy making by comparing New York Mayor Bloomberg's plan to prohibit sales of large-size soft drinks by force of law with a health care institution's development of a hiring policy—public law and private policy have very different ethical implications.

Interestingly, both essayists claim that the no-smokers policy is aimed at the public image of the health care institution, but each sees its purpose in an entirely different light. Jones describes this aspect of the policy as the institution maintaining "its health-promoting image to secure the trust of patients," an altogether praiseworthy objective. Novick understands this facet of the policy completely differently, seeing it as merely another sales pitch aimed at the public, "which is constantly deluged by marketing and public relations firms to 'buy' their product." [...]

The number of companies, including many health-related companies, that have adopted a no-hiring-of-smokers policy is said to be over 6,000 and increasing.[25] The facts that 65% oppose policies that ban the hiring of smokers and 29 states have already passed laws prohibiting such policies[26] suggest that the contest between supporters and opponents of smoker hiring bans is likely to continue for the foreseeable future. It also seems likely that no clear winner will emerge any time soon.

References

1. Asch DA, Muller RW, Volpp KG. Conflicts and compromises in not hiring smokers. *N Engl J Med*. 2013;368:1371–3.
2. Ten leading causes of death and injury. Injury Prevention and Control: Data and Statistics. Atlanta: Centers for Disease Control and Prevention. http://www.cdc.gov/injury/wisqars/leadingcauses.html. Accessed December 3, 2013.
3. Englehardt H. *The Foundations of Bioethics*. New York: Oxford University Press; 1986.

4. Jones JW, Novick W, Sade RM. Should a medical center deny employment to a physician because he smokes tobacco products? *Ann Thorac Surg.* 2014;98(3):799–805.

5. Llewellyn DJ, Lang IA, Langa KM, et al. Exposure to secondhand smoke and cognitive impairment in non-smokers: national cross sectional study with cotinine measurement. *BMJ* 2009;338:b462.

6. Pipe A, Sorensen M, Reid R. Physician smoking status, attitudes toward smoking, and cessation advice to patients: an international survey. *Patient Educ Couns.* 2009;74:118–23.

7. Mill J. *On Liberty.* London: John W. Parker and Son; 1859:34.

8. Code of Ethics. Chicago: Society of Thoracic Surgeons; 2009. http://www.sts.org/about-sts/policies/code-ethics. Accessed December 3, 2013.

9. Schmidt H, Voigt K, Emanuel EJ. The ethics of not hiring smokers. *N Engl J Med.* 2013;368:1369–71.

10. Satcher D. Surgeon general's column. *Commissioned Corps Bull.* 2002; 16(2):1–2.

11. Johannes L, Stecklow S. Dire warnings about obesity rely on slippery statistic. *The Wall Street Journal.* February 9, 1998:B1.

12. Allison DB, Fontaine KR, Manson JE, et al. Annual deaths attributable to obesity in the United States. *JAMA.* 1999;282:1530–8.

13. Ogden CL, Carroll MD, Kit BK, Flegal KM. Prevalence of Obesity in the United States, 2009–2010. NCHS Data Brief, No. 82. Atlanta: National Center for Health Statistics; January 2012.

14. White IR, Altmann DR, Nanchahal K. Alcohol consumption and mortality: modeling risks for men and women at different ages. *BMJ.* 2002; 325:191–8.

15. US Census. Transportation: motor vehicle accidents and fatalities. http://www.census.gov/compendia/statab/cats/transportation/motor_vehicle_accidents_and_fatalities.html. Accessed December 3, 2013.

16. Kolata G. Data on deaths from obesity is inflated, U.S. agency says. *The New York Times.* November 24, 2004. http://www.nytimes.com/2004/11/24/health/24obese.html. Accessed December 3, 2013.

17. Nelson DE, Giovino GA, Emont SL, et al. Trends in cigarette smoking among US physicians and nurses. *JAMA.* 1994;271(16);1273–5.

18. Schmidt H, Voight K, Emanuel EJ. The ethics of not hiring smokers. *N Engl J Med.* 2013;15:1369–71.

19. Tobacco Treatment Center. http://my.clevelandclinic.org/tobacco/default.aspx. Accessed December 3, 2013.

20. Editorial: Not hiring smokers crosses privacy line. *USA Today.* January 29, 2012. http://usatoday30.usatoday.com/news/opinion/editorials/story/2012-01-29/not-hiring-smokers-privacy/52874348/1. Accessed December 3, 2013.

21. The American Presidency Project. Richard Nixon. Statement about signing the Equal Employment Opportunity Act of 1972. http://www.presidency.ucsb.edu/ws/?pid=3358. Accessed December 3, 2013.

22. US Bill of Rights, Fourth Amendment. http://www.archives.gov/exhibits/charters/bill_of_rights_transcript.html. Accessed December 3, 2013.

23. Grynbaum MM. New York soda ban to go before state's top court. *The New York Times.* October 18, 2010. http://www.nytimes.com/2013/10/18/nyregion/new-york-soda-ban-to-go-before-states-top-court.html?_r=0. Accessed December 3, 2013.

24. Grynbaum MM, Connelly M. 60% in city oppose Bloomberg's soda ban, poll finds. *The New York Times*. August 23, 2012. http://www.nytimes.com/2012/08/23/nyregion/most-new-yorkers-oppose-bloombergs-soda-ban.html. Accessed December 3, 2013.

25. Homans MD. Banning smokers may harm your company's health. *The Legal Intelligencer*. 2012;245(92). http://www.flastergreenberg.com/media/article/383_Michael%20Homans%20Byline%20Article_May%202012.pdf. Accessed December 3, 2013.

26. More workplaces don't allow employees to smoke at work, anywhere. WFMY News. January 6, 2012. http://www.digtriad.com/news/article/207243/8/Experimental%20Severe%20Weather%20Warnings%20To%20Motivate%20Response. Accessed December 3, 2013.

INDEX

AANS (American Association of Neurological Surgeons), 100
AATS (American Association for Thoracic Surgery), 27, 276, 287, 338
ABTS (American Board of Thoracic Surgery), 27, 29
Accola, Kevin, 61–5, 66, 67
accountability, 5, 144
Accreditation Council for Graduate Medical Education (ACGME)
  and eighty-hour work week, 69, 74, 80
  guidelines for presentations, 9
  policies regarding conflicts of interest, 262
ACGME (Accreditation Council for Graduate Medical Education), *see* Accreditation Council for Graduate Medical Education
ACRE (Association of Clinical Researchers and Educators), 289–90
ACS (American College of Surgeons), *see* American College of Surgeons
addiction, 168; *see also* substance abuse
addicts, 163–71
administrators, surgeons as, 3
advance directives, 104, 107, 116, 120, 122, 123, 124, 125, 126
adversity, ability to cope with, 165
advocacy, restricted *vs.* unrestricted, 153
age
  and adoption of technology, 197, 198, 200–1
  and cognitive function, 198
  and manual dexterity, 7
air pollution, 331
AKA (Anti-Kickback Act), 277–8
American Academy of Pain Medicine, 168
American Association for Thoracic Surgery (AATS), 27, 276, 287, 338
American Association of Neurological Surgeons (AANS), 100
American Board of Surgery, 198
American Board of Thoracic Surgery (ABTS), 27, 29
American College of Cardiology Foundation–The Society of Thoracic Surgeons Collaboration on the Comparative Effectiveness of Revascularization Strategies (ASCERT), 218

American College of Physicians Ethics Manual, 143, 149
American College of Surgeons (ACS), 74
  Code of Conduct, 60, 97
  mission statement, 199
  motto, 199
  standards of behavior for expert witnesses, 98
American Medical Association (AMA)
  Code of Medical Ethics (*see* Code of Medical Ethics (AMA))
  Council on Ethical and Judicial Affairs, 60, 270
  Jehovah's Witnesses's view of, 109
  on obligation to assist in administration of justice, 97
  Principles of Medical Ethics, 60
  standards of behavior for expert witnesses, 98
  on tobacco cessation, 338
American Pain Society, 168
American Society of Addiction Medicine, 168
American Society of Transplant Surgeons, 257
American Thoracic Society, 125–6
Angell, Marcia, 281
Annals of Thoracic Surgery, The (ATS), 26, 27, 28, 29, 291
Anti-Kickback Act (AKA), 277–8
aortic valve replacement (AVR) surgery
  in noncompliant patients, 163–72
  outcome-volume relationship in, 206
apology, 134
Araujo, Katia, 168–71
Aristotle, 37–8, 77, 96, 133
Armey, D., 96
ASCERT (American College of Cardiology Foundation–The Society of Thoracic Surgeons Collaboration on the Comparative Effectiveness of Revascularization Strategies), 218
Association of American Medical Colleges, 3
Association of Clinical Researchers and Educators (ACRE), 289–90
ATS (Annals of Thoracic Surgery, The), *see* *Annals of Thoracic Surgery*
attentional failures, 83–4

Auburn University, 226
authority
    argument from, 12
    of physicians, 24
autonomy, behavioral, 337–8
autonomy, patient
    balance with paternalism, 50
    of death row inmates, 256–7
    described, 243
    emphasis on, 19, 61
    and impending loss of insurance, 155
    implications of, 104
    and incentives for organ donation, 241, 244–5
    and informed consent, 84, 85
    new emphasis on, 38
    and refusal of blood transfusions, 107–16
    and refusal of treatment, 111
    respect for, 12, 156–7
    social context of, 245
    undermining of, 115
    understanding of, 115
aviation, 89–90
AVR (aortic valve replacement) surgery, *see*
    aortic valve replacement surgery

Bakken, Earl, 292
bankruptcy, 155
Bavaria, Joseph E., 204–7
Beauchamp, Tom, 12, 159, 243
Beecher, Henry, 184, 192
behavioral freedoms, 337
Belmont Report, 159
beneficence, 12, 156, 159
    concept of, 151
    described, 243
    and disclosure of HCV status, 49–50
    and impending loss of insurance, 155
    and market for organs, 245
    and providing treatment, 123
    and refusal of treatment, 111
    and refusal to testify, 97
    and treatment goals, 126
benefits, 42, 136, 137, 139
Bentham, J., 96
Bernstein, Ron, 168–71
best interests, patient's
    determining, 151
    and gifts from industry, 268
    guidance for, 3
    and industry gifts, 268
    and new technologies, 196
    and rationing, 221
    and regionalization, 321
    responsibility to, 261
    vs. social responsibility, 309
    and surgeon-industry relationships, 282

best interest standard, 127; *see also* best
    interests, patient's
Bigger, Thomas, 81
bioethics
    Beauchamp-Childress framework for, 12, 159,
        243–4
    diversity of viewpoints in, 11
    foundation of, 133
    and law, 176–7
    principles in, 243–4 (*see also* autonomy;
        beneficence; justice; nonmaleficence)
    see also ethical analysis; ethics
Birkmeyer, J. D., 313, 320
blame, 144
blood transfusions, 104–5, 107–16
Bok, Sissela, 38
Bolam principle, 66
Bolling, S. F., 209
Bosk, Charles, 5
brain death, 232, 234, 256
Brett, A. S., 155
Bridges, Charles R., 107, 112–15, 116
business, 282; *see also* industry

CABG (coronary artery bypass graft
    surgery), *see* coronary artery bypass graft
    surgery
capital punishment, moral justifications
    of, 253–4
Cardiothoracic Ethics Forum, *see* Ethics Forum
cardiothoracic surgery, and need for knowledge
    about ethical challenges, 28
Cardiovascular Patient Outcomes Research
    Team– Elective Angioplasty Study
    (CPORT-E), 208
Cardozo, Benjamin, 113
care
    appropriateness of, determining, 147–8,
        153–61
    futile care, 126
    informed care, 142–3
    quality of, 321–2
    refusal of, 19
career, 7, 197, 199
Carrel, Alexis, 75
Cassell, Eric, 153
CDC (Centers for Disease Control and
    Prevention), *see* Centers for Disease
    Control and Prevention
CEJA (Council on Ethical and Judicial
    Affairs), 60, 270
Centers for Disease Control and Prevention (CDC)
    on causes of death, 336
    and guidelines for surgeons with HCV, 47, 53
    recommendations for health care providers
        with HBV, 51

CER (cost-effective ratio), 221
Cerfolio, Robert James, 270–3, 274
Cherry, Mark J., 329–33
Childress, James, 12, 159, 243
Chisolm, Guy, 289
choice, process of, 73
Choudhry, N. K., 198
Chu, M. W., 87
Churchill, Winston, 75
cigarettes, *see* tobacco
Cleveland Clinic, 337, 338–9, 340
clinical studies, 8–10; *see also* randomized
    controlled trial; research
Code of Medical Ethics (AMA), 2
  description of informed consent in, 60
  and disclosure of other surgeons' errors,
    142–3, 149
  honesty in, 40
  marketing in, 202
  and patient self-determination, 38
  resource allocation in, 171–2
  on surrogate/proxy, 128
Code of Professional Conduct (American
    College of Surgeons), 60, 97
coercion
  influence on decision making, 115
  and organ donation, 253, 256–7
  in public health measures, 328, 329, 332
COIs (conflicts of interest), *see* conflicts of
    interest
compassion, 2, 3
competence, 2, 6–7, 195
competition
  and disclosure, 33
  and informed consent, 58–67
  and quality of care, 321–2
Concept of the Corporation, The (Drucker), 283
conduct, professional standards of, 97–8
conflict, surgeon-family, 118–28
conflicts of interest (COIs)
  articles on, 283–4
  corruption narrative of, 279
  difficulties in studying, 288, 293
  disclosure of, 263, 278–9
  evidence of effects of, 290–4
  gifts from industry, 265–74
  laws and regulations regarding, 262, 263
  misuse of term, 281
  policies regarding, 262
  recognizing, 261–2
  resolutions of, 262, 278–9
  secondary interests, 286–7
  see also surgeon-industry relationships
Congress, U. S., 276–7
Conklin, Lori D., 74–6, 78
consent, *see* informed consent

consequentialism, 12, 136–7, 138
consulting, *see* surgeon-industry relationships
continuing medical education events, 9
coronary artery bypass graft surgery (CABG)
  regionalization of, 299, 311–22
  volume-outcome effect in, 205–6, 312–14,
    316, 318
Coselli, Joseph S., 74–6, 77, 78
cost-effective ratio (CER), 221
Council on Ethical and Judicial Affairs
    (CEJA), 60, 270
courage, 135
CPORT-E (Cardiovascular Patient Outcomes
    Research Team– Elective Angioplasty
    Study), 208
Crawford, F. A., 319
Cruzan, Nancy Beth, 177
CSRS (New York Cardiac Surgery Reporting
    System), 313
customers, 282
Czeisler, Charles A., 81–6, 90

D'Amico, Thomas A., 120–3, 127, 128
Daniels, Norman, 153
DCD (donation after cardiac death)
    protocol, 232, 233, 252–3, 257–8
Dead Donor Rule (DDR), 228, 231–6, 253, 255
death
  accepted definitions of, 255–6
  brain death, 232, 234, 256
  causes of, 336, 339
  determination of, 228, 232–3, 234
  Uniform Determination of Death Act, 228,
    232–3, 256
  and withdrawal of LST, 235–6
DeBakey, Michael E., 74
debate format, 11, 17
deception
  benefits and harms of, 42–5
  in Code of Ethics, 38
  early views of, 38–9
  by insurance companies, 41
  of insurance companies, 32, 37–45
  and long-term harm, 43–5
  vs. lying, 38, 134
  of patients, 38–9
  as self-serving, 41–2
decision making, 2, 5–6, 305
  about end-of-life care, 120
  and authority of physicians, 24
  considering society's good in, 220
  freedom in, 115
  and lack of advance directive, 122
  motivations in, 182
  risk-benefit ratio in, 336–7
  social worth in, 171–2

decision making (*cont.*)
  and UHCDA, 108, 111, 116
  unconscious bias in, 279
  see also autonomy
decision-making, shared, 61, 159
decision-making, surgeon-patient, 52
decision-making, surrogate/proxy
  and advance directives, 104, 114, 115–16
  ATS statement on, 125–6
  authority of, 127–8
  and lack of advance directive, 122
  and overriding of advance directives, 111–12
  and rejection of treatment, 107
  standard for, 127
  in study on ethics gap, 20–4
  and surgeon-family conflict, 120
Declaration of Helsinki, 192
Denlinger, Chadrick E., 145–9
deontology, 12
destination therapy, 303; *see also* left ventricular
  assist device
detailing, 265–74
deterrence function of capital punishment, 254
Deveney, Karen E., 197–200, 201
devices, 7–8
  approval of, 190
  availability of, and disclosure, 58–67
  development of, 304
  efficacy of, 216
  efficiency of, 216–17
  research on, 8–10
  use of in history, 176
  see also technologies, surgical
Dewey, T. M., 209
Dickey, Jamie, 70–4, 77
dignity, and refusal of treatment, 111
DiMaio, J. Michael, 164–8
Dimick, J. B., 320
disability, and treatment withdrawal
  decisions, 22–3
discrimination, 340, 341
diseases, communicable
  guideline for physicians with, 50–1
  and vaccinations, 332
  see also hepatitis C virus
diseases, self-inflicted, 106; *see also* smoking;
  substance abuse
donation after cardiac death (DCD)
  protocol, 232, 233, 252–3, 257–8
Dorotheus of Gaza, 45
Dresler, Carolyn, 48–52, 55, 56, 325–9, 333
Drucker, Peter, 282, 283
drug companies
  advertising in journals, 269–70
  banning of representatives of, 274
  gifts from, 265–74

marketing by, 268
regulation of, 270
see also industry
drugs, 7, 8–10
drug samples, 269
drug use, 72, 163–72
duress, giving consent under, 110

Eagle, Kim A., 312–16
economic issues
  in refusal to operate on noncompliant
    patient, 167
  and treatment, 154–61
Edmunds, L. Henry, xvii
Edwards, Lowell, 280, 292
effectiveness, *vs.* efficacy, 216–17
egalitarian principle, 220, 244, 246
eighty-hour work week, 33, 69, 73–4, 87
Eisenhower, Dwight D., 75
end-of-life care, 118–28
Engelhardt, H., 336
equipoise, 8
errors
  and blame, 144
  disclosure of, 3, 105, 130–40, 141, 145
  disclosure of, manner of, 134, 150
  disclosure of, rates of, 144
  *To Err is Human: Building a Safer Health
    System,* 105, 130, 141
  nondisclosure of, 135–8
  other surgeons', disclosure of, 141–50
  and well-being of surgeon, 139, 144, 145
errors, other surgeons', 141–50
Estrera, Anthony L., 152–5, 160, 161
"ethical," concepts of, 96
ethical acceptability, 20, 21, 22
ethical analysis
  difficulties in using prescriptive
    analysis, 159
  models of, 1, 12, 20, 49–50, 133, 136, 138–9
ethical obligations, 75, 76
ethics
  foundations of, 96
  need to know about, 28
  and public decision making, 305, 306
  relation with law, 101
  research ethics, 8–10
  surgical ethics, 4–10, 15, 16
  in surgical literature, 20
  values in, 111
ethics committee, 124–5
ethics education, 16–17, 26–30
Ethics Forum, xvii, xx, 10, 26–30
ethics gap, xvii, 16, 20–5
evidence, types of, 293
evidence-based medicine, 62

excellence, and volume-outcome relationship debate, 210
execution, and organ donation, 252, 256, 257
expertise, transmission of, 208–9

FAA (Federal Aviation Administration), 89–90
False Claims Act, 277
FDA (Food and Drug Administration), 189–90, 216, 217
Federal Aviation Administration (FAA), 89–90
Ferraris, Victor A., 316–21
fidelity to patient's interests, *see* best interests, patient's
fiduciary duty, 337; *see also* best interests, patient's
Fitzgerald, Faith, 165
Fogarty, Tom, 280
Food and Drug Administration (FDA), 189–90, 216, 217
Frater, Robert, 166
fraud, 43
freedoms, behavioral, 337
free market, 244–5
Freidman, Richard, 81
futility, 126

Gallagher, T. H., 134, 144, 149, 150
Gaudiani, Vincent, 277, 280–3
Gawande, Atul, 199
Georgetown Mantra, 159
Gibbon, John, 280, 292
gifts, from industry, 262–3, 267–8, 270, 272; *see also* conflicts of interest
Gilbert, J. A., 81
"Giving Life After Death Row" (Longo), 250–1
Goethe, Johann von, 308
Gorney, Mark, 100
GRADE (Grading of Recommendations Assessment, Development and Evaluation) Working Group, 293
Grassley, Charles, 276–7
Green, Philip, 204, 207–9
Greenwood, James, 247
group learning, 208–9

Halm, E. A., 318
harms
    balancing with benefits, 42
    and behavioral autonomy, 337–8
    and disclosure of error, 136, 137, 139
Harvard Medical Practice Study, 147
HCV (hepatitis C virus), *see* hepatitis C virus
health
    definition of, 165, 306
    maximizing, 308
    responsibility for, 165

Health and Human Services, Department of, 270
health care
    access to, 316
    availability of, 316
    cost of, 74, 301, 303–4, 338
    distribution of, 157–8, 244 (*see also* regionalization)
    inequalities in, 220
    payors, 298, 302, 306
    priorities in, 307, 308, 309
    rationing of (*see* rationing)
    right to, 309
    sustainable limits of, 215
health care policy
    concerns of, 306–8
    and ethics, 297, 305, 306
    physicians in development of, 297–8
health care reform
    and miscoding, 44
    Patient Protection and Affordable Care Act, 222, 289
    and rationing, 220, 222
    and reporting of industry payments to physicians, 276–7, 289
health information, privacy of, 54–5, 85
health law, understanding of, 25; *see also* legal acceptability
Health Savings Accounts, 309
Helsinki, Declaration of, 192
hemodialysis, 176
hepatitis C virus (HCV), 32–3
    guidelines for health care workers with, 50–1, 53, 54
    incidence of, 55–6
    lack of guidelines for surgeons with, 47
    stigma of, 55
    transmission of, 52–3, 55
    treatment of, 53
heroic measures, 118–28
Himmelstein, D. U., 155
Hippen, Benjamin, 240–3, 247
Hippocrates, 123
Hippocratic Oath, 49, 60–1, 97, 165, 303; *see also* nonmaleficence
Holmes, Oliver Wendell, 244
honesty, 2, 3, 4
    and character, 43
    in Code of Medical Ethics, 40
    and deception of insurance companies, 37–45
    and disclosure of HCV status, 51–2, 56
    history of, 32
    in professional integrity, 32
house officers, *see* residents
human rights, 327–8
Hume, David, 43

IDE (Individual Device Exemption), 190
Ikonomidis, John S., 155–8, 160, 161, 210
Ikonomidis, Sharon, 155–8, 160, 161
illnesses, medical
    cost of, 338
    and regionalization, 319
    see also disease
Immelt, Stephen J., 277–9
impairment, performance, 82–3
Individual Device Exemption (IDE), 190
industry
    benefits of medicine's relationship with, 270–1
    calls to remove from medicine, 272
    gifts from, 262–3, 267–8, 270, 272
    and innovation, 64–5
    see also drug companies; surgeon-industry
        relationships
infection
    by bloodborne pathogen, 47 (*see also*
        hepatitis C virus)
    of health care workers, 166
informed consent
    basic conditions of, 104
    for clinical studies, 8–10
    in Code of Medical Ethics, 60
    and cognitive understanding, 113
    and communication, 124
    complexity of, 104
    and comprehension, 110–11
    by death row inmates, 256–7
    disclosure during process of, 33
    disclosure of all options in, 58–67
    and disclosure of other surgeons' errors,
        142–4
    disclosure of sleep deprivation in, 33–4, 82–91
    under duress, 110
    ethical principles of, 161
    explicit consent, 123–4, 125
    focus on, 50
    implied consent, 125
    importance of, 103
    informational requirements for, 65–7
    legal definition of, 113
    management of perioperative complications
        in, 125
    newness of, 19
    and patient autonomy, 84, 85
    physician's obligation in, 60
    preconditions of, 103–4
    "reasonable patient" standard, 66–7, 84, 85
    "reasonable physician" standard, 66, 84
    reporting innovation during process of, 175
    and respect for autonomy, 115
informed refusal of care, 19, 111
injustice, 157–8
innovation, 7

adoption of, 63–4
distinguished from research, 175, 177, 188
downside of, 184
FDA's role in, 189–90
innovation review committee, 184–8, 190,
    191, 192
introduction into surgery, 188
Law of Diffusion of Innovation, 63–4
reducing risks of, 184
regulation of, 177, 181–93
reporting during informed consent
    process, 175
see also devices; procedures; technologies,
    surgical
innovation review committees (IRC), 184–8,
    190, 191, 192
Institute of Medicine (IOM)
    on conflicts of interest, 278–9, 286–7
    on disclosure of financial relationships, 288
    To Err is Human, 105, 130, 141
    on studies of volume-outcome effect, 318
insurance companies
    deceiving, 32, 37–45
    deception by, 41
insurance coverage, impending loss of, 151–61
integrity, 2, 4
    and disclosure of other surgeons' errors,
        142–3
    honesty in, 32
    meaning of, 31
intentionality, 115
International Council of Medical Editors, 9
International Covenant on Civil and Political
    Rights, 328
International Covenant on Economic, Social,
    and Cultural Rights, 328
internists, in study on ethics gap, 23, 24
interpretation, and ethical analysis, 159
IOM (Institute of Medicine), *see* Institute of
    Medicine
Iran, 242
IRBs, 189
IRC (innovation review committees), 184–8,
    190, 191, 192
Iserson, Kenneth V., 267–70, 271, 274

Jackson, J., 134
JAMA *(Journal of the American Medical
    Association),* 272
Jehovah's Witness, 104–5, 107–16
Jones, James W., 336–9, 342
Jones, R. S., 74
Jonsen, A., 153, 244
Journal of Bone and Joint Surgery, 288
*Journal of the American Medical Association
    (JAMA),* 272

Journal of Thoracic and Cardiovascular Surgery (JTCVS), 26, 27, 28, 29, 287, 291
journals
advertising in, 269–70
articles on conflict of interest in, 283–4
JTCVS *(Journal of Thoracic and Cardiovascular Surgery)*, 27, 28, 29, 291
JTCVS *(Journal of Thoracic and Cardiovascular Surgery)*, 26
judgments, in surgeon-family conflict, 118–28
justice, 12
administration of, 97
described, 244
egalitarian justice, 244, 246
and health care distribution, 157–8
and impending loss of insurance, 155
in professional's moral role, 153
in rationing health care, 220, 221
and refusal of treatment, 111
and resource allocation, 244
and Utilitarianism, 245–6

Kant, I., 96, 133, 156
Kassirer, Jerome, 290
Kaul, S., 197
Kent, Michael S., 52–5, 56
kidneys, supply of, 240; *see also* organ donation/transplantation
Kornfield, Donald, 81
Krasna, Diane M., 123–7, 128
Krasna, Mark J., 123–7, 128
Krause, E. A., 217
Krizek, T. J., 134

Lamm, Richard, 301, 303, 304, 305–10
law
and informational requirements for informed consent, 66–7
relation with ethics, 101
Law of Diffusion of Innovation, 63–4
lawsuits
and disclosure of errors, 131, 137
effects of, 94
monetary awards in, 138
number of, 94
surgeons' testimony in, 34, 94–102
threats of, 34
lawyers, 94
Leapfrog Group, 187, 318, 320
left ventricular assist device (LVAD), 298, 301–10
legal acceptability, 20–1, 22–3
Leon, Martin B., 204, 207–9
letters of recommendation (LOR), 48–56
liability, and apology, 134

lifestyle
and disease, 106, 339
of physicians, 337, 340
of surgeons, 72–3, 76
see also eighty-hour work week; smoking; substance abuse
life support, withdrawal of, 118–28, 235–6
Lin, Shu S., 251–5, 258
litigation, *see* lawsuits
living will, 120; *see also* advance directives
lobotomy, prefrontal, 176
Longo, Christian, 250–1, 253, 256
LOR (letters of recommendation), 48–56
Luft, H. S., 312
lung cancer, 336
LVAD (left ventricular assist device), 298, 301–10
lying, 37–8
vs. deception, 38, 134
justified, 40
and sense of wrongdoing, 45
see also deception

Mack, Michael J., 187–91, 192
malpractice litigation, *see* lawsuits
manipulation, 115
manual dexterity, 6–7
marketing
in Code of Ethics, 202
by drug companies, 268, 269–70
of robotic surgery, 202
smoke-free policies as, 341, 342
usefulness of, 282
Marshall, George, 305
Mavroudis, Constantine, 132–5, 138
Mavroudis, Constantine D., 132–5, 138
maximizing principle, 220
Mayer, John E. Jr., 214, 215–18, 221, 222
Mazor, K. M., 134
McCarthy, Patrick, 301, 303–5, 308–10
McKneally, Martin, 184
Medical School Graduation Questionnaire, 3
medicine, evidence-based, 62
medicine, foundational moral principles in, 97
Medtronic, 288, 292
Menke, T. J., 318
Mill, J. S., 96, 337–8
Miller, Franklin G., 233–6
miscoding, 39–45
misdiagnosis, and previous miscoding, 43
mistakes, *see* errors
Moffatt-Bruce, Susan D., 142–5, 148–9
money, saving, 167
Moniz, Egas, 176
Moore, Francis D., 189
morality, 133
moral obligations, 75

morbidity and mortality conferences, 130, 136
Morreim, Haavi, 183–7, 190, 191, 192
mortality
    and blood transfusions, 112
    from drug abuse, 166
    and volume, 205
Murphy, J. Peter, 286–90, 291, 293

Nallamothu, Brahmajee K., 312–16
National Agenda to Improve Patient Safety, 207
National Institutes of Health (NIH)
    and academic-industry relationships, 271, 272
    on coercion of prisoners, 257
National Organ Transplant Act (NOTA), 225, 243, 251
National Sleep Foundation, 85
Naunheim, Keith, 107, 108–12, 116, 135–8
need principle, 219
negligence, 147; *see also* lawsuits
New England Journal of Medicine, 284
New York Cardiac Surgery Reporting System (CSRS), 313
New York Review of Books, 281
New York Times, 281
"no heroic measures," 118–28
noncompliance, 163–72
nondisclosure, of errors, 135–8
nonmaleficence, 12, 156, 159
    concept of, 49–50
    described, 243–4
    and impending loss of insurance, 155
    and market for organs, 245
    and providing treatment, 123, 124
    and refusal to testify, 97
    and treatment goals, 126
NOTA (National Organ Transplant Act), 225, 243, 251
Novick, William M., 339–41, 342
Nuremberg Code, 192
Nuremberg trials, 192, 327

obesity, 339–40
obligations
    ethical obligations, 75, 76, 95–8, 101, 141
    moral obligations, 75
    personal obligations, 75
    of physicians, 139, 171
    professional obligations, 142–3, 167–8
On the Take (Kassirer), 290
open heart surgery, 280
operative notes, dictation of, 39, 42
Oregon, 307
Organ Donation Breakthrough Collaborative, 226, 240

organ donation/transplantation
    and autonomy, 244–5, 256–7
    and coercion, 253, 256–7
    compensation for, 240–7
    Dead Donor Rule, 228, 231–6, 253, 255
    by death row inmates, 228, 250–9
    distribution of available organs, 226–7
    distribution of organs, 244
    donation after cardiac death protocol, 232, 233, 252–3, 257–8
    incentives to donate, 228, 238–47
    laws and regulations, 226, 243, 247, 251, 256
    market in organs, 240–7
    and method of execution, 252, 256, 257
    need to rethink ethics of, 234
    number of deceased donors, 238
    organ trafficking, 241
    policy on, 225
    procuring organs before withdrawal of LST, 235–6
    prohibition of valuable considerations for, 225, 226
    rates of, 226
    supply of organs, 225, 233, 238–47
    waiting lists, 238
Organ Donor Clarification Act, 247
Organ Procurement and Transplantation Network, 225, 226, 257
Osmon, S., 134
outcomes, surgical
    in investigations of effects conflicts of interest, 294
    relationship with volume (*see* volume-outcome effect)

Paget, Stephen, 76
Pal, Jay D., 255–8, 259
PARTNER (Placement of Aortic Transcatheter Valve) trial, 209, 215
paternalism, 50, 52, 60–1, 325, 332, 335, 341
patient, noncompliant, 163–72
patient-physician relationship, 4–5; *see also* autonomy; informed consent
Patient Protection and Affordable Care Act, 222, 289; *see also* health care reform
patients
    best interests of (*see* best interests, patient's)
    as customers, 282
    privacy of, 54–5
    serving good of, 2–3
    solicitation of, 202
Patrick, G. T. W., 81
PCI (percutaneous coronary intervention), outcome-volume relationship in, 207
pediatricians, in study on ethics gap, 23, 24
Pellegrini, Carlos A., 86–90, 91

Pellegrino, E. D., 96
Percival, Thomas, 38, 197
perfection, 135–6, 195
performance impairment, 82–3
personal obligations, 75
persuasion, 115
Petersen, L. A., 317
Peterson, E. D., 318
pharmaceutical companies, *see* drug companies
phronesis, 77
physician, compromised, 50–1; *see also*
    hepatitis C virus
physician harm, 136, 137, 139
physician-industry relationships, *see*
    surgeon-industry relationships
Physician Payments Sunshine Act, 276, 289
physicians
    as customers, 282
    as educators, 3
    obligations of (*see* obligations)
    as policymakers, 297–8
    responsibilities of, 217, 218, 261 (*see also* best
        interests, patient's)
    roles of, 1–2, 3–4
    and social responsibility, 309
    see also surgeons
pilot fatigue, 90
placebo, surgery as, 184
Placement of Aortic Transcatheter Valve
    (PARTNER) trial, 209, 215
Plato, 37, 38, 40, 96, 133
policy, defined, 297
policy, health care, *see* health care policy
political correctness, 96, 98
poverty, and market for organ donation, 241–2,
    245, 246
prefrontal lobotomy, 176
prescriptions, information on, 269
presentations, and disclosure of financial
    interactions, 286–94
preventive ethics, 114
"Principles of Medical Ethics, The" (AMA), 60
principlism, 12
prisoners
    organ donation by, 250–9
    spending on, 304
privacy, 4–5, 54–5, 85
private goods, 330–1
procedures
    acceptance of, 63–4
    access to, 178
    see also technologies, surgical; specific
        procedures
profession, defined, 32
professional, defined, 32
professionalism, and malpractice testimony, 101–2

prudence, 77
publications, and disclosure of financial
    interactions, 286–94
public goods, 331
public health, coercion in, 328, 329, 332

Quinlan, Karen Ann, 177

randomized controlled trial (RCT), 8, 9–10, 181,
    189, 293
Randomized Evaluation of Mechanical
    Assistance in Treatment of Chronic Heart
    Failure (REMATCH), 303
rationing, 214–22, 298, 301–10
RCT (randomized controlled trial), 8, 9–10, 181,
    189, 293
"reasonable patient" standard, 66–7, 84, 85
"reasonable physician" standard, 66, 84
reciprocity, 265, 286
referral system, 311; *see also* regionalization
regionalization
    alternatives to, 320
    consequences of, 319
    of coronary artery bypass graft surgery, 311–22
    and cost savings, 318–19
    defined, 298–9
    described, 316–17
    evidence supporting, 313–14
    and medical illnesses, 319
    and patient's best interests, 321
    recommendations for, 314–15
    and referral system, 311
    and volume-outcome effect, 317
REMATCH (Randomized Evaluation of
    Mechanical Assistance in Treatment of
    Chronic Heart Failure), 303
reputation, 56
research, 3–4
    cardiothoracic surgical studies, 181
    conflicts of interest in, 262
    defined, 181–2
    distinguished from innovation, 175
    and introduction of new technology, 175
    and physician-industry relationships,
        271–2, 273
    recognition of need for oversight in, 192
    in surgery, 189
    see also randomized controlled trial
research ethics, 8–10
residency programs, unfilled, 76
residents
    readiness of, 7
    work hours of, 33, 69, 73–4, 87
resource allocation, 8, 167, 171–2, 216, 244;
    see also organ donation/transplantation;
    rationing

respect, 2, 3
retribution function of capital punishment, 254
Ricci, Marco, 168–71
Rich, Lauren, 251–5, 258
Richardson, J. David, 75, 76
rights
  human rights, 327–8, 329
  legal rights, 327, 329
  and smoking bans, 337
risk-to-benefit ratio, 156, 336–7
Robicsek, Francis, 95, 98–100, 101
Rosner, Gregg F., 204, 207–9
Ross, Lanie Friedman, 243–7
Rothschild, J. M., 87
rules, 12
rules of rescue, 219
Russell, Charles Taze, 108, 109

Sade, Robert M., 290–4
Salerno, Tomas A., 168–71
samples, of medications, 269
SAPIEN Aortic Bioprosthesis European
    Outcome (SOURCE) Registry, 208
SAPIEN Transcatheter Heart Valve, 207
Satir, Virginia, 73
*Schloendorff v. The Society of New York
    Hospital,* 113
Schwartz, Allan, 204, 207–9
scientists, 3–4
secondary interests, 286–7
self-awareness, 5–6
self-determination, of patients, *see* autonomy
self-interest, 199
SHEA (Society for Healthcare Epidemiology
    of America), 50–1
Silen, William, 7
Skipper, Eric, 59–61
sleep deprivation, 6
  disclosure of, 33–4, 80–91
  effects of, 80, 81–4, 86
  mitigating risk of, 88–90
  studies on, 81–2, 86–7
  and surgical outcomes, 81–2, 87, 90
sleep inertia, 83
Sleep Research Society, 85
smoke, secondhand, 325, 326, 328, 330, 331,
    332; *see also* smoking
smoking
  banning of in public places, 324–34
  as cause of death, 336
  and denial of employment, 299, 335–42
  effects of, 324, 325, 326
  as moral failure, 336
  prohibition of, 299
  risk-benefit ratio, 336–7

secondhand smoke, 325, 326, 328, 330,
    331, 332
  see also tobacco
Smoking: The Opinions of Physicians (STOP)
    study, 337
Smyth, Jessica K., 195–7, 200
social contract, 76
social justice, 157
social responsibility, 165, 309
social welfare, 309
social worth, in decision making, 171–2
society, 326–7
society, good of, 166–7, 305
Society for Healthcare Epidemiology of America
    (SHEA), 50–1
Society for Thoracic Surgery National Cardiac
    Database, 313
Society of Thoracic Surgeons (STS)
  Code of Ethics, 338
  on physician-industry interactions, 276, 287
  position statement on off-label use of
    coronary artery stents, 61
  standards of behavior for expert witnesses, 98
  in study on ethics gap, 27
socioeconomic status, and market for organ
    donation, 241–2, 245, 246
solicitation, of patients, 202
Sollano, J. A., 320
SOURCE (SAPIEN Aortic Bioprosthesis
    European Outcome) Registry, 208
specialty, choice of, 76
Specter, Arlen, 247
standards of professional conduct, 97–8
Starr, Albert, 280, 292
stents, off-label use of, 61
STOP (Smoking: The Opinions of Physicians)
    study, 337
Stossel, Thomas P., 272, 284, 290
structural variables, 317–18
STS (Society of Thoracic Surgeons), *see* Society
    of Thoracic Surgeons
students, medical, 3; *see also* residents
substance abuse
  by physicians, 72
  and treatment, 163–72
substituted judgment standard, 127
suicide, physicians' risk of, 72
surgeon-family conflict, 118–28
surgeon-industry relationships, 263–4
  articles on conflict of interest in, 283–4
  benefits of, 280, 288, 292–3
  corruption narrative of, 278, 279, 281
  disclosure of financial interactions, 276–7,
    286–94
  effects of financial motives, 287–8

evidence of effects of, 274, 284, 288, 290–4
institutional oversight of, 279
investigations of effects of, 293–4
and patient's best interests, 282
regulation of financial interactions, 276–84
transparency in, 288
surgeons
as authoritarian, 20
career peak of, 199
roles of, 1–2, 3–4
in study on ethics gap, 23, 24
training of, 15–16
well-being of, 144, 145
work environment of, 89
work hours of, 80(*see also* sleep deprivation)
surgery
image problem of, 15
lack of understanding of, 15–16
as placebo, 184
refusal to perform, 163–72
and risk of transmission of HCV, 52–3
surgery, preemptive, 151–61
surgery, robotic, 177
adoption of, 194–202
advantages of, 196–7
development of, 196
disadvantages of, 198
effectiveness of, 200, 201
learning curve of, 199
and marketing, 202
prevalence of, 200
surrogate decision-making, *see* decision-making,
surrogate/proxy
survival, meaningful, 126
Synergy between Percutaneous Coronary
Angioplasty with Taxus and Cardiac
Surgery (SYNTAX) trial, 208
system congruence, 73
system esteem, 73

TAVI (transcatheter aortic valve
implantation), 178, 214–22
TAVR (transcatheter aortic valve
replacement), 177–8, 204–11, 218
teaching, conflicts of interest in, 262
techniques, introduction of into surgery, 188
technologies, surgical, 7–8
acceptance of, 63–4
access to, 204–11
adoption of, 188, 194–202
and best interests of patients, 196
diffusion of, 218
focus of ethical concerns about, 62
history of, 176
industry perspective on, 64–5

motivations for adopting, 199, 201
opportunities for learning, 198–9
promotion of, 65
rationing of, 178, 214–22, 301–10
and research, 175
robotic surgery, 194–202
surgeon's responsibility to, 62–3
see also devices; innovation; procedures;
specific procedures
teleological ethics, 12
Terpeluk, Paul, 337
testimony, expert, 94–102; *see also* lawsuits
thoracic aortic aneurysm surgery,
outcome-volume relationship in, 206
Thoracic Surgical Directors Association
(TSDA), 28
tobacco, 304; *see also* smoke, secondhand;
smoking
To Err is Human: Building a Safer Health System
(Institute of Medicine), 105, 130, 141
tort system, 132, 138; *see also* lawsuits
trainees, 3; *see also* residents
training, of surgeons, 15–16
transcatheter aortic valve implantation
(TAVI), 178, 214–22
transcatheter aortic valve replacement
(TAVR), 177–8, 204–11, 218
transparency
and disclosure of HCV status, 51–2, 56
in surgeon-industry relationships, 288, 289
trauma care, 317
treatment
outside of standards, 105–6, 151–61
refusal of, 107 (*see also* blood transfusions)
treatment withdrawal decisions, 22–3, 118–28
trust
and decision making, 67
and full disclosure, 134
loss of, 43
and miscoding, 44
in physician-patient relationship, 4–5
trustworthiness, 3
truth, 37–8, 94–102; *see also* deception; errors;
honesty
truthfulness, and refusal of treatment, 111
TSDA (Thoracic Surgical Directors
Association), 28

UAGA (Uniform Anatomical Gift Act),
251, 256
UDDA (Uniform Determination of Death
Act), 228, 232–3, 234, 256
UHCDA (Uniform Health Care Decisions
Act), 108, 111, 115, 116
uncertainty, 5

Ungerleider, Ross M., 70–4, 77
Uniform Anatomical Gift Act (UAGA), 251, 256
Uniform Determination of Death Act
   (UDDA), 228, 232–3, 234, 256
Uniform Health Care Decisions Act
   (UHCDA), 108, 111, 115, 116
United Nations Charter, 328
United Network for Organ Sharing, 225, 226,
   257
US Preventive Services Task Force
   (USPSTF), 293
Utilitarianism, 133, 137, 166–7, 245–6

VA (Veterans Affairs), 317
values, 111
ventilation, artificial, 176
Veterans Affairs (VA), 317
virtue ethics, 12
virtues, 2, 3, 4, 96
volume-outcome effect
   concerns about studies of, 210–11, 313–14,
      317–18, 321–2
   debate on, 204–11
   evidence supporting, 312–13, 316
   and excellence, 210
   and regionalization, 317

studies of effects of in CABG, 313–14
see also regionalization

Wall Street Journal, 288
Watson, Donald, 95–8, 100, 101
Watson, Thomas, 280, 292
well-being, patient's, 153
Wheatley, Grayson H. III, 214, 219–21
Whyte, Richard, 52–5, 56
Wilper, A. P., 154
wisdom, practical, 77
witch hunt, 272
Witman, A. B., 137
witness, expert, 94–102; *see also* lawsuits
work environment, 89
work ethic, 69, 77; *see also* work week
work-life balance, 72–3, 74
work shifts, 82
work week, eighty-hour, 33, 69, 73–4, 87
World Health Organization, 255, 306
World Medical Association, 255
Wray, N. P., 318
Wu, Y., 221

Zion, Libby, 69, 86
Libby Zion Law, 80